EPIDEMIOLOGY IN MEDICINE

EPIDEMIOLOGY IN MEDICINE

CHARLES H. HENNEKENS, M.D., Dr.P.H.
Professor of Medicine and Preventive Medicine,
Department of Medicine and Preventive Medicine,
Harvard Medical School, Brigham and Women's
Hospital; Adjunct Professor of Epidemiology and
Biostatistics, Boston University School of Public
Health, Boston

JULIE E. BURING, Sc.D.
Associate Professor, Department of Preventive
Medicine, Harvard Medical School, Brigham and
Women's Hospital; Adjunct Associate Professor of
Epidemiology and Biostatistics, Boston University
School of Public Health, Boston

EDITED BY
SHERRY L. MAYRENT, Ph.D.
Associate in Medicine (Epidemiology), Harvard
Medical School, Brigham and Women's Hospital,
Boston

FOREWORD BY
SIR RICHARD DOLL, F.R.S.
Regis Professor Emeritus of Medicine, Oxford
University, Oxford, England

LITTLE, BROWN AND COMPANY
BOSTON/TORONTO

TO THE MEMORY OF C.H.H. AND M.E.B.

Contents

Foreword

Like Moliere's *bourgeois gentilhomme* who eventually discovered that he had been speaking prose without knowing it for more than 40 years, there are, I suspect, many inquisitive people who are interested in the prevention of disease who have practiced epidemiology in the same way. For epidemiology is the simplest and most direct method of studying the causes of disease in humans, and many major contributions have been made by studies that have demanded nothing more than an ability to count, to think logically, and to have an imaginative idea. With the accumulation of knowledge, however, it has become harder for individuals working alone to make effective contributions, and epidemiological research is becoming increasingly a matter of teamwork, not only because of the large number of people that may have to be studied and the large amount of data that have to be collected and analyzed, but also because of the need to bring together for the design and conduct of the study, clinical experience, biological understanding, statistical expertise, and many other special skills that vary from one study to another. But if, in this sense, epidemiological research is becoming more complex, the core of the subject remains essentially simple, and a good epidemiological study should be capable of description in such a way that all who are interested in the cause of disease can follow the argument and decide for themselves on the validity of the conclusions.

This is just as well, for the results of epidemiological research are often of immediate concern to the individual in the way he conducts his daily life, and to society in the way its activities are controlled. The media in consequence give the results wide publicity, and hardly a day passes without some reference being made to the hazards associated with radioactivity, chemical waste, food additives, contraceptives, medicines, the so-called drugs of solace, or new sources of infection. Unfortunately, claims about the existence of hazards are often based on half-baked and preliminary findings without adequate allowance for the vagaries of chance, bias in reporting, and the complexity caused by the way different social and environmental factors are interrelated. They may consequently cause much unnecessary work for professional epidemiologists and much unnecessary anxiety for the public, which could be avoided if there were more general understanding of the power and limitations of epidemiological investigation. Dr. Hennekens' and Dr. Buring's book will, therefore, be welcome, not only to those who bring special skills to the epidemiological team and want to learn how they can most effectively be used, but also to the wide range of health workers who are called on to help others assess the relevance to their own lives of the most recent epidemiological report.

SIR RICHARD DOLL

Preface

The impetus for writing this textbook arose from our teaching experiences in epidemiology at Harvard Medical School and Boston University School of Public Health as well as at other schools of medicine and public health, both in the United States and abroad. Our students have consistently suggested that their learning would be enhanced by the availability of an accompanying textbook, to serve both as an aid during the course and, subsequently, as a reference resource. We have also delivered lectures and conducted seminars with groups ranging from predominantly health professionals, such as the American Heart Association and the American Cancer Society, to media representatives, to meetings of biochemists, pharmacologists, nutritionists and other investigators whose primary interest is in basic science or clinical research. The universal concerns expressed by all these diverse groups have been how to evaluate what they read in the medical literature, and how to determine its value to their particular areas. We believe these concerns to be both important and timely. The importance of gaining such insights is borne out by the fact that much of continuing medical and public health education is derived from current literature. The timeliness is reflected in the large quantity of information from the medical literature which is now widely and daily disseminated to the general public by the media.

Careful application of epidemiologic principles and methods requires the development of a particular way of thinking, which we have attempted to incorporate into this textbook. Our major objective in writing this book is to enable all readers, be they medical or public health students, clinicians, or other health professionals, to interpret and apply the principles of epidemiology to their own particular needs.

For some readers, we hope this textbook will facilitate their collaboration with epidemiologists by providing a better understanding of the methods employed in the pursuit of valid results for each of several different types of research questions. For the smaller subgroup of all readers who will pursue epidemiology as a career, we hope this book will provide a useful bridge to more advanced concepts and textbooks.

This textbook is divided into four sections. Part I (Chapters 1–4) considers the definition, scope, and history of epidemiology; the fundamental strategies of epidemiologic research; the framework for assessing valid statistical associations and making judgments of causality; and basic measures of disease frequency and association. This section is a general overview of all the basic principles and methods used in epidemiologic research. Part II (Chapters 5–8) consists of detailed discussions of the various types of study design as well as their particular strengths and limitations. Part III (Chapters 9–12) addresses issues in the analysis and interpretation of epidemiologic data, including use of descriptive statistics as well as methods for the evaluation and control of chance, bias, and confounding in assessing the presence of a valid statistical association. Part IV (Chapter 13) provides an example of the application of epidemiologic principles and methods to disease control in the context of screening programs.

We have particularly tried to present the principles and methods of epidemiology in as clear and concise a manner as possible. To do so, we have used extensively examples from our own work as well as that of our colleagues and others in the fields in which we have the most direct knowledge and experience. We have also chosen, so far as possible, illustrations of current public health importance.

We have attempted to achieve a balanced perspective between an exposition of epidemiologic methods and their application by relying on our own different yet complementary backgrounds and experiences. One of us (C.H.) has an M.D. and has trained in internal medicine and subsequently spent 2 years as an EIS medical epidemiologist and later received master's and doctoral degrees in epidemiology; J.B. received a bachelor's degree in mathematics, a master's degree in biostatistics and a doctorate in epidemiology. Our combined perspective, therefore, includes the understanding and application of epidemiologic principles and methods from the viewpoints of both clinical medicine as well as mathematics and biostatistics.

C.H.H.

J.E.B.

Acknowledgments

Throughout our careers we have profited immensely from the exchange of epidemiologic concepts with teachers, colleagues, and students. We are privileged to have experienced the vision and leadership of Richard Doll. In addition, George B. Hutchison and Richard Peto have particularly nurtured and inspired us. While steadfastly adhering to seemingly unachievable standards of excellence for anyone but themselves, they have shared with us the priceless gifts of their time and wisdom. By doing so, they have led us to the thresholds of our own minds.

We have also been strongly influenced by our experiences in the classroom, both as students and teachers. As students, we have had the privilege to learn epidemiology and biostatistics from some truly outstanding teachers, including Elizabeth Barrett-Connor, Phil Cole, Ted Colton, Marge Drolette, John Fox, Alex Langmuir, Ken Rothman, and Noel Weiss. As teachers ourselves, we have had the good fortune to encounter many students who have been extremely interested and enthusiastic as well as challenging and stimulating.

We are indebted to our many colleagues who have read our early drafts with care. The comments and suggestions of Ted Colton on biostatistical issues, Fran Cook on confounding, and Larry Friedman on clinical trials have been especially helpful.

Within our own research group, all our colleagues have provided support and encouragement. In particular, we thank Trish Alexander, Charlene Belanger, Nancy Cook, Kim Eberlein, Denis Evans, Georgina Friedenberg, Sam Goldhaber, Dave Gordon, Pat Hebert, Janet Lang, Gerry O'Connor, Suzanne Satterfield, Meir Stampfer, Jim Taylor, and Walt Willett. In addition, major and crucial input on specific chapters has been provided by Georgina Friedenberg (Chapter 7), Pat Hebert (Chapters 6 and 13) and Janet Lang (Chapters 10 and 12). Michael Jonas has given valuable editorial assistance throughout this project.

Finally, it is not possible to enumerate the dedicated, conscientious, tireless, and outstanding efforts of Sherry Mayrent, without whom this book could not have been completed.

I. Basic Concepts

1

Definition and Background

Epidemiology may be viewed as based on two fundamental assumptions: first, that human disease does not occur at random, and second, that human disease has causal and preventive factors that can be identified through systematic investigation of different populations or subgroups of individuals within a population in different places or at different times. This leads directly to a useful and comprehensive definition of epidemiology: "the study of the distribution and determinants of disease frequency" in human populations [16]. These three closely interrelated components—distribution, determinants, and frequency—encompass all epidemiologic principles and methods.

The first component to be considered is measurement of disease frequency, which involves quantification of the existence or occurrence of disease. The availability of such data is a prerequisite for any systematic investigation of patterns of disease occurrence in human populations. The second, the distribution of disease, considers such questions as who is getting the disease within a population, as well as where and when the disease is occurring. Such questions may involve comparisons between different populations at a given time, between subgroups of a population, or between various periods of observation. Knowledge of such distributions is essential to describe patterns of disease as well as to formulate hypotheses concerning possible causal or preventive factors. The third component, the determinants of disease, derives from the first two, since knowledge of frequency and distribution of disease is necessary to test an epidemiologic hypothesis.

As suggested by consideration of the three components of this definition, there is a natural progression in epidemiologic reasoning. The process begins with a suspicion concerning the possible influence of a particular factor on the occurrence of disease. This suspicion may arise from clinical practice, examination of disease patterns, observations from laboratory research, or even from theoretic speculation, and leads to the formulation of a specific hypothesis. This hypothesis is tested in epidemiologic studies of individuals that include an appropriate comparison group. The systematic collection and analysis of data involves the determination of whether a statistical association exists—in other words, whether the probability of developing a particular outcome in the presence of a given factor or exposure is different from the corresponding probability in its absence. It is then necessary to assess the validity of any observed statistical association by excluding possible alternative explanations, such as the luck of the draw (chance), systematic errors in collecting or interpreting data (bias), as well as the effects of additional variables that might be responsible for the observed association (confounding). Finally, a judgment is made as to whether that statistical association represents a cause-effect relationship between exposure and disease. Such a judgment requires inferences far beyond the data from any single study and involves consideration of criteria that include the magnitude of the association, the consistency of findings from all other studies, and biologic credibility. This progression, which represents the usual pattern of reasoning in epidemiology, in many ways parallels its historical development.

HISTORY OF EPIDEMIOLOGY

In one sense, epidemiology is as old as medicine itself. Hippocrates, considered the father of modern medicine, first suggested in the fifth century B.C. that the development of human disease might be related to the external as well as personal environment of an individual [13].

Whoever wishes to investigate medicine properly should proceed thus: in the first place to consider the seasons of the year, and what effects each of them produces. Then the winds, the hot and the cold, especially such as are common to all countries, and then such as are peculiar to each locality. In the same manner, when one comes into a city to which he is a stranger, he should consider its situation, how it lies as to the winds and the rising of the sun; for its influence is not the same whether it lies to the north or the south, to the rising or to the setting sun. One should consider most attentively the waters which the inhabitants use, whether they be marshy and soft, or hard and running from elevated and rocky situations, and then if saltish and unfit for cooking; and the ground, whether it be naked and deficient in water, or wooded and well watered, and whether it lies in a hollow, confined situation, or is elevated and cold; and the mode in which the inhabitants live, and what are their pursuits, whether they are fond of drinking and eating to excess, and given to indolence, or are fond of exercise and labor.

For the next 2000 years, such causes of disease were considered, but without any attempt to measure their impact. Then, in 1662, a London haberdasher named John Graunt published *The Nature and Political Ob-*

servations Made Upon the Bills of Mortality, in which he analyzed the weekly reports of births and deaths in London and, for the first time, quantified patterns of disease in a population [10]. He noted an excess of men compared with women for both births and deaths, the high infant mortality rate, and the seasonal variations in mortality alluded to by Hippocrates. Graunt also attempted to provide a numerical assessment of the impact of plague on the population of the city and examined characteristics of the years in which such outbreaks occurred. His recognition of the value of routinely collected data in providing information about human illness forms the basis of modern epidemiology.

These new techniques saw little further application for almost two centuries, until William Farr, a physician, was given responsibility in 1839 for medical statistics in the Office of the Registrar General for England and Wales. Farr set up a system for routine compilation of the numbers and causes of deaths, and his Annual Reports of the Registrar General during the next 40 years established a tradition of careful application of vital statistical data to the evaluation of health problems of the general public. Like Graunt, Farr recognized that data collected from human populations could be used to learn about illness. He compared mortality patterns of married and single persons, as well as those of workers in different occupations, such as metal mines and the earthenware industry. He noted the association between elevation above sea level and deaths from cholera, and attempted to ascertain the effect of imprisonment on mortality [14]. In doing this, he had to address many major methodologic issues relevant to modern epidemiologic studies, such as defining the exact population at risk, choosing an appropriate comparison group, and considering whether other factors could affect the results, such as age, duration of exposure, or general health status.

Hippocrates, Graunt, and Farr each contributed to an increasing sophistication in the understanding of disease frequency and distribution—two of the three components of the definition of epidemiology. Two decades after Farr began his work, the availability of routinely collected data on the population and mortality patterns of England enabled another British physician, John Snow, to formulate and test a hypothesis concerning the origins of an epidemic of cholera in London [20]. On the basis of the available descriptive data, including the observations made by Farr, Snow postulated that cholera was transmitted by contaminated water through a then unknown mechanism. He observed that death rates from cholera were particularly high in areas of London that were supplied with water by the Lambeth Company or the Southwark and Vauxhall Company, both of which drew their water from the Thames River at a point heavily polluted with sewage. Between 1849 and 1854, the Lambeth Company changed its source to an area of the Thames where the water was "quite free from the sewage of London." The rates of cholera declined in those areas of the city supplied by the

Table 1-1. Death rates from cholera, 1853–1854,
according to water company supplying subdistrict of London

Water company	Population in 1851	Cholera deaths in 1853–1854	Deaths per 100,000 living
Southwark and Vauxhall	167,654	192	114
Both companies	301,149	182	60
Lambeth	14,632	0	0

Source: J. Snow, *On the Mode of Communication of Cholera* (2nd ed). London: Churchill, 1855. Reproduced in *Snow on Cholera.* New York: Hafner, 1965.

Lambeth Company, while there was no change in those areas receiving water from the Southwark and Vauxhall Company.

In 1854, Snow [20] noted that "the most terrible outbreak of cholera which ever occurred in this kingdom, is probably that which took place in Broad Street, Golden Square and the adjoining streets, a few weeks ago. Within two hundred and fifty yards of the spot where Cambridge Street joins Broad Street, there were upwards of five hundred fatal attacks of cholera in ten days." As shown in Table 1-1, Snow tabulated the number of deaths from cholera that occurred from the commencement of the epidemic in August 1853 to January 1854 according to the two water companies supplying the various subdistricts of London. The areas of London supplied entirely by the Southwark and Vauxhall Company experienced a rate of 114 deaths from cholera per 100,000 persons, whereas there were no deaths from cholera during that time in the districts supplied entirely by the Lambeth Company. A large area supplied by both companies experienced a rate midway between those for the districts supplied by either alone.

These observations were consistent with Snow's hypothesis that drinking water supplied by the Southwark and Vauxhall Company increased the risk of cholera compared with water from the Lambeth Company. Snow also recognized the possibility that many factors other than the water supply differed between the two geographic areas and thus could account for the observed variation in cholera rates. His unique contribution to epidemiology lies in his recognition of an opportunity to test the hypothesis implicating the water supply. Snow [20] outlined his natural experiment in his book *On the Mode of Communication of Cholera:*

In the subdistricts enumerated in the above table as being supplied by both Companies, the mixing of the supply is of the most intimate kind. The pipes of each Company go down all the streets, and into nearly all the courts and alleys. A few houses are supplied by one Company and a few by the other, according to the decision of the owner or occupier at that time when the Water Companies were

Table 1-2. Death rates from cholera in London, 1853–1854, according to water company supplying actual house

Water company	Number of houses	Deaths from cholera	Deaths per 10,000 houses
Southwark and Vauxhall	40,046	1263	315
Lambeth	26,107	98	37
Rest of London	256,423	1422	59

Source: J. Snow, *On the Mode of Communication of Cholera* (2nd ed). London: Churchill, 1855. Reproduced in *Snow on Cholera*. New York: Hafner, 1965.

in active competition. In many cases a single house has a supply different from that on either side. Each company supplies both rich and poor, both large houses and small; there is no difference either in the condition or occupation of the persons receiving the water of the different Companies. Now it must be evident that, if the diminution of cholera, in the districts partly supplied with the improved water, depended on this supply, the houses receiving it would be the houses enjoying the whole benefit of the diminution of the malady, whilst the houses supplied with the water from Battersea Fields [the Southwark and Vauxhall Company] would suffer the same mortality as they would if the improved supply did not exist at all. As there is no difference whatever, either in the houses or the people receiving the supply of the two Water Companies, or in any of the physical conditions with which they are surrounded, it is obvious that no experiment could have been devised which would more thoroughly test the effect of water supply on the progress of cholera than this, which circumstances placed ready made before the observer.

The experiment, too, was on the grandest scale. No fewer than three hundred thousand people of both sexes, of every age and occupation, and of every rank and station, from gentlefolks down to the very poor, were divided into two groups without their choice, and, in most cases, without their knowledge; one group being supplied with water containing the sewage of London, and amongst it, whatever might have come from the cholera patients, the other group having water quite free from such impurity.

To turn this grand experiment to account, all that was required was to learn the supply of water to each individual house where a fatal attack of cholera might occur.

Within the area supplied by both companies, Snow walked from house to house and, for every dwelling in which a cholera death had occurred, was able to determine which company supplied the water. The death rates from cholera according to source of water supply are shown in Table 1-2. These data provided Snow with convincing evidence that water supplied by the Southwark and Vauxhall Company was responsible for the outbreak of cholera in London. Thus, Snow charted the frequency and distribution of cholera and also ascertained a cause, or determinant, of the outbreak. In so doing, he was perhaps the first investigator to draw together all three components of the definition of epidemiology.

John Snow's investigation of the cholera epidemic of 1853 to 1854 utilized the approach that epidemiologists still use today. Both his clinical knowledge and observations concerning the distribution of cholera rates helped formulate the hypothesis that the disease was spread through the water supply. He then proceeded to test this hypothesis, while recognizing the need to allow for evaluation of alternative explanations for his observations. This approach was applied primarily to outbreaks of infectious diseases throughout the nineteenth and early twentieth centuries. Thus, the term *epidemiology* was originally used almost exclusively to mean the study of epidemics of infectious disease. Over the past 80 years, patterns of mortality in developed countries have changed markedly, with chronic diseases assuming increasing importance. As a consequence, the concept of an epidemic has become much broader and more complex, necessitating more advanced methods than those first developed by Snow.

CHANGING PATTERNS OF MORTALITY

Until the latter part of the nineteenth century, the chief causes of death in all parts of the world were tuberculosis, smallpox, dysentery, typhoid, and diphtheria [1], infectious diseases characterized by relatively short latency periods between exposure and the onset of illness. For any population, 80 percent or more died in early childhood from these diseases, and a large proportion of the survivors succumbed to famine or pestilence before reaching middle age [11]. In 1900 in the United States, for example, the average life expectancy for newborns was about 50 years [1, 11], a figure comparable to that in 1985 for newborns in developing countries. Since that time, in the U.S. industrialization has been accompanied by many profound improvements in nutrition, housing conditions, sanitation, and water supply. Vastly improved methods of treatment, such as antibiotics, were also developed, and widespread immunization programs were implemented by the Centers for Disease Control (CDC), which also monitored trends in the incidence of disease through the systematic collection, consolidation, and evaluation of morbidity and mortality reports and other relevant data [3, 15]. Together, these factors have virtually eliminated infectious diseases as major causes of death in the U.S. and are reflected in an increase in life span to an average of nearly 74 years in 1984 [24].

The control of infectious diseases in the United States and other developed nations has been paralleled by the emergence of chronic diseases, which are characterized by latency periods of 10 to 20 years or more, as the major causes of mortality. Table 1-3 illustrates the marked

Table 1-3. Chief causes of death in the United States, 1900 and 1982

1900		1982	
Pneumonia/influenza	11.8%	Heart disease	34.4%
Tuberculosis	11.2%	Cancer	23.9%
Heart disease	9.4%	Accidents	6.6%
Stroke	7.6%	Stroke	6.5%
Diarrhea/enteritis	6.3%	Chronic lung disease	2.9%
Nephritis	5.9%	Suicide	2.1%
Cancer	4.5%	Pneumonia/influenza	2.0%
Accidents	4.2%	Chronic liver disease	1.9%
Diphtheria	1.9%	Diabetes mellitus	1.7%
Other	37.2%	Other	18.0%
	100.0%		100.0%

Source: U.S. D.H.H.S., *Prevention '84/'85*. Washington, D.C.: Public Health Service Office, 1985.

shift in causes of death in the U.S. from 1900 to 1982. Coronary heart disease now accounts for over 34 percent of mortality in the United States; cancer is responsible for almost 24 percent of fatalities, and cerebrovascular disease, or stroke, causes 6.5 percent of all deaths. By contrast, pneumonia and influenza, the chief contributors to mortality from infectious diseases, now account for about 2 percent of all deaths in the U.S. [25]. This pattern holds true for other developed countries as well, while for developing nations, the chief causes of death continue to be malnutrition and infections due to bacteria such as tuberculosis, viruses such as measles, and parasites such as malaria.

This change in mortality patterns for developed countries has had far-reaching implications for epidemiology. First, there has been a dramatic shift in the subgroup of the population to whom public health interventions are primarily directed. During the first 70 years of the twentieth century, any overall increase in life expectancy was due almost exclusively to improvements in infant and childhood mortality rates. In contrast, during the last 15 years, increases have resulted primarily from the prevention of premature death among middle-aged people, chiefly due to steadily declining rates of death from coronary heart disease.

Second, during the twentieth century, these changes in disease distributions have resulted in a broadening of the term *epidemic* to include any disease, infectious or chronic, occurring at a greater frequency than usually expected. By this definition, coronary heart disease in the U.S. is clearly epidemic. Despite a recent period of decline, mortality from this disease remains the chief cause of death among both men and women, occurring at one of the highest rates in the world. Lung cancer in the

United States today is also epidemic, since the overall mortality rate from this disease tripled between 1950 and 1983, rising from 12.8 to 38.1 per 100,000, even after taking into account the increasing age of the general population [24]. Similarly, the occurrence of vaginal cancer among young women whose mothers took diethylstilbestrol (DES), a drug used to prevent miscarriage, represents an epidemic, as otherwise this exceedingly rare disease occurs almost exclusively in women over 50 years of age [12].

Third, the increased importance of chronic disease has necessitated the development of new methodology. For example, investigators of an outbreak of an infectious disease such as diphtheria would know to pursue sources of exposure that occurred 1 to 3 days prior to the development of the illness by questioning affected individuals about that short and well-defined period of time. With chronic diseases, the exposure of interest could have occurred many years prior to the onset of disease. Specifically, while investigation of the etiologies of colon cancer would include dietary factors, it would not be the foods consumed yesterday, a week ago, or even a year prior to diagnosis that would be most relevant, but rather the food consumption patterns of perhaps 10 to 20 years before. Such information is far more difficult to assess precisely and accurately. Moreover, in addition to the problem of long latency periods between exposure and disease occurrence, the expected magnitudes of effect for most determinants of chronic diseases are likely to be small to moderate in size. Few exposures have effects on the risk of a chronic disease as large as the 20-fold increase in lung cancer for heavy cigarette smoking [22]. A more typical finding is the approximately twofold increase in risk of coronary heart disease seen among current smokers [23]. If studies are not carefully designed, conducted and interpreted, effects of this size can easily be missed, even if they truly exist. Conversely, an association can be observed when in fact there is none. Consequently, the increasing importance of chronic diseases as a cause of mortality has required the development of methodology specifically designed to address the problems resulting from longer latency periods and small to moderate magnitudes of effect.

DEVELOPMENTS IN MODERN EPIDEMIOLOGY

The early evolution of epidemiology took place very slowly and sporadically over several centuries. Interestingly, the time interval between the contributions of Hippocrates and Graunt spanned 2000 years, whereas that between Graunt and Farr was about 200 years, and that between Farr and Snow was only about 20 years. This trend has continued into the present; since World War II, there has been an unparalleled period of rapid and systematic progress in the development of both principles and methods of epidemiologic research.

The first major development was the design of studies and techniques for collecting and analyzing data to facilitate the evaluation of risk factors for chronic diseases. One such strategy, developed specifically to address the problem of long latency periods, was to assemble a group of individuals with a particular disease as well as a comparable group of subjects without it and obtain information about their previous medical history and health habits. This approach, referred to as the case-control study, allowed investigators to look backward in time to assess quickly the effect of a relevant exposure without having to wait many years for the disease to develop. Among the first investigations of this kind was the classic study of cigarette smoking and lung cancer published by Doll and Hill [5] in 1950. They obtained information on smoking history and other health-related variables from over 700 men and women with lung cancer and a similar number of patients hospitalized for nonmalignant conditions. Using this design, Doll and Hill were able to evaluate the hypothesis in a valid as well as rapid and efficient manner.

While the case-control study successfully addressed the problem of having to wait many years for an outcome to develop, other techniques were developed to address the need to obtain accurate and precise exposure information for a period of years prior to the event. One such strategy was the cohort study, which assembles a group of individuals without the disease of interest, classifies them with respect to their exposure status at the start of the study, and monitors the subsequent development of the disease in exposed and nonexposed subjects over time. An early and important study of this kind was the Framingham Heart Study, in which a group of almost 5200 residents of Framingham, Massachusetts was assembled and has since been followed for over 35 years to explore the relationships of a wide variety of risk factors with coronary heart disease [4]. Another early cohort study assembled over 20,000 male physicians in Great Britain who have been followed since 1951 to assess the health effects of cigarette smoking and other exposures [6, 7]. The investigators conducting these and similar studies have had to establish means to identify large numbers of subjects, collect accurate and precise exposure information, and maintain regular contact with participants over long periods of time so that complete follow-up data can be obtained.

A relatively recent development has been the application of epidemiologic principles and methods to the design, conduct, and analysis of clinical trials, studies in which the investigators themselves allocate to participants the exposures being studied. Since Snow first published the results of his "natural experiment," epidemiologists have recognized the potential importance of manipulating the human environment much as basic researchers control conditions in the laboratory. The largest formal human experiment ever conducted was the field trial of the poliomyelitis vaccine in the early 1950s [9], in which nearly a million school children were assigned at random to receive either the experimental vaccine or an inert placebo. This trial clearly demonstrated the efficacy and safety of the vaccine. Since that time, clinical trials have become an integral part of the evaluation of new preventive therapeutic agents and procedures.

One asset in the management of large data bases has been the invention and continued evolution of computer technology. Snow went from house to house, collecting a single piece of information on each person who had died from cholera, and the tabulation of his data was a relatively simple matter. In contrast, many studies conducted today involve tens of thousands of individuals, and each participant may provide data periodically over 10 or more years. In addition, because the etiologies of chronic diseases are many and complex, it may be necessary to obtain information on a large number of variables. Such investigations would clearly be far less feasible without the use of computer technology to process, analyze and summarize the data.

THE UNIQUE CONTRIBUTION OF EPIDEMIOLOGY

In this chapter, we have emphasized three essential components of the definition of epidemiology: disease distributions, disease determinants, and disease frequency. A fourth aspect of the definition, which is the unique contribution of this discipline, is the fact that epidemiologic studies are conducted in human populations. While basic laboratory and animal research can achieve virtually complete control of exposures, environment, and sometimes even genetics, their results may differ so greatly from those that apply to people as to render them of no direct relevance to humans. The inability to predict the applicability of findings from a particular species of animals to humans is underscored by Cairns [2], who has observed: "Who could have guessed that *Homo sapiens* would share with the humble guinea pig the unenviable distinction of being incapable of synthesizing ascorbic acid, or share with armadillos a susceptibility to the bacterium that causes leprosy, or that intestinal cancer usually occurs in the large intestine of humans and the small intestine of sheep?"

Another major concern about the extrapolation of animal studies to humans relates to differences in dosages and routes of administration. For example, in animal experiments, permanent hair dyes have been associated with the development of cancers of the skin, lymph glands, and thyroid [18]. However, exposures in these studies were frequently administered at dosages far out of proportion to any plausible human exposure over a lifetime. Furthermore, the route of administration was through a nasogastric tube for the entire life of the animal rather than occasional topical application to the scalp. Because of such problems, the results from animal research are unlikely to provide any reliable quantitative estimate of human risk. Such research, however, can provide useful information to set priorities for epidemiologic research [8].

Thus while basic research may add to our biologic understanding of why an exposure causes or prevents disease, only epidemiology allows the quantification of the magnitude of the exposure-disease relationship in humans and offers the possibility of altering the risk through intervention. Indeed, epidemiologic research has often provided information that has formed the basis for public health decisions long before the basic mechanism of a particular disease was understood. For example, epidemiologic findings led to the judgment by the U.S. Surgeon General in 1964 [21] that there was proof beyond a reasonable doubt that cigarette smoking caused lung cancer years before there was any clear understanding of alterations in DNA by initiators or promoters of cancer, let alone of the physiologic effects of tobacco or its individual constituents [8]. Similarly, the large increase in cases of toxic shock syndrome among young women [19] was attributed to the use of superabsorbent tampons through a number of epidemiologic observations. Based on this evidence, but without an understanding of any biologic mechanism, such products were removed from the market in 1980, with a resultant marked decrease in the development of the disease. It would be another 5 years before it was postulated that an interaction among superabsorbent tampon fibers, magnesium, and bacterial growth was the mechanism responsible for development of this disease [17]. In striving to identify factors that cause or prevent disease, laboratory testing and theoretic speculation about possible mechanisms are important, but no more so than direct, straightforward observation of what actually happens in human populations. If epidemiologic studies are well designed and conducted, and if the data are properly analyzed and interpreted, they can provide strong and reliable evidence on which to base policy and ultimately decisions affecting the health of the general public.

STUDY QUESTIONS

1. Discuss the chief causes of death in the United States in 1900 and today, and explain the accompanying changes in life expectancy.
2. Compare and contrast the utility of findings from epidemiologic research in humans and studies in experimental animals.

REFERENCES

1. Cairns, J. *Cancer: Science and Society*. San Francisco: Freeman, 1978.
2. Cairns, J. The treatment of diseases and the war against cancer. *Sci. Am.* 253:51, 1985.
3. Centers for Disease Control. *Morbidity and Mortality Weekly Reports*. Atlanta: U.S. D.H.H.S., Public Health Service.
4. Dawber, T. R. *The Framingham Study: The Epidemiology of Atherosclerotic Disease.* Cambridge, MA: Harvard University Press, 1980.
5. Doll, R., and Hill, A. B. Smoking and carcinoma of the lung: Preliminary report. *Br. Med. J.* 2:739, 1950.
6. Doll, R., and Hill, A. B. Lung cancer and other causes of death in relation to smoking: A second report on the mortality of British doctors. *Br. Med. J.* 2:1071, 1956.
7. Doll, R., and Peto, R. Mortality in relation to smoking: Twenty years' observations on male British doctors. *Br. Med. J.* 2:1525, 1975.
8. Doll, R., and Peto, R. *The Causes of Cancer*. New York: Oxford University Press, 1981.
9. Francis, T., Jr., Korns, F. T., Voight, R. B., et al. An evaluation of the 1954 poliomyelitis vaccine trials: Summary report. *Am. J. Public Health* 45:1, 1955.
10. Graunt, J. *Natural and Political Observations Made Upon the Bills of Mortality: London, 1662.* Baltimore: Johns Hopkins Press, 1939.
11. Gwatkin, D. R., and Brandel, S. K. Life expectancy and population growth in the Third World. *Sci. Am.* 246(5):62, 1982.
12. Herbst, A. L., and Scully, R. E. Adenocarcinoma of the vagina in adolescence: A report of 7 cases including 6 clear-cell carcinomas (so-called mesonephromas). *Cancer* 25:745, 1970.
13. Hippocrates. On airs, waters, and places. *Med. Classics* 3:19, 1938.
14. Humphreys, N. A. (ed). *Vital Statistics: A Memorial Volume of Selections from the Reports and Writings of William Farr, 1807–1883.* London: Sanitary Institute of Great Britain, 1885.
15. Langmuir, A. D. The surveillance of communicable diseases of national importance. *N. Engl. J. Med.* 268:182, 1963.
16. MacMahon, B., and Pugh, T. F. *Epidemiology: Principles and Methods*. Boston: Little, Brown, 1970.
17. Mills, J. T., Parsonnet, J., Tsai, Y-C., et al. Control of production of Toxic-Shock-Syndrome Toxin-1 (TSST-1) by magnesium ion. *J. Infect. Dis.* 151:1158, 1985.
18. National Cancer Institute. *Carcinogenesis Testing Program*. Washington, D.C.: Government Printing Office, 1978.
19. Reingold, A. L., Hargrett, N. T., Shand, K. N., et al. Toxic shock syndrome surveillance in the United States, 1980 to 1981. *Ann. Intern. Med.* 96:875, 1982.
20. Snow, J. *On the Mode of Communication of Cholera* (2nd ed.). London: Churchill, 1855. Reproduced in *Snow on Cholera*. New York: Hafner, 1965.
21. U.S. D.H.E.W. *Smoking and Health. Report of the Advisory Committee to the Surgeon General of the Public Health Service.* P.H.S. Publication No. 1103. Washington, D.C.: Government Printing Office, 1964.

22. U.S. D.H.H.S. *The Health Consequences of Smoking: Cancer. A Report of the Surgeon General.* Rockville, MD: Office on Smoking and Health, 1982.
23. U.S. D.H.H.S. *The Health Consequences of Smoking: Cardiovascular Disease. A Report of the Surgeon General.* Rockville, MD: Office on Smoking and Health, 1983.
24. U.S. D.H.H.S. *Health United States 1984.* D.H.H.S. Publication No. (P.H.S.) 85-1232. Hyattsville, MD: National Center for Health Statistics, 1984.
25. U.S. D.H.H.S. *Prevention '84/'85.* Washington, D.C.: Public Health Service Office, 1985.

2

Design Strategies in Epidemiologic Research

As discussed in Chapter 1, epidemiology is concerned with the distributions and determinants of disease frequency in human populations. The basic design strategies used in epidemiologic research can be broadly categorized according to whether such investigations focus on describing the distributions of disease or elucidating its determinants. Descriptive epidemiology is concerned with the distribution of disease, including consideration of what populations or subgroups do or do not develop a disease, in what geographic locations it is most or least common, and how the frequency of occurrence varies over time. Information on each of these characteristics can provide clues leading to the formulation of an epidemiologic hypothesis that is consistent with existing knowledge of disease occurrence. Analytic epidemiology focuses on the determinants of a disease by testing the hypotheses formulated from descriptive studies, with the ultimate goal of judging whether a particular exposure causes or prevents disease.

Each descriptive and analytic study design has its unique strengths and limitations. In Part II of this textbook, we will discuss in detail the issues to be considered in the design and conduct of each type of study. At this stage, however, a broad understanding of the types of studies and their interrelationships is important to provide both theoretic and practical foundations for later concepts. Thus, in this chapter, we provide a brief overview of the various design strategies used in epidemiologic research.

DESCRIPTIVE STUDIES

As the name implies, descriptive epidemiology is concerned with describing the general characteristics of the distribution of a disease, particularly in relation to person, place, and time. Indices of person include basic demographic factors, such as age, sex, race, marital status, or occupation, as well as life-style variables such as the consumption of various foods or medication use. Characteristics of place refer to the geographic distribution of a disease, including variation among countries or within countries, such as between urban and rural areas. With regard to time, descriptive studies may examine seasonal patterns in disease onset or compare the frequency today with that of 5, 10, 50, or 100 years ago. Information on many characteristics of person, place, and time are readily available, so that descriptive studies can be done fairly quickly and easily. Descriptive data provide valuable information to enable health care providers and administrators to allocate resources efficiently and to plan effective prevention or education programs. In addition, descriptive studies have often provided the first important clues about possible determinants of a disease. Due to limitations inherent in their design, however, descriptive studies are primarily useful for the formulation of hypotheses that can be tested subsequently using an analytic design.

Correlational Studies

There are three main types of descriptive studies, which are listed in Table 2-1. The first type, the correlational study, uses data from entire populations to compare disease frequencies between different groups during the same period of time or in the same population at different points in time.

As an example of the former, correlational studies have suggested that various dietary components may be risk factors for colon cancer. Figure 2-1 shows the correlation between per capita daily consumption of meat and rates of colon cancer in women from a large number of countries [1]. There is a very striking positive relationship. Countries with the lowest meat intakes have the lowest rates of colon cancer, and correspondingly, those with the highest intake of meat experience the highest frequency of this disease.

As regards changes in disease frequency within the same population over time, Figure 2-2 illustrates the difference between the approximately 820,000 deaths from coronary heart disease that would have been expected in the United States in 1977 if the 1968 rates had continued to apply and the approximately 630,000 deaths actually observed [13]. Such data suggest two possible explanations: (1) that the decline in deaths from coronary heart disease could be due to its prevention through improvements in life-style habits and consequent risk factor reduction, and (2) that while the rates of development of coronary heart disease did not decline, fewer people with the disease were dying from it due to improvements in the treatment of this condition. Thus, these data have raised numerous hypotheses concerning the respective roles of prevention and treatment in the overall decline in coronary disease mortality during this period [12].

While such correlational studies are useful for the formulation of hy-

Table 2-1. Overview of epidemiologic design strategies

Descriptive studies
Populations (correlational studies)
Individuals
Case reports
Case series
Cross-sectional surveys
Analytic studies
Observational studies
Case-control studies
Cohort studies—retrospective and prospective
Intervention studies (clinical trials)

potheses, they cannot be used to test them because of a number of limitations inherent in their design. Since correlational studies refer to whole populations rather than to individuals, it is not possible to link an exposure to occurrence of disease in the same person. For example, from the data in Figure 2-1, it is not possible to tell whether the women who develop colon cancer in any particular country are in fact those with the highest mean intakes, only that on average, populations with the highest per capita consumption of meat also have the highest rates of the disease. Moreover, there may be other differences between countries in factors that are associated with level of meat consumption that might in themselves account for the observed variations in disease frequency. Populations with high meat consumption might also tend to have diets high in saturated fat or low in fiber, both of which may affect risks of colon cancer. Thus, observed differences in colon cancer rates between countries may be due not to varying levels of meat consumption, but rather to the independent effects of these other variables on risk of colon cancer. These differences cannot be taken into account using data on populations. Thus, correlational data can only raise the hypothesis that meat consumption increases the risk of developing colon cancer. Testing this hypothesis would require the design and conduct of analytic studies among individuals, which could account for the effects of other risk factors.

Case Reports and Case Series

The case report is the most basic type of descriptive study of individuals, consisting of a careful, detailed report by one or more clinicians of the profile of a single patient. For example, in 1961 a case report was published of a 40-year-old premenopausal woman who developed a pulmonary embolism 5 weeks after beginning to use an oral contraceptive preparation to treat endometriosis [16]. Since pulmonary embolism is

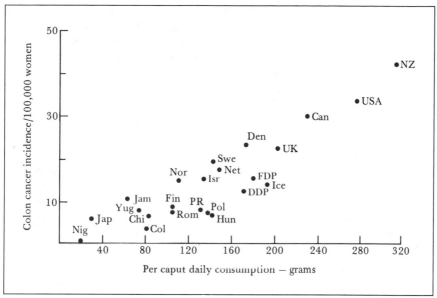

Fig. 2-1. Correlation between per capita meat consumption and colon cancer among women in various countries. (From B. K. Armstrong and R. Doll, Environmental factors and cancer incidence and mortality in different countries, with special reference to dietary practices. *Int. J. Cancer* 15:617, 1975.)

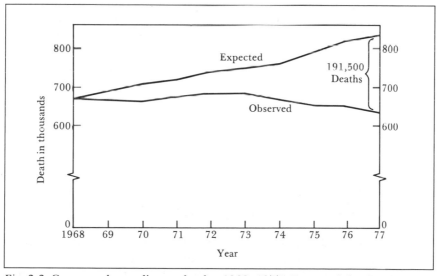

Fig. 2-2. Coronary heart disease deaths, 1968–1977: Expected deaths based on 1968 mortality rates compared with observed deaths. (From R. J. Havlik and M. Feinleib [eds.], *Proceedings of the Conference on the Decline in Coronary Heart Disease Mortality.* U.S. D.H.E.W., N.I.H. Publication No. 79–1610, 1979.)

far more common in older, postmenopausal women, the investigator postulated that the drug may have been responsible for this rare occurrence. On the other hand, since the use of oral contraceptives is not an unusual occurrence among women in this age group, it was, of course, also possible that some other characteristic of the patient or her medical history could have accounted for this outcome, in which case it would have been merely a coincidence that she had also used oral contraceptives. The crucial question is whether women who develop pulmonary embolism are more likely to have used oral contraceptives than women who did not develop the disease. Thus, although this case report of the experience of a single patient was suggestive, it was not possible to differentiate between various alternative explanations in the absence of studies of an adequate sample of individuals using an appropriate comparison group. Parenthetically, such studies were subsequently undertaken and have consistently shown an association between use of oral contraceptives and risk of this disease [23].

The individual case report can be expanded to a case series, which describes characteristics of a number of patients with a given disease. Routine surveillance programs often use accumulating case reports to suggest the emergence of new diseases or epidemics [17]. For example, five young, previously healthy homosexual men were diagnosed as having *Pneumocystis carinii* pneumonia at three Los Angeles hospitals during a 6-month period in 1980 to 1981 [6]. This clustering of cases was striking in that, until then, this form of pneumonia had been seen almost exclusively among older men and women whose immune systems were suppressed. This unusual circumstance suggested that these individuals were actually suffering from a previously unknown disease, subsequently called Acquired Immunodeficiency Syndrome (AIDS). Moreover, the fact that these cases were all identified in young homosexual men raised the hypothesis that some aspect of sexual behavior could be related to risk of the disease. As was true with the case-report, however, to test the hypothesis would require a study that evaluated whether the risk of disease is different among individuals exposed or not exposed to a factor of interest.

Cross-Sectional Surveys

The third type of descriptive epidemiologic study design in individuals is the cross-sectional survey, in which the status of an individual with respect to the presence or absence of both exposure and disease is assessed at the same point in time. For example, the Health Interview Survey (HIS) is a national cross-sectional study that periodically collects extensive information by questionnaire from a representative sample of over 100,000 individuals throughout the United States. Participants are asked to record their current status, as of the date of the questionnaire, with respect to personal and demographic characteristics, illnesses, health habits, and utilization of health care resources [25]. The frequencies of various diseases, injuries, and other health outcomes are calculated and examined in relation to age, sex, race, socioeconomic variables, medication use, cigarette smoking, and other risk factors. Such data are of great value to public health administrators in assessing the health status and health care needs of the U.S. population.

Since exposure and disease are assessed at the same point in time, cross-sectional surveys cannot always distinguish whether the exposure preceded the development of the disease or whether presence of the disease affected the individual's level of exposure. For example, it has been observed in cross-sectional studies that individuals with cancer have significantly lower levels of serum beta-carotene, a vitamin A precursor, than healthy individuals of the same age and sex. However, it is not possible to determine from such a design whether the observed low beta-carotene levels preceded the development of cancer, which might suggest a possible etiologic role, or whether the low beta-carotene levels were in fact a result of the disease itself due to dietary changes or the general debilitating effects of cancer. For factors that remain unaltered over time, such as sex, race, or blood group, the cross-sectional survey can provide evidence of a valid statistical association. Such instances are rare, however, and for the vast majority of associations evaluated, the temporal relationship between exposure and disease cannot be clearly determined. Thus, cross-sectional studies are, in general, useful for raising the question of the presence of an association rather than for testing a hypothesis.

ANALYTIC EPIDEMIOLOGY

All study designs involve some implicit (descriptive) or explicit (analytic) type of comparison of exposure and disease status. In a case report, for example, where a clinician observes a particular feature of a single case, a hypothesis is formulated based on an implicit comparison with the "expected" or usual experience. In analytic study designs the comparison is explicit, since the investigator assembles groups of individuals for the specific purpose of systematically determining whether or not the risk of disease is different for individuals exposed or not exposed to a factor of interest. It is the use of an appropriate comparison group that allows testing of epidemiologic hypotheses in analytic study designs.

There are a number of specific analytic study design options that can be employed. These can be divided into two broad design strategies: observational and intervention (see Table 2-1). The major difference between the two lies in the role played by the investigator. In observational studies, the investigator simply observes the natural course of events, noting who is exposed and nonexposed and who has and has not developed the outcome of interest. In intervention studies, the investigators themselves allocate the exposure and then follow the subjects for the subsequent development of disease.

Observational Studies

There are two basic types of observational analytic investigation: the case-control and the cohort study. In theory, it is possible to test a hypothesis using either design strategy. In practice, however, each design offers certain unique advantages and disadvantages, discussed in detail in Chapters 6 and 7. In general, the decision to use a particular design strategy is based on features of the exposure and disease, the current state of knowledge, and logistic considerations such as available time and resources.

In a case-control study, a case group or series of patients who have a disease of interest and a control, or comparison, group of individuals without the disease are selected for investigation, and the proportions with the exposure of interest in each group are compared. For example, to evaluate the possible association between consumption of artificial sweeteners and risk of bladder cancer, investigators [19] examined 592 patients hospitalized in the Boston area with a primary cancer of the lower urinary tract and 536 control subjects without bladder cancer who were selected at random from the general population. All participants were interviewed to obtain information on their history of consumption of artificially sweetened beverages and foods, use of sugar substitutes, and a number of other possible risk factors for bladder cancer, including smoking, medication use, and coffee consumption. The investigators found a similar proportion of individuals who had used artificial sweeteners among cases of bladder cancer and controls.

In contrast, in a cohort study, subjects are classified on the basis of the presence or absence of exposure to a particular factor and then followed for a specified period of time to determine the development of disease in each exposure group. In most instances, the follow-up period must be at least several years in duration to allow for an adequate number to develop the outcome, so that meaningful comparisons of disease frequency between exposed and nonexposed individuals can be made. For example, one large ongoing cohort study, the Nurses' Health Study [14], enrolled over 120,000 married female nurses, aged 30 to 55 years, who were registered in one of 11 U.S. states at the time of the initial mail survey in 1976. On a baseline questionnaire, participants provided information on a number of demographic, reproductive, medical history, and life-style variables. The enrolled nurses then completed, at 2-year intervals, follow-up questionnaires that asked about the development of outcomes during that period, updated the exposure information that had been collected on the baseline questionnaire, and obtained data on new variables of interest. By comparing those classified as exposed or nonexposed to a particular risk factor, such as use of oral contraceptives, postmenopausal hormones, or hair dyes, consumption of dietary fat, age at first birth and menopause, and family history of disease, the Nurses' Health Study has provided important data about the relationship of these variables with the development of cancer [3, 5, 14, 18, 27] and cardiovascular disease [7, 8, 9, 22].

Retrospective and Prospective Studies

Considerable confusion has arisen concerning the terms *retrospective* and *prospective* as applied to epidemiologic studies. Some investigators have used these terms synonymously with *case-control* and *cohort*, respectively, reasoning that the former looks backward from a disease to a possible cause, while the latter looks forward from an exposure to an outcome. We believe it is more informative to use these terms to refer to the temporal relationship between initiation of the study by the investigator and the occurrence of the disease outcomes being studied. Thus, while this terminology is theoretically applicable to case-control studies, it has the greatest practical utility for differentiating two main types of cohort studies, i.e., retrospective cohort and prospective cohort studies.

Figure 2-3 illustrates the interrelationship of the exposure, the disease, and the time of initiation of the investigation for case-control, prospective cohort, and retrospective cohort study designs. As shown in the top diagram, in a case-control study, the investigator selects individuals on the basis of whether or not they have the disease and then determines their previous exposure. In contrast, as shown in the next two diagrams, for all cohort studies, the subjects are selected according to whether they are exposed or nonexposed to the factor under investigation, and their subsequent disease status is ascertained.

The feature that distinguishes a prospective from a retrospective cohort is simply and solely whether the outcome of interest has occurred at the time the investigator initiates the study. Thus, as shown in the middle diagram, at the beginning of a prospective cohort study, the groups of exposed and unexposed subjects have been assembled, but the disease has not yet occurred, so that the investigator must conduct follow-up during an appropriate interval to ascertain the outcome of interest. For example, between 1950 and 1952, investigators from the Framingham Heart Study [10] identified and examined 5127 men and women from the community, aged 30 to 59 years, who were free from coronary heart disease. Information was collected on demographic variables, medical history, cigarette smoking, and a number of clinical and laboratory parameters. Members of the cohort have been followed and reexamined at regular intervals since that time to monitor the development of cardiovascular events. From these prospective data, it has been

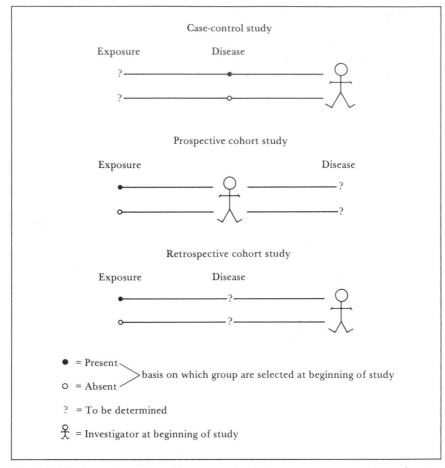

Fig. 2-3. Timing of case-control, prospective cohort, and retrospective cohort studies in relation to exposure and outcome.

possible to identify numerous risk factors for cardiovascular disease including the major determinants: cigarette smoking, level of blood cholesterol, and hypertension.

In contrast, as shown in the bottom diagram, in a retrospective cohort study, the investigation is initiated at a point in time after both the exposure and disease have already occurred. For example, to assess whether workers in shipyards building nuclear submarines were at increased risk of dying from leukemia or other cancers, personnel records of the Portsmouth Naval Shipyard in Portsmouth, New Hampshire, were reviewed [21]. A cohort was formed consisting of all 24,545 white males employed in the shipyard at any time during 1952 to 1977. Information on length of employment and annual radiation exposure was used to classify each worker with respect to total exposure during his period of employment. Information on vital status as of August 15, 1977 was then obtained for all cohort members, and for all those who had died, cause of death was ascertained from death certificate review. These data were used to compare the mortality experience of shipyard workers exposed to radiation with that of workers with no such exposure. This study used a cohort design, since participants were classified on the basis of exposure to radiation resulting from working in a nuclear shipyard and then followed to determine their subsequent mortality experience. It is a retrospective cohort study because at the time the investigation began, both the exposures and outcomes of interest had already occurred. The conduct of the study involved compiling existing information on mortality rather than awaiting any further deaths.

Choice of Observational Study Design

It is often possible to investigate a particular hypothesis using either a case-control or cohort study design. For example, the hypothesis that oral contraceptive use increases the risk of breast cancer has been evaluated in a number of case-control studies [2, 4, 26] that identified women with and without breast cancer and compared the proportions who were users of oral contraceptives. In addition, the question has been examined using a cohort design as in the Nurses' Health Study [18], where women initially free from disease were classified according to their use of oral contraceptives and then followed forward over time to compare the development of breast cancer in the two groups.

The choice of which type of design to use to study a particular exposure-disease relationship depends on the nature of the disease under investigation, the type of exposure, and the available resources. For example, the case-control design is particularly efficient for investigation of a relatively rare disease since it selects a group of individuals who have already developed the outcome. In the previous example of artificial sweeteners and bladder cancer, it would have been much more costly and time-consuming to use a cohort approach involving identification of a necessarily very large group of individuals who used artificial sweeteners and a comparable group of nonusers and follow them to compare how many would subsequently develop bladder cancer over the next 10 to 20 years. Conversely, since cohort studies enroll individuals who are initially healthy and observe the subsequent development of disease over time, this design is best suited to investigations of relatively common outcomes that will accrue in sufficiently large numbers over a reasonably short period of follow-up. In general, therefore, cohort studies of rare diseases are far less feasible. For example, since the frequency of liver cancer among women in the U.S. is so low (1.2/100,000/year) [24], even the cohort of 120,000 participants in the Nurses' Health Study had not accrued a sufficient number of cases after 8 years of follow-up to test adequately the hypothesis that oral contraceptive use increases the risk of hepatocellular carcinoma. In contrast, the cohort study design is uniquely well suited to the study of the risks associated with rare exposures, such as a specific occupational factor like employment in a naval shipyard [21]. The relative advantages and disadvantages of the case-control and cohort approaches are discussed more fully in Chapters 6 and 7.

Intervention Studies

Intervention studies, also referred to as experimental studies or clinical trials, may be viewed as a type of prospective cohort study, because participants are identified on the basis of their exposure status and followed to determine whether they develop the disease. The distinguishing feature of the intervention design is that the exposure status of each participant is assigned by the investigator. For example, in the Hypertension Detection and Follow-up Program [15], nearly 8000 men and women with diastolic blood pressures of 90 mm Hg or higher were assigned at random by the investigators either to a program of intensive treatment in special clinics (stepped care) or to their usual source of medical care (referred care). At the end of 5 years, those assigned to stepped care had experienced 17 percent fewer deaths than those assigned to referred care, a finding indicative of a marked benefit from the stepped-care approach to the treatment of hypertension.

Intervention studies are often considered as providing the most reliable evidence from epidemiologic research. This is due to the unique strength of randomization as a means of determining exposure status in a trial. When participants are allocated to a particular exposure group at random, such a strategy achieves, on average, control of all other factors that may affect disease risk. While such variables, if they are known to the investigators, could be controlled in the design and analysis of observational studies, the unique feature of randomization is that it also, on average, controls the effects of risk factors that are unrecognized at the time the study is designed. It is this ability to control both known and unknown influences that makes the randomized trial such a powerful epidemiologic strategy, especially for studying small to moderate effects. Of course, ethical concerns preclude the allocation of exposures that are known to be hazardous. Such exposures can properly be assessed in intervention studies only by attempts to eliminate them, as in the Multiple Risk Factor Intervention Trial [20], which was designed to evaluate the effects of smoking cessation, blood pressure reduction, and cholesterol lowering on decreasing risk of coronary heart disease. There are also particular concerns of costs and feasibility for intervention studies. Nevertheless, when well designed and conducted, intervention studies can indeed provide the most direct epidemiologic evidence on which to judge whether an exposure causes or prevents a disease.

CONCLUSION

In this chapter, we have presented a general overview of the various design strategies that can be used to formulate or test epidemiologic hypotheses. While distinctions are not always clear-cut, in general descriptive studies are useful primarily for describing patterns of disease occurrence and for allowing the formulation of etiologic hypotheses. Similarly, while data from analytic studies can certainly be used to generate additional research questions, their chief contribution is to test epidemiologic hypotheses.

It is important to remember that a particular research question may be addressed using different approaches. The choice of study design best suited for investigation of an issue at a given time is influenced by particular features of the exposure and disease, logistic considerations of time and resources, as well as results from previous studies and gaps in knowledge that remain to be filled. For most epidemiologic hypotheses, it is necessary and desirable to employ both descriptive and analytic design strategies. For example, an investigator wondering about a possible and previously uninvestigated relationship between consumption of a particular nutrient and cancer risk might begin by compiling available data on trends in per capita consumption and frequency of the disease to see whether there is any basis for formulating a hypothesis. If, on the other hand, intake of that particular nutrient had already been found to be associated with a decreased risk of cancer in both case-control and cohort studies, especially if the postulated effect is small or moderate in size, the investigators might propose to conduct an intervention study to provide clearer and more conclusive evidence as to whether the nutrient itself actually reduces cancer risk. Judging the existence of a cause-effect relationship is then based on evaluation of the totality of available data. The approach to making such a judgment will be considered in Chapter 3.

STUDY QUESTIONS

1. To evaluate the role of hard contact lens wear as an environmental risk factor in the development of keratoconus, a group of 162 keratoconus patients from a hospital in Florida were studied [11]. The authors chose a comparison group of 1248 individuals of approximately the same age and refractive error (a measure of visual acuity)

who were fitted for soft contact lenses. The latter group was observed over a period of time ranging from 1 to 6 years. The investigators found that 43, or 26.5 percent, of the keratoconus patients wore hard contact lenses before their diagnosis and that only one patient in the comparison group of soft lens wearers developed keratoconus. The authors concluded that these data supported the hypothesis that use of hard contact lenses was a risk factor for keratoconus.

What study design does this investigation utilize? Comment on your interpretation of the study results.

2. It has been asserted that the best observational design option for investigating an epidemiologic hypothesis is the prospective cohort study. Explain why you agree or disagree with this statement.

REFERENCES

1. Armstrong, B. K., and Doll, R. Environmental factors and cancer incidence and mortality in different countries, with special reference to dietary practices. *Int. J. Cancer* 15:617, 1975.
2. Arthes, F. G., Sartwell, P. E., and Lewison, E. F. The pill, estrogens, and the breast: Epidemiologic aspects. *Cancer* 28:1391, 1971.
3. Bain, C. J., Speizer, F. E., Rosner, B., et al. Family history of breast cancer as a risk indicator for the disease. *Am. J. Epidemiol.* 111:301, 1980.
4. Boston Collaborative Drug Surveillance Programme. Oral contraceptives and venous thromboembolic disease, surgically confirmed gallbladder disease, and breast tumors. *Lancet* 1:1399, 1973.
5. Buring, J. E., Hennekens, C. H., Lipnick, R. J., et al. A prospective study of postmenopausal hormone use and risk of breast cancer in U.S. women. *Am. J. Epidemiol.*, 1987. In press.
6. Centers for Disease Control. *Pneumocystis* pneumonia—Los Angeles. *M.M.W.R.* 30:250, 1981.
7. Colditz, G. A., Stampfer, M. J., Willett, W. C., et al. A prospective study of parental history of myocardial infarction and coronary heart disease in women. *Am. J. Epidemiol.* 123:48, 1986.
8. Colditz, G. A., Willett, W. C., Stampfer, M. J., et al. A prospective study of age at menarche, parity, age at first birth, and coronary heart disease in women. *Am. J. Epidemiol.* In press, 1987.
9. Colditz, G. A., Willett, W. C., Stampfer, M. J., et al. Menopause and risk of coronary heart disease in women. *N. Engl. J. Med.* 316:1105, 1987.
10. Dawber, T. R. The Framingham Study: The Epidemiology of Atherosclerotic Disease. Cambridge, MA: Harvard University Press, 1980.
11. Gasset, A. R., Houde, W. L., and Garcia-Bengochea, M. Hard contact lens wear as an environmental risk in keratoconus. *Am. J. Ophthalmol.* 85:339, 1978.
12. Goldman, L., and Cook, E. F. The decline in ischemic heart disease mortality rates: An analysis of the comparative effects of medical interventions and changes in lifestyle. *Ann. Intern. Med.* 101:825, 1984.

13. Havlik, R. J., and Feinleib, M. (eds.). *Proceedings of the Conference on the Decline in Coronary Heart Disease Mortality.* U.S. D.H.E.W., N.I.H. Publication No. 79-1610, 1979.
14. Hennekens, C. H., Speizer, F. E., Rosner, B., et al. Use of permanent hair dyes and cancer among registered nurses. *Lancet* 1:1390, 1979.
15. Hypertension Detection and Follow-up Program Cooperative Group. Five-year findings of the Hypertension Detection and Follow-up Program: I. Reduction in mortality of persons with high blood pressure, including mild hypertension. *J.A.M.A.* 242:2562, 1979.
16. Jordan, W. M. Pulmonary embolism. *Lancet* 2:1146, 1961.
17. Langmuir, A. D. The surveillance of communicable diseases of national importance. *N. Engl. J. Med.* 268:182, 1963.
18. Lipnick, R. J., Buring, J. E., Hennekens, C. H., et al. A prospective study of oral contraceptives and risk of breast cancer. *J.A.M.A.* 255:58, 1986.
19. Morrison, A. S., and Buring, J. E. Artificial sweeteners and cancer of the lower urinary tract. *N. Engl. J. Med.* 302:537, 1980.
20. Multiple Risk Factor Intervention Trial Research Group. Multiple Risk Factor Intervention Trial: Risk factor changes and morbidity results. *J.A.M.A.* 248:1465, 1982.
21. Rinsky, R. A., Zumwalde, R. D., Waxweiler, R. J., et al. Cancer mortality at a naval nuclear shipyard. *Lancet* 1:231, 1981.
22. Stampfer, M. J., Willett, W. C., Colditz, G. A., et al. A prospective study of postmenopausal hormones and coronary heart disease. *N. Engl. J. Med.* 313:1044, 1985.
23. Stead, R. B. The Hypercoagulable State. In S. Z. Goldhaber (ed.), *Pulmonary Embolism and Deep Venous Thrombosis.* Philadelphia: Saunders, 1985. Pp. 161–178.
24. U.S. D.H.H.S. *Surveillance, Epidemiology, and End Results: Incidence and Mortality Data, 1973–77.* N.I.H. Publication No. 81-2330. Bethesda, MD: National Cancer Institute, 1981.
25. U.S. D.H.H.S. *Health United States 1984.* D.H.H.S. Publication No. (P.H.S.) 85-1232. Hyattsville, MD: National Center for Health Statistics, 1984.
26. Vessey, M. P., Doll, R., and Jones, K. Oral contraceptives and breast cancer: Progress report of an epidemiologic study. *Lancet* 1:941, 1975.
27. Willett, W. C., Stampfer, M. J., Colditz, G. A., et al. Dietary fat and risk of breast cancer. *N. Engl. J. Med.* 316:22, 1987.

3

Statistical Association and Cause-Effect Relationships

In the previous chapter, we presented a general overview of various strategies used in epidemiologic research, ranging from an individual case report to a randomized clinical trial of large sample size. As we discussed, the formulation of etiologic hypotheses most often occurs through the use of descriptive studies, while testing them is the primary function of the analytic study designs. Testing an epidemiologic hypothesis first involves consideration of the concept of "association" between a particular exposure and a disease. Association refers to the statistical dependence between two variables, that is, the degree to which the rate of disease in persons with a specific exposure is either higher or lower than the rate of disease among those without that exposure. The presence of an association, however, in no way implies that the observed relationship is one of cause and effect. The often asked question "What does that have to do with the price of eggs?" refers to an observed association between two variables that has no known logical causal basis. Nonetheless, our primary objective in epidemiology is to judge whether an association between exposure and disease is, in fact, causal. To do this is neither simple nor straightforward and requires a judgment based on the totality of evidence, of which the result of any single study is only one component.

A causal association is one in which a change in the frequency or quality of an exposure or characteristic results in a corresponding change in the frequency of the disease or outcome of interest. Making judgments about causality from epidemiologic data involves a chain of logic that addresses two major areas: first, whether, for any individual study, the observed association between an exposure and disease is valid; and second, whether the totality of evidence taken from a number of sources supports a judgment of causality. Assessing whether the results observed in any individual study represent a valid association—that is, whether the particular study findings reflect the true relationship between the exposure and the disease—is a matter of determining the likelihood that alternative explanations such as chance, bias, or confounding could account for the findings. Judging whether the association is causal extends beyond the validity of the results of any single study and includes consideration of other epidemiologic data as well as the biologic credibility of the hypothesis.

In this chapter, we first present a framework that can be used to evaluate the presence of a valid statistical association in any analytic study design. Second, we consider the criteria used to judge whether a cause and effect relationship exists for a particular hypothesis. Third, this dual process of assessing the validity of an association and the presence of a cause-effect relationship is illustrated in an evaluation of the specific hypothesis that smoking causes lung cancer.

EVALUATION OF THE PRESENCE OF A VALID STATISTICAL ASSOCIATION

Since epidemiologic research is conducted among free-living humans, epidemiologists can never achieve the degree of control that is possible in a laboratory. Thus, while the results of any epidemiologic study may reflect the true effect of an exposure on the development of disease, it is also possible that the findings may have an alternative explanation. One possibility is that the observed association is due to the play of chance, or the "luck of the draw," which can occur any time a sample of a population is examined. A second explanation is that the findings result from some bias or systematic error in the way individuals were selected into the study or the way in which information was obtained or reported. Finally, an observed association between an exposure and disease could, in fact, be due totally or in part to the effect of other baseline differences between the groups that were unmeasured or uncontrolled, or confounding. All three of these alternative explanations must be considered before we can conclude the presence of a valid statistical association. In this section, we provide an overview of the approach used in assessing these possibilities; a detailed discussion of each will be provided in Chapters 10, 11, and 12.

The Role of Chance

A principal assumption underlying the use of measures of disease frequency in any epidemiologic study is that we can draw an inference about the experience of an entire population based on an evaluation of only a sample. For example, if we wish to know the frequency of obesity among men aged 45 to 65 years in a community, measurements of height and weight would, in theory, have to be made on each and every man in that age range in the entire population. In practice, however, we usually evaluate a sample, and based on that estimate, we make an inference about the frequency of obesity in the whole population.

One of the major problems in drawing such an inference is that the play of chance may always affect the results observed simply because of random variation from sample to sample. In other words, because of chance variation, it is very unlikely that the proportion of obese individuals will be identical in any two samples drawn from the same total population and the estimate of the frequency of obesity in the total population based on a study sample will always reflect, to some extent, the play of chance. One of the major determinants of the degree to which chance affects the findings in any particular study is sample size. If we had obtained heights and weights on a random sample of 10 men aged 45 to 65, the resultant estimate might differ substantially from the true frequency of obesity among all men of that age in the community as a whole, simply as a result of chance. If we had obtained data from a random sample of 1000 men, there would be less variability in our estimate, and we would consequently be much more likely to draw a valid inference about the experience of the total population. Thus, in general, the smaller the sample from which our inference is made, the more variability there will be in the estimates and the less likely the findings will reflect the experience of the total population. Conversely, the larger the sample on which the estimate is based, the less variability and the more reliable the inference.

There is a clear need to quantify the degree to which chance variability may account for the results observed in any individual study. This is done by performing an appropriate test of statistical significance (such as a t test or chi-square test, which will be discussed in detail in Chap. 10). A measure that is often reported from all tests of statistical significance is the P value, which is defined as the probability that an effect at least as extreme as that observed in a particular study could have occurred by chance alone, given that there is truly no relationship between the exposure and disease. By convention, in medical research, if the P value is less than or equal to 0.05, meaning that there is no more than a 5-percent, or 1 in 20, probability of observing a result as extreme as that observed due solely to chance, then the association between the exposure and disease is considered statistically significant. Alternatively, if the P value is greater than 0.05, by convention we consider that chance cannot be excluded as a likely explanation, and the findings are stated to be not statistically significant at that level.

One problem inherent in the interpretation of the P value results from the fact that it is a composite measure that reflects both the magnitude of the difference between the groups and the sample size. Consequently, even a small difference may be statistically significant, or deemed unlikely to be due to chance, if the sample size is sufficiently large and, conversely, a larger effect may not achieve statistical significance if the sample size is insufficient. To overcome this problem, a related but far more informative measure of the role of chance is the confidence interval, or the range within which the true magnitude of effect lies with a certain degree of assurance. The confidence interval can provide all the information of the P value in terms of deciding whether an association is statistically significant at a specified level. In addition, the effect of sample size can also be ascertained from the width of the confidence interval itself. The narrower the confidence interval, the less variability was present in the estimate of the effect, reflecting a larger sample size. The wider the confidence interval, the greater the variability in the estimate of effect, and the smaller the sample size. When interpreting data that are not statistically significant, or null results, the width of the confidence interval can be particularly informative. Specifically, a narrow interval implies that there is most likely no real effect of exposure, whereas a wide interval suggests that the data are also compatible with a true harmful (or beneficial) effect and that the sample size was simply not adequate to have sufficient statistical power to conclude that chance was not a likely explanation of the findings.

The statistical significance of an association is very often misinterpreted by both authors and readers. First, as seen from the discussion above, statistical significance should never be viewed as a clearcut yes or no statement, but rather merely as a guide to action. A statistically significant result does not mean that chance cannot have accounted for the findings, only that such an explanation is unlikely. Similarly, a result that is not statistically significant does not mean that chance is responsible for the results—only that it cannot be excluded as a likely explanation. The absolute magnitude of the P value, as well as the contribution of sample size as seen from the confidence interval, must be considered in interpreting the utility of the results. Second, the presence of a statistically significant association provides no information about whether the exposure under study is itself responsible for the observed effect. While a significant P value indicates that chance is an unlikely explanation of the findings, it cannot assess the adequacy of the study design or evaluate the possibility that the results may be attributable to bias or confounding. Conversely, the absence of statistical significance does not imply that the association cannot be one of cause and effect. As has been stated above, it may merely mean that the sample size was inadequate to exclude chance as a likely explanation of the findings. Finally, statistical significance cannot address whether the differences observed are important for health or longevity—in other words, whether they have any biologic importance. The British statistician Sir Austin Bradford Hill [14] referred to such undue emphasis on the results of tests of statistical significance when he stated that all too often "the glitter of the t-table diverts attention from the inadequacy of the fare."

The Role of Bias

A second and equally important alternative explanation for an observed relationship of an exposure with a disease is the possibility that some aspect of the design or conduct of a study has introduced a systematic error, or bias, into the results. In general, the key word in the understanding of the concept of bias is "different." If the way in which participants are selected into the study is different for cases and controls, for example, and that difference is related to their exposure status, then the possibility of a bias exists in assessment of the association between the exposure and disease. Similarly, if the manner in which information is obtained, reported, or interpreted is different between groups in the study, then an inaccurate impression of the true relationship may be obtained. Although a number of specific types of bias will be considered in detail in Chapters 6, 7, 8, and 11, we shall briefly discuss here the sources from which they may arise.

One general type of bias can result when noncomparable criteria are used to enroll participants in an investigation (selection bias). This can be a particular problem in case-control studies, where presence or absence of the exposure may influence which particular diseased or nondiseased individuals are entered into the study. For example, when the now well-established positive association between oral contraceptive use and thromboembolism was first postulated in the medical community, physicians were more likely to hospitalize women presenting with symptoms of thromboembolism if they currently used oral contraceptives than if they did not. As a result, any case-control investigation of the relationship between this exposure and disease that utilized only hospitalized cases could overestimate the true relationship, since the proportion of exposed women would be artificially high among those hospitalized with thromboembolism compared with all cases of thromboembolism [37].

A second general type of bias may arise whenever noncomparable information is obtained from the different study groups (observation bias). This may arise from either the investigators eliciting or interpreting the information differentially (interviewer bias) or the study subjects themselves reporting events in a non-comparable manner (recall bias). As regards the former, in a case-control study evaluating the possible role of moderate alcohol consumption in decreasing risk of myocardial infarction (MI) if the interviewer knew the disease status of the participants and was also aware of the hypothesis, he or she might probe for a history of the exposure differentially among cases and controls. In this circumstance, an association between the exposure and disease might, in theory, result from or be obscured by this kind of systematic error. Specifically, if alcohol consumption were thought by the interviewer to be beneficial, such probing might lead to an inflated estimate of drinking among controls, while if alcohol were believed detrimental, observation bias could produce an inflated estimate of drinking among the cases. In either circumstance, the estimate of the effect of alcohol consumption on risk of MI in the study data would be neither valid nor accurate.

Recall bias may arise because individuals with a particular exposure or adverse health outcome are likely to remember their experiences differently from those who are not similarly affected. For example, in a study of occupational exposure to anesthetic gases and risk of spontaneous abortion among hospital personnel in Sweden, comparison of hospital records with questionnaire data revealed that 70 percent of all miscarriages in the nonexposed groups were reported, compared with 100 percent of miscarriages reported in the group of exposed women [1]. Similarly, in studies of exposures widely believed to be detrimental, such as cigarette smoking, individuals with a particular disease or other adverse health outcome might, consciously or unconsciously, tend either to exaggerate their actual level of exposure if they believe it to have caused their illness, or to minimize their exposure to appear more acceptable to the interviewers or investigators. In either event, any observed result, whether positive, inverse, or null, would not reflect the true effect of that exposure.

In any study, inaccuracies in the collection of data are inevitable, and it is quite possible that only a fraction of the relevant exposures in a case-control study or outcomes among a cohort may be reported. When this proportion is the same in both study groups, then the effect of such random misclassification will only minimize the differences between the groups, resulting in an underestimate of the true association. In contrast, if the proportions of incorrect data are different in the various study groups, for any of the reasons outlined above, the estimate of effect can be biased in the direction of being either more or less extreme than the true association. (It is even possible that the estimate will be correct due solely to the play of chance.) Although it is very difficult to determine precisely the impact a potential source of bias actually has on an estimate of effect, it remains crucial to attempt to identify the magnitude as well as the direction of the bias for any estimate.

The Role of Confounding

The third alternative explanation that must be considered is that an observed association (or lack of one) is in fact due to a mixing of effects between the exposure, the disease, and a third factor that is associated with the exposure and independently affects the risk of developing the disease. This is referred to as confounding, and the extraneous factor is called a confounding variable.

Confounding can lead to either the observation of apparent differences between study groups when they do not truly exist or, conversely, the observation of no differences when they do exist. For example, a number of observational epidemiologic studies have shown an inverse relationship of consumption of vegetables rich in beta-carotene with risk of cancer [26]. While it may be the beta-carotene itself that is responsible for this lower risk, it is also possible that the association is confounded by other differences between consumers and nonconsumers of vegetables. It may not be the beta-carotene at all, but rather another component of vegetables such as fiber, which is known to reduce cancer risk. In addition, those who eat vegetables might also be younger or less likely to eat fat or to smoke cigarettes, all of which in themselves might reduce cancer risk. Thus, the observed decreased risk of cancer among those consuming large amounts of vegetables rich in beta-carotene may be due, either totally or in part, to the effect of these confounding factors.

Similarly, an observed association between consumption of coffee and increased risk of myocardial infarction could be due, at least in part, to the effect of cigarette smoking, since coffee drinking is associated with smoking and, independent of coffee consumption, smoking is a risk factor for MI [3]. On the other hand, any true effect of coffee on risk of death from coronary heart disease (CHD) may be underestimated by a failure to address the negative confounding effect of prior MI. Specifically, coffee consumption is less frequent among those who have previously experienced a myocardial infarction because many doctors prescribe abstinence for their patients. Further, prior myocardial infarction is a strong and independent risk factor for death from CHD. Consequently, coffee drinkers will, as a group, have a lower frequency of history of MI and, therefore, an observed lower risk of CHD that is due to the confounding effects of this risk factor.

These examples illustrate the basic characteristics of a confounder, that it must be associated with both the exposure and, independent of that exposure, be a risk factor for the disease. If the variable is associated with the disease but not with the exposure, or vice versa, it cannot be confounding. Thus, in an investigation of oral contraceptive use and CHD, religion would not be a potential confounding factor even though religious beliefs are known to be associated with oral contraceptive use, unless there is also an independent relationship of religion with risk of CHD.

There are numerous approaches to the control of confounding that can be utilized in both the design and analysis of analytic studies. All techniques for the control of confounding are based on an understanding of the characteristics of a confounder. If the confounding factor does not vary between those exposed and nonexposed, or those diseased or nondiseased, by definition there can be no confounding by that variable. Thus if, in either the design or analysis, the association between the exposure and disease is evaluated only among those who are similar with respect to the confounding factor, there can be no confounding. Specific methods for the evaluation and control of confounding, which include restriction of the study population, matching, randomization of exposure, stratification, and multivariate analysis, will be discussed in detail in Chapter 12.

Validity and Generalizability

In this chapter, we have emphasized that the evaluation of chance, bias, and confounding as alternative explanations for research findings can lead us to conclude that an observed association between an exposure and disease is valid. A related issue that must be considered, but only subsequently, is whether the findings are generalizable, that is, whether the results are applicable to other populations. Since any individual study is conducted on a particular sample of persons with certain characteristics, it is necessary to ask whether there are other groups of individuals to whom the results might apply. For example, numerous case-control and cohort studies among white males in developed countries have shown that current cigarette smoking increases risk of fatal CHD [36]. It is reasonable to assume that current smoking is likely to be equally harmful for other populations, including nonwhite males, females, or individuals in developing countries. Based on the known or postulated mechanisms of tobacco smoke constituents, we must judge whether the findings in the population of white males can be generalized to these other groups. As such questions become addressed directly in subsequent studies, there can be increasing certainty that the observed effect of an exposure in one population is applicable to others. This situation with respect to cigarettes is reflected in the increasing generalization of the risks associated with smoking to a wide variety of subgroups of individuals in successive Surgeon General's Reports between 1964 and 1984.

It is crucial to remember that the validity of the study results must always be the primary objective, because it is clearly not possible to generalize an invalid finding. In the design of a study, it may be tempting to try to select study subjects who are representative of an entire population, to allow the greatest degree of generalizability. Such attempts, however, may only increase the likelihood that any estimate of effect will be affected by bias or confounding, since it is so much more difficult to gain the cooperation of a random sample of participants and collect complete and accurate information from them. It is far more important to restrict admissibility to individuals who are comparable with respect to other risk factors for the outcome under study, as well as on whom complete and accurate information can be obtained. This issue can be further clarified by considering that a laboratory researcher wishing to determine the risk of bladder cancer associated with saccharin consumption in rats would certainly not select the animals at random from the city dump to represent the entire rat community. In fact the very opposite is true, in that the rats used are chosen from the same litters, so that they are genetically similar and have been exposed to the same environmental factors.

For example, when a large-scale prospective cohort study [11] was initiated in 1976 to evaluate the health effects of various contraceptive practices among women, one approach could have been to select a large random sample of all women in the United States in the appropriate age range. The investigators, however, were concerned about such a design because they felt, first, that it might not be possible to obtain detailed and accurate medical information by mail questionnaires alone from women in the general population and, second, that complete, long-term follow-up of more than 100,000 women from 50 states would be logistically unfeasible. Consequently, the study population chosen consisted of all married, female registered nurses between the ages of 30 and 55 years who resided in one of the 11 states with the largest number of registrants. The choice of nurses increased the likelihood of obtaining accurate medical data by mail, while the chances of achieving complete follow-up were increased by limiting follow-up procedures to participants living in only 11 states and by selecting a group who were likely to continue to provide updated demographic information to the American Nurses' Association. In fact, the 94-percent morbidity and 97-percent mortality follow-up rates achieved after 8 years [30, 31] reflect the wisdom of these choices. Thus, confidence in the validity of the findings from this study was enhanced by selecting a study population on which accurate and complete information could be obtained. The question then is whether results coming from this specified population can be generalized. Specifically, it is necessary to consider whether there is any reason to believe that the finding in this population of an inverse association between postmenopausal hormone use and risk of CHD [30], an increased risk of MI among women with a parental history [31], or the lack of an association between use of hair dyes and risk of breast cancer [11] would not also apply to nurses in the other 39 states, to women in the U.S. who were not nurses, or to women in other countries. The answer to this question involves a judgment based on an understanding of the basis on which the cohort was formed as well as the particular research hypothesis at issue. However, it is important to keep in mind that validity should not be compromised in an effort to achieve generalizability, because generalizability can be inferred only for a valid result.

JUDGMENT OF A CAUSE-EFFECT RELATIONSHIP

In a given study, if chance, bias, and confounding are all determined to be unlikely alternative explanations of the findings, we can then conclude that a valid statistical association exists between the exposure and disease in these data. It is then necessary to consider whether this relationship can be judged one of cause and effect, since the presence of a valid statistical association in no way implies causality. Such a judgment can only be made in the context of all evidence available at that moment and as such must be reevaluated with each new finding. There are positive criteria that can aid in the judgment concerning causality, including strength of the association, biologic credibility of the hypothesis, consistency of the findings, as well as other information concerning the temporal sequence and the presence of a dose-response relationship.

Strength of the Association

For epidemiologic hypotheses, the magnitude of the observed association is useful to judge the likelihood that the exposure itself affects the risk of developing the disease and, therefore, the likelihood of a cause-effect relationship. Specifically, the stronger the association—that is, the greater the magnitude of the increased (or decreased) risk observed—the less likely that the relationship is due merely to the effect of some unsuspected or uncontrolled confounding variable. For example, individuals who smoke heavily (20+ cigarettes per day) have a risk of mortality from laryngeal cancer that is 20 times higher than that of nonsmokers [35]. This strong relationship remains even after control for other known confounding factors, such as age, sex, and alcohol consumption. To account for such a great increase in risk, there would have to be another factor that is present among smokers at an extraordinarily higher rate than among nonsmokers and is also an independent risk factor for laryngeal cancer. Since it seems unlikely that such a powerful but as yet undiscovered determinant of cancer of the larynx could exist (or else it would have been controlled), the finding of this strong association with cigarette smoking increases the likelihood that it is one of cause and effect.

This line of reasoning does not imply that an association of small magnitude cannot be judged to be one of cause and effect—only that in such cases it is more difficult to exclude alternative explanations. For example, in the late 1950s, the data from one study [32] suggested that children who had been exposed to x-rays in utero had a 90-percent increased risk of death from leukemia or other cancers compared with children without this exposure. Since exposure status had been determined by interviewing mothers of the children selected for study, it was possible that those whose children had died of cancer might be more likely to remember being x-rayed during a pregnancy several years previously than mothers of healthy children. Such recall bias would have led to a false positive association, that is, an overestimate of any true effect of prenatal x-ray exposure on childhood cancer. To take this into account, a subsequent study [20] was conducted that identified intra-uterine x-ray exposure solely from prenatal medical records. Moreover, this study attempted to account for a variety of factors that had been identified in previous reports as possible confounders, including birth order, twin status, and age at death. After these potential sources of bias and confounding were considered, a statistically significant 40-percent excess risk persisted. Since that time, there have been a number of additional studies that have consistently shown this increased risk. Thus, this small, 40-percent increase in risk of childhood cancer among those receiving prenatal x-ray seems most likely to be one of cause and effect [21].

Biologic Credibility

The belief in the existence of a cause and effect relationship is enhanced if there is a known or postulated biologic mechanism by which the exposure might reasonably alter risk of developing the disease. For example, belief that the daily consumption of small to moderate amounts of alcohol reduces risk of CHD is enhanced by the fact that there is a plausible biologic mechanism, in particular that alcohol raises high-density lipoprotein (HDL) cholesterol, increased levels of which decrease risk of CHD [12]. Similarly, support for a causal interpretation of the association between use of postmenopausal hormones and increased risk of uterine cancer derives from the fact that estrogens cause endometrial proliferation, an early stage of carcinogenesis [2].

Since what is considered biologically plausible at any given time depends on the current state of knowledge, the lack of a known or postulated mechanism does not necessarily mean that a particular relationship is not causal. For example, John Snow demonstrated that water was the source of cholera epidemics in London long before the identification of *Vibrio cholerae*. Similarly, the British Navy reduced the risk of scurvy among their sailors by providing diets containing fresh fruits and vegetables hundreds of years before the identification of vitamin C. More recently, when the now generally regarded causal association between oral contraceptive use and circulatory disease was first observed, there was no physiologic mechanism known or postulated by which such hormones could act so profoundly. Only later were the production of a hypercoagulable state, increased platelet adhesiveness, and changes in the arterial wall identified as effects of oral contraceptive use [8]. Similarly, the epidemiologic evidence that smoking is a major cause of CHD had been compelling for many years before the understanding of basic mechanisms began to emerge [15]. While there are several plausible biologic mechanisms by which cigarette smoking might directly increase risk of CHD, including observed effects on blood lipids, ventricular premature beats, and platelet function, as well as the enhancement of atherosclerosis, the precise cellular and molecular mechanisms of tobacco-related CHD have not yet been completely elucidated. In fact, there is still no consensus even as to which component(s) of tobacco smoke are responsible [36]. Thus, as these numerous examples illustrate, while the presence of a known or postulated biologic mechanism certainly strengthens belief in causality, the lack may merely reflect current limitations of knowledge. A statistical association that does not appear biologically credible at one time may eventually prove to be so, and indeed the observation of a seemingly implausible association may sometimes represent the beginning of the advancement of knowledge of mechanisms.

Consistency with Other Investigations

Since epidemiology is by its nature inexact, and it is never possible to achieve the degree of control possible in a laboratory, perhaps the most persuasive evidence to support a judgment of a cause-effect relationship arises when a number of studies, conducted by different investigators at various times using alternative methodology in a variety of geographic or cultural settings and among different populations, all show similar results. For example, the judgment of a cause effect relationship between current cigarette smoking and CHD risk has been greatly strengthened by the fact that a large number of case-control and cohort studies have been conducted over the last 30 years in a wide range of cultural settings and involving millions of person-years of observation, all of which have consistently demonstrated an increased risk [13].

In the same way, a lack of consistency in the evidence concerning a particular hypothesis should result in a high degree of caution in any causal interpretation of the findings. For example, with respect to a possible association between the consumption of artificial sweeteners and risk of bladder cancer, the evidence has been conflicting. The majority of the many studies conducted in humans have shown no overall effect. Further, among those that have shown a positive relation among certain groups within a single population, the particular subgroups of users at increased risk have not been consistent from study to study. In one investigation [24], a moderately increased risk of bladder cancer among long-term users of sugar-free beverages was confined to women; moreover, in both sexes, nonsmokers had higher relative risks than smokers.

In another [17, 23], a positive association between use of artificial sweeteners and risk of bladder cancer was present only in men and, furthermore, was somewhat stronger in heavy smokers than in light or nonsmokers. A third study [16] found that risk appeared to rise moderately with increasing frequency of use of artificial sweeteners in women who did not smoke and among heavy smokers of both sexes. This lack of consistency in the observation of increased risks in various subgroups suggests that such results are more likely to represent chance fluctuations in the data than true increased susceptibility. Such consistency is analogous to the replication of results in laboratory experiments. While it might be suspected that some type of systematic error or uncontrolled confounding has affected the results of any individual epidemiologic study, it seems far less likely that the same kind and degree of bias or uncontrolled confounding occurred in a number of studies. Consequently, the criterion of consistency with other investigations provides perhaps the firmest foundation on which to base a belief in the existence of a cause and effect relationship.

Additional Positive Criteria for Assessing Causality

Taken together, the magnitude of the association, the biologic credibility of the hypothesis, and the consistency of findings are the strongest criteria by which to judge that a relationship is causal. There are, however, two additional criteria that are often cited: an appropriate time sequence of the association and the presence of a dose-response relationship.

Time Sequence

It appears obvious that for a judgment of causality to be reasonable, it should be clear that the exposure of interest preceded the outcome by a period of time consistent with any proposed biologic mechanism. Unfortunately, the existence of an appropriate time sequence can sometimes be difficult to establish. Many life-style variables, such as physical activity, smoking, or the consumption of particular foods and beverages, are very likely to be altered after the first symptoms of a disease appear, either deliberately or as a biologic consequence of the disease process itself. For example, in studying a possible protective association between physical activity level and risk of CHD, it would be very important to distinguish whether a lower level of activity among individuals with the disease relative to a group of healthy persons reflected effects of an exposure that preceded the onset of disease or whether it in fact resulted because individuals with CHD reduced their ordinary exercise levels in response to their early symptoms.

The evidence that the exposure precedes the development of the disease is most direct in data from a prospective cohort study or randomized trial, because exposure status is defined prior to the development of disease. Nonetheless, there can still be problems in interpretation when the time period between the postulated cause and effect is short. For example, a number of studies [6, 10] have shown higher lung cancer death rates among former cigarette smokers during the first year after cessation than among those who continue to smoke. The most likely explanation is not that continuing to smoke decreases the risk of lung cancer, but that a substantial proportion of those who voluntarily stop smoking at any given time do so because of early symptoms or signs of the already existing but as yet undiagnosed preclinical fatal illness. Thus, as these examples illustrate, while a clearly appropriate time sequence supports the judgment of a cause-effect relationship, it may not always be easy to establish in any particular study.

Dose-Response Relationship

One factor that is commonly considered as evidence supporting causality is the presence of a dose-response relationship; that is, the observation of a gradient of risk associated with the degree of exposure. The fact that those who smoke moderate amounts of cigarettes have a death rate from CHD intermediate between the rates of nonsmokers and heavy smokers adds credibility to the hypothesis that cigarette smoking causes CHD [36]. Similarly, the hypothesis that use of postmenopausal hormones causes endometrial cancer is supported by evidence showing that risk of disease increases with dosage, with duration, and with increasing duration of use within each dose level [38].

The difficulty in using this criterion in judging causality lies in the fact that the presence of a dose-response relationship does not mean that the association is one of cause and effect and conversely, the absence of a dose-response gradient does not mean that a cause-effect relationship does not exist. An observed dose-response relationship may merely reflect the effect of an uncontrolled confounding factor. For example, alcohol consumption causes hepatic cirrhosis, and there is a strong dose-response relationship between cigarette smoking and alcohol consumption. Thus, the apparent dose-response relationship between cigarette smoking and hepatic cirrhosis is due solely to the effect of heavy alcohol consumption [34]. On the other hand, a dose-response relationship can frequently be masked by an inability to quantitate exposure sufficiently to distinguish between risks associated with different levels. Moreover, it is not unusual for biologic factors to demonstrate a threshold phenomenon, where no effect is present until a certain level of the exposure is reached. Consequently, the presence or absence of a dose-response gradient must always be carefully evaluated in the context of the other alternative explanations and positive criteria that have been discussed.

THE EVALUATION OF A HYPOTHESIS: SMOKING AND LUNG CANCER

In this chapter, we have proposed a framework that can be used to evaluate any epidemiologic hypothesis (Table 3-1): first, to assess whether the data from a specific study represent a valid statistical association and second, to decide whether the observed relationship can be judged to be one of cause and effect. The application of this framework can be illustrated in the context of evaluating the specific hypothesis that smoking causes lung cancer.

During the twentieth century, vital statisticians, first in Great Britain and later in the United States, began to note rapid increases in the numbers of deaths attributed to cancer of the lung, far out of proportion to the changes in the population at risk. Concomitantly, over the previous several decades, smoking rates in men had also been noted to have greatly increased. These descriptive studies of trends by person, place, and time were certainly suggestive [4], but until the 1950s, there was little more direct evidence about the possible role of tobacco in the etiology of lung cancer. One of the first tests of this hypothesis was conducted in England and published by Sir Richard Doll and Sir Austin Bradford Hill in 1950 [4]. This study remains a classic epidemiologic investigation of this important public health issue.

In this case-control design, 649 male and 60 female patients with lung cancer were identified from 20 London hospitals and matched to an equal number of control patients of the same age and sex who were admitted to the same hospital with a disease other than cancer. A detailed smoking history was obtained from each patient, including whether they had ever smoked at any period of their lives, ages at starting and stopping, amount smoked before onset of current illness, maximum amount ever smoked, type of tobacco, changes in smoking history, and whether or not they inhaled.

As shown in Table 3-2, most men, both cases and controls, reported that they had smoked at some time in their lives. However, the proportion of those with lung cancer who had never smoked (0.3%) was significantly less than the corresponding proportion in the control group (4.2%) ($P = 0.00000064$). Although smoking was far less common among women overall, the proportion of nonsmokers was again significantly less among those with cancer (31.7%) than among controls (53.3%) ($P = 0.016$). When level of tobacco consumed was considered, there was a significantly higher proportion of heavy smokers among those with lung cancer: 26 percent of the male and 14.6 percent of the female lung cancer patients who smoked reported consuming 25 or more cigarettes per day, while only 13.5 percent of the male and none of the female controls smoked that amount. Similar differences were found for maximum and total amounts ever smoked. As a group, the

Table 3-1. Framework for the interpretation of an epidemiologic study

Is there a valid statistical association?
  Is the association likely to be due to chance?
  Is the association likely to be due to bias?
  Is the association likely to be due to confounding?
Can this valid statistical association be judged as cause and effect?
  Is there a strong association?
  Is there biologic credibility to the hypothesis?
  Is there consistency with other studies?
  Is the time sequence compatible?
  Is there evidence of a dose-response relationship?

Table 3-2. Proportion of smokers and nonsmokers in lung cancer cases and controls with diseases other than cancer

Disease status	Number of smokers	Number of nonsmokers	P-value
Males			
Lung cancer cases	647 (99.7%)	2 (0.3%)	
Controls	622 (95.8%)	27 (4.2%)	0.00000064
Females			
Lung cancer cases	41 (68.3%)	19 (31.7%)	
Controls	28 (46.7%)	32 (53.3%)	0.016

Data from R. Doll and A. B. Hill, Smoking and carcinoma of the lung: Preliminary report. *Br. Med. J.* 2:739, 1950.

lung cancer patients appeared to have a tendency to begin smoking earlier, continue longer, and stop less frequently than the controls, although none of these differences achieved statistical significance.

Overall these data indicated a strong positive association between smoking and lung cancer. In determining whether this finding was valid, however, three alternative explanations must be considered. First, the observed differences in smoking habits between those with lung cancer and controls might have been merely a result of chance. Second, such differences might have been due to a bias in the way the particular subjects were selected for the study, the way in which the interviewers asked or interpreted the smoking histories, or the way in which patients who thought they had an illness that could be attributed to smoking reported their smoking habits. Third, the association might have been due to some unknown or uncontrolled confounding variables.

Chance is a very unlikely explanation of the study results, since the findings were highly statistically significant for men and achieved significance for women, although less strongly because of the much smaller sample size. With respect to bias, both selection and observation bias were potential problems. As regards selection of study subjects, the method of identifying lung cancer cases varied from hospital to hospital and was believed to have resulted in less than complete notification. However, since at the time the study was conducted the potential carcinogenic effect of tobacco was not generally recognized, it is unlikely that those identified were selected on the basis of their smoking history. For the same reason, and because at the time of interview lung cancer patients were largely unaware that they were suffering from cancer, it is unlikely that cases would have tended to exaggerate their smoking habits, so that the increased rate of smoking reported among lung cancer patients cannot be attributed to recall bias.

Observation bias might have arisen from the interviewers' knowledge of the diagnosis when the exposure information was obtained. Fortunately, in this study there was a method to assess this directly. A number of patients were interviewed who were thought at the time to have lung cancer but were subsequently determined to have another condition. The smoking histories of those incorrectly thought to have lung cancer were in fact significantly different from those with lung cancer but were similar to the non-cancer controls interviewed. Thus, it is not possible to attribute the increased rate of smoking recorded among lung cancer patients to this type of bias.

The cases and controls were compared with respect to four potential confounding factors: age, sex, social class, and place of residence. The main difference observed was that a higher proportion of lung cancer patients than of controls were from the rural districts. However, consumption of tobacco was known to be less in rural areas than in London. Consequently, this difference in residence would, in fact, only lead to an underestimate of the true effect of smoking on risk of lung cancer and could not have accounted for the observation that the cancer patients smoked more than did the controls. Thus, it can be concluded that the findings of this study could not be reasonably attributed to the effects of chance, bias, or confounding, and therefore reflect a valid statistical association between smoking and lung cancer. To judge whether this represents a cause-effect relationship, however, requires an evaluation of considerations far beyond the findings from this particular study. At the time these results were published, there were relatively few other data available from either epidemiologic or laboratory studies, so that a judgment of cause and effect was not yet supportable. At that time, there was not even a potential biologic mechanism that could be invoked. In fact, Doll and Hill state that "the only carcinogenic substance which has been found in tobacco smoke is arsenic" and suggest that use by tobacco growers of insecticides containing arsenic could be a source of increased lung cancer risk rather than components of the tobacco itself [4]. Moreover, even within their own data, there were apparently anomalous results. The fact that there was no difference between cases and controls with regard to inhaling did not appear consistent with the logical assumption that, whatever the carcinogenic component, if smoking is harmful to the lungs, the detrimental effect should, in theory, be enhanced if the smoke were inhaled. Thus, while Doll and Hill demonstrated a valid statistical association between smoking and lung cancer, they were severely limited in the inferences they could draw from their data by the state of knowledge at the time of their study. Nevertheless, based on the strength of the association, the time sequence, the observed dose-response relationship, and the general compatibility with all the available evidence on the distribution of lung cancer by person, place and time, Doll and Hill stated their belief that smoking was a cause of lung cancer.

During the next several years, evidence began to accumulate so rapidly on the smoking and lung cancer question that by 1957, the U.S. Surgeon General made a preliminary judgment of causality [29]. However, the bulk of that report still concentrated on the numerous major areas of uncertainty that remained, including several possible alternative explanations of the association between cigarettes and lung cancer. It was not until the 1964 Surgeon General's Report [33] that there was enough diverse information to address all the positive criteria for assessing cause-effect relationships that have been outlined in this chapter.

The first, and perhaps most important, positive criterion addressed by the report was the overwhelming consistency of findings. Suspicions were first raised by descriptive epidemiologic studies, such as case reports and case series as early as 1939 [25, 27] by physicians who observed that the lung cancer patients they saw were almost exclusively heavy smokers. There were also reports of the increasing prevalence of lung cancer in case series of autopsies. In addition, the dramatic increase in cigarette consumption by men after World War I, when large numbers switched from chewing tobacco to smoking preformed cigarettes, was quantified and correlated with lung cancer rates. Specifically, annual per capita cigarette consumption in the U.S. rose from 49 in 1900 to 1365 in 1930, 3322 in 1950, and 3758 in 1962. Mortality from lung cancer exhibited a similar rise, but with a time lag reflecting the approximately 20-year latent period of the disease, with lung cancer death rates among men rising from 5 per 100,000 in 1930, to 30 per 100,000 in 1955, and about 42 per 100,000 in 1962 [28]. This pattern is illustrated in Figure 3-1 which presents the relationship between per capita cigarette consumption in 11 countries in 1930 and lung cancer mortality rates in 1950 [33].

During the postwar period, these descriptive data had prompted the initiation of the first analytic studies to test the hypothesis, specifically, the large case-control investigations conducted by Doll and Hill in Eng-

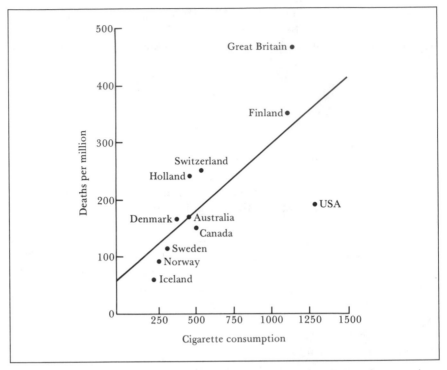

Fig. 3-1. Crude death rate for lung cancer among men in 1950 and per capita consumption of cigarettes in 1930 in various countries. (From U.S. D.H.E.W. *Smoking and Health: Report of the Advisory Committee to the Surgeon General of the Public Health Service.* P.H.S. Publication No. 1103. Washington, D.C.: U.S. Government Printing Office, 1964.

land [5] and Wynder and Graham in the U.S. [39]. By the time of the 1964 Surgeon General's Report [33], there had been 29 case-control studies published that used various methodologic approaches and were conducted in diverse geographic locations such as Australia, Finland, France, Germany, Great Britain, Japan, the Netherlands, Switzerland, and the U.S. Without exception, they all demonstrated a strongly positive and highly significant statistical association between cigarette smoking and lung cancer in men. In addition, even though the sample sizes were small, all but one of the studies among women reported statistically significant positive associations. The 1964 report also included data from seven prospective cohort studies, all of which showed an "impressively high" increase in risk of mortality from lung cancer among cigarette smokers [33].

As regards strength of the association, the published prospective studies reported an average 9- to 10-fold increase in risks among all current smokers and a 20-fold increase among heavy smokers. There was also a significant dose-response relationship, with the risk of developing lung cancer increasing with the number of cigarettes smoked per day and even more strongly with duration of the habit.

With respect to biologic credibility, by 1964 knowledge of possible mechanisms had advanced considerably. In 1959, a comprehensive review of the constituents of cigarette smoke [18] identified over 200 different compounds in seven chemical classes that were known carcinogens and cocarcinogens or cancer promoters including the alkaloid nicotine and polycyclic hydrocarbons. Arsenic content of tobacco, derived from insecticides used by tobacco growers, was by then dismissed as an important carcinogenic component of cigarette smoke. In 1964, it was not yet possible, on the basis of available data, to identify one or more specific biologic mechanisms, or even to differentiate between the contributions of the gaseous component of cigarette smoke and the particulate matter. Nevertheless, biologic knowledge of the carcinogenic potential of the chemical components of cigarettes was compatible with and contributed to the judgment that smoking causes lung cancer [33].

Finally, strong evidence concerning the temporal relationship between the purported cause and effect was derived from changes over time in risk of developing lung cancer following cessation of smoking [5]. Ex-smokers were consistently found to have lower risks of lung cancer than those who continued to smoke, with risks generally starting to decline 2 years after stopping and then decreasing further with increasing interval since smoking cessation (although never to that of the lifelong nonsmokers). The differential effects of cigarette smoking among men and women similarly supported a temporal relationship between smoking and lung cancer In the U.S., women did not begin to smoke cigarettes in large numbers until after World War II; even in 1955, the rate of current smokers was only 32 percent, compared with 65 percent among men [9]. Based on available data, the 1964 Surgeon General's Report [33] could only judge the evidence of a causal association among women to be suggestive but not yet conclusive. If correct, however, an epidemic of lung cancer among women would have been predicted to begin to emerge in the 1970s. The truth of that prediction is clearly evident today, as currently in the U.S. lung cancer has surpassed breast cancer as the leading cause of cancer mortality among women over the age of 55 [28].

On the basis of all these considerations, the committee who prepared the 1964 U.S. Surgeon General's Report [33] judged that "cigarette smoking is causally related to lung cancer in men; the magnitude of the effect of cigarette smoking far outweighs all other factors. The data for women, though less extensive, point in the same direction." They further stated that "cigarette smoking is a health hazard of sufficient importance in the U.S. to warrant appropriate remedial action," even though there remained gaps in knowledge, especially concerning effects among women and the exact biologic mechanism(s) of carcinogenesis.

The framework we have presented in this chapter for assessing causality provides a strong and cohesive basis for these conclusions. In fact, the conclusive nature of the available evidence concerning the deleterious health consequences of smoking was emphasized in the preface to the 1979 Surgeon General's Report [34] by Joseph A. Califano, Jr., Secretary of the Department of Health, Education and Welfare, who stated that: "In truth, the attack upon the scientific and medical evidence about smoking is little more than an attack upon science itself: an attack upon the epidemiological, clinical, and experimental research disciplines upon which these conclusions are based."

CONCLUSION

In epidemiologic research, causation must always remain a matter of belief or judgment based on all available evidence in accordance with the framework and criteria discussed in this chapter. In a field characterized by as much uncertainty as epidemiology, however, it is rare for the evidence on the presence of a cause-effect relationship to be as unequivocal as that for cigarette smoking and lung cancer. In chronic disease, there has never been as firm an epidemiologic basis to judge a cause-effect relationship. Thus, there must often come a point at which it becomes prudent to act on the premise that a causal relationship exists rather than await further evidence. In fact, acting on the judgment of proof beyond a reasonable doubt in a cause-effect relationship may well precede by years a complete understanding of the disease or its biologic mechanism. As Bradford Hill [14] cautioned: "All scientific work is incomplete—whether it be observational or experimental. All scientific work is liable to be upset or modified by advancing knowledge. This does not confer upon us a freedom to ignore the knowledge we already have, or to postpone the action that it appears to demand at a given time. Who knows, asked Robert Browning, but that the world may end tonight? True, but on available evidence most of us make ready to commute on the 8.30 next day."

STUDY QUESTIONS

1. Many hair dyes contain substances that are suspected human carcinogens. Consequently, several investigations have attempted to assess the risk of cancer among beauticians and others frequently exposed to hair dyes. One study [7] based on death certificate data found that among a group of cases who died of lung cancer and a set of controls,

matched on age, sex, and race, who died of causes other than cancer, beauticians had six times the risk of dying of pulmonary malignancy. In a subsequent study [22], based on data from a countywide cancer surveillance program in which it was possible to control for the effects of social class, beauticians were found to have approximately twice the risk of developing lung cancer.

Based on the reported results of these studies, how do you interpret the association between exposure to hair dyes and risk of lung cancer?

2. Recently, findings have been reported from a prospective cohort study [19] that demonstrated a significant positive association between coffee consumption and increased risk of coronary heart disease. Specifically, the authors reported a 2½-fold increased risk among those drinking five or more cups of coffee daily, with a 95% confidence interval from 1.08 to 5.77. Based on these data, the public health recommendation was made that people limit their coffee consumption to two cups or less per day. On what basis do you agree or disagree with this recommendation?

3. Explain why, in epidemiology, statistical association is often said to be considered a matter of fact (like death or taxes in the U.S.), whereas causality must remain a matter of judgment (like truth or beauty).

REFERENCES

1. Axelsson, G., and Rylander, R. Exposure to anaesthetic gases and spontaneous abortion: Response bias in a postal questionnaire study. *Int. J. Epidemiol.* 11:250, 1982.
2. Buring, J. E., Bain, C. J., and Ehrmann, R. L. Conjugated estrogen use and risk of endometrial cancer. *Am. J. Epidemiol.* 124:434, 1986.
3. Dawber, T. R., Kannel, W. B., and Gordon, T. Coffee and cardiovascular disease: Observations from the Framingham study. *N. Engl. J. Med.* 291:871, 1974.
4. Doll, R., and Hill, A. B. Smoking and carcinoma of the lung: Preliminary report. *Br. Med. J.* 2:739, 1950.
5. Doll, R., and Hill, A. B. Lung cancer and other causes of death in relation to smoking: A second report on the mortality of British doctors. *Br. Med. J.* 2:1071, 1956.
6. Doll, R., and Peto, R. Mortality in relation to smoking. Twenty years' observations on male British doctors. *Br. Med. J.* 2:1525, 1976.
7. Garfinkel, J., Selvin, S., and Brown, S. M. Possible increased risk of lung cancer among beauticians. *J.N.C.I.* 58:141, 1977.
8. Goldhaber, S. Z., Buring, J., and Hennekens, C. H. Epidemiologic Concepts and Strategies. In S. Z. Goldhaber (ed.), *Pulmonary Embolism and Deep Vein Thrombosis: Epidemiology and Pathophysiology.* Philadelphia: Saunders, 1985. Pp. 3–9.
9. Haenszel, W., Shimkin, M. B., and Miller, H. P. Tobacco smoking patterns in the United States. *Public Health Monogr.* 45:1, 1956.

10. Hammond, E. C. Smoking in relation to the death rates of one million men and women. In W. Haenszel (ed.), Epidemiological Approaches to the Study of Cancer and Other Chronic Diseases. *N.C.I. Monogr.* 19:127, 1966.
11. Hennekens, C. H., Speizer, F. E., Rosner, B., et al. Use of permanent hair dyes and cancer among registered nurses. *Lancet* 1:1390, 1979.
12. Hennekens, C. H. Alcohol. In N. Kaplan and J. Stamler (eds.), *Prevention of Coronary Heart Disease.* Philadelphia: Saunders, 1983. Pp. 130–138.
13. Hennekens, C. H., Buring, J. E., and Mayrent, S. L. Smoking and Aging in Coronary Heart Disease. In R. Bosse and C. L. Rose (eds.), *Smoking and Aging.* Lexington, MA: D. C. Health, 1984. Pp. 95–115.
14. Hill, A. B. The environment and disease: Association or causation? *Proc. R. Soc. Med.* 58:295, 1965.
15. Holbrook, J. H., Grundy, S. M., Hennekens, C. H., et al. Cigarette smoking and cardiovascular diseases: A statement for health professionals by a task force appointed by the Steering Committee of the American Heart Association. *Circulation* 70:1114A, 1984.
16. Hoover, R., and Strasser, P. H. Artificial sweeteners and human bladder cancer: Preliminary results. *Lancet* 1:837, 1980.
17. Howe, G. R., Burch, J. D., Miller, A. B., et al. Artificial sweeteners and human bladder cancer. *Lancet* 2:578, 1977.
18. Johnstone, R. A. W., and Plimmer, J. R. The chemical constituents of tobacco and tobacco smoke. *Chem. Rev.* 59:885, 1959.
19. LaCroix, A. Z., et al. Coffee consumption and incidence of coronary artery disease. *N. Engl. J. Med.* 315:977, 1986.
20. MacMahon, B. Prenatal x-ray exposure and childhood cancer. *J.N.C.I.* 28:1173, 1962.
21. MacMahon, B., and Hutchison, G. B. Prenatal x-ray and childhood cancer: A review. *Acta Un. Int. Cancer* 20:1172, 1964.
22. Menck, H. R., Pike, M. C., Henderson, B. E., et al. Lung cancer risk among beauticians and other female workers. *J.N.C.I.* 59:1423, 1977.
23. Miller, A. B., and Howe, G. R. Artificial sweeteners and bladder cancer. *Lancet* 2:1121, 1977.
24. Morrison, A. S., and Buring, J. E. Artificial sweeteners and cancer of the lower urinary tract. *N. Engl. J. Med.* 302:537, 1980.
25. Muller, F. H. Tabakmissbrauch und Lungencarcinom. *Z. Krebsforsch.* 49:57, 1939.
26. Peto, R., Doll, R., Buckley, J. D., et al. Can dietary beta-carotene materially reduce human cancer rates? *Nature* 290:201, 1981.
27. Schairer, E., and Schoeniger, E. Lungenkrebs und Tabakverbrauch. *Z. Krebsforsch.* 54:261, 1943.
28. Silverberg, E., and Lubera, L. Cancer statistics, 1987. *CA* 37:2, 1987.
29. Smoking and Health. Joint Report of the Study Group on Smoking and Health. *Science* 125:1129, 1957.
30. Stampfer, M. J., Willett, W. C., Colditz, G. A., et al. A prospective study of postmenopausal hormones and coronary heart disease. *N. Engl. J. Med.* 313:1044, 1985.
31. Stampfer, M. J., Willett, W. C., Rosner, B., et al. A prospective study of parental history of myocardial infarction and coronary heart disease in women. *Am. J. Epidemiol.* 123:48, 1986.

32. Stewart, A., Webb, J., Giles, D., et al. Malignant disease in childhood and diagnostic irradiation in utero: Preliminary communication. *Lancet* 2:447, 1956.

33. U.S. D.II.E.W. *Smoking and Health: Report of the Advisory Committee to the Surgeon General of the Public Health Service.* P.H.S. Publication No. 1103. Washington, D.C.: U.S. Government Printing Office, 1964.

34. U.S. D.H.E.W. *Smoking and Health: A Report of the Surgeon General.* D.H.E.W. Publication No. (P.H.S.) 7-50066. Rockville, MD: U.S. D.H.E.W., 1979.

35. U.S. D.H.H.S. *The Health Consequences of Smoking: Cancer. A Report of the Surgeon General.* Rockville, MD: Office on Smoking and Health, 1982.

36. U.S. D.H.H.S. *The Health Consequences of Smoking: Cardiovascular Disease. A Report of the Surgeon General.* Rockville, MD: Office on Smoking and Health, 1983.

37. Vessey, M. P., and Doll, R. Investigation of relation between use of oral contraceptives and thromboembolic disease: A further report. *Br. Med. J.* 2:651, 1969.

38. Weiss, N. S., Syckely, D. R., English, D. R., et al. Endometrial cancer in relation to patterns of menopausal estrogen use. *J.A.M.A.* 242:261, 1979.

39. Wynder, E. L., and Graham, E. A. Tobacco smoking as a possible etiologic factor in bronchiogenic carcinoma. A study of six hundred and eighty-four proved cases. *J.A.M.A.* 143:329, 1950.

4

Measures of Disease Frequency and Association

In the previous chapters, we have emphasized that the discipline of epidemiology encompasses both the description of the distribution of patterns of disease occurrence in human populations and the identification of disease determinants. To achieve either of these objectives, it is first necessary to measure the frequency of a disease or other outcome of interest. Such measures serve as basic tools for hypothesis formulation and testing by permitting comparison of frequencies of disease between different populations, as well as among individuals with and without a particular exposure or characteristic within a population. The various types of information provided have different uses, some for public health administrators and others for epidemiologic researchers.

In this chapter, we first outline the basic measures of disease frequency, how they are calculated, and their strengths and limitations. We then describe the various measures of association between exposure and disease and the type of information they each provide.

MEASURES OF DISEASE FREQUENCY

A prerequisite for any epidemiologic investigation is the ability to quantify the occurrence of disease. The most basic measure of disease frequency is a simple count of affected individuals. Such information is essential for public health planners and administrators who wish to determine the allocation of health care resources in a particular community. However, count data alone have very limited utility for epidemiologists. To investigate distributions and determinants of disease, it is also necessary to know the size of the source population from which affected individuals were derived, as well as the time period during which the data were collected. The use of such measures allows direct comparisons of disease frequencies in two or more groups of individuals.

The need for measures of disease frequency that take into account not

Table 4-1. Hypothetical data on the frequency of hepatitis in two cities

Location	New cases of hepatitis	Reporting period	Population
City A	58	1985	25,000
City B	35	1984–1985	7000

Annual rate of occurrence of hepatitis:

City A: 58/25,000/1 year = 232/10^5/year

City B: 35/7000/2 years = 17.5/7000/1 year

  = 250/10^5/year

only the numbers of affected individuals but also the size of the source populations from which they were derived can be illustrated by the data presented in Table 4-1, which shows the number of cases of hepatitis diagnosed in each of two hypothetical cities. In City A, 58 new cases were reported during 1985, while in City B, there were 35 cases during a 2-year period from 1984 to 1985. This information would be sufficient for health care administrators in the two cities to plan for the personnel and services necessary to treat affected individuals. These count data alone, however, would erroneously suggest that hepatitis is much more common in City A than in City B, since there were more reported cases in 1 year in the former than were reported in the latter in twice that time. Some might even falsely conclude that City A was experiencing an epidemic of hepatitis. The fallacy in this line of thinking is that, as shown in the table, the population of City A is much larger than that of City B. To compare the frequency of hepatitis in these two populations, it is necessary to account for both the difference in population size and the different lengths of the reporting periods. In this example, the annual rate of occurrence of hepatitis in City A is 58 per 25,000, while the comparable rate for City B is 35 per 7000 for 2 years, or 17.5 per 7000 per year.

For ease of comparing two rates directly, the same unit of population in the denominator of each rate is often used. This is usually expressed as a power of 10; that is, the number of events is expressed per population of 100 (10^2), 1000 (10^3), 10,000 (10^4), 100,000 (10^5), or 1 million (10^6). In general, it is preferable to maintain integers or whole numbers in the numerator of a rate. For example, 6 cases per 100,000 per year seems more understandable and easier to communicate than the equivalent 0.06 cases per 1000 per year. Similarly, for convenience, it is not necessary to write out "per," so that 6 cases per 100,000 per year can be expressed more succinctly as 6/10^5/year. Using 100,000 as the common unit of population in the example in Table 4-1, the annual rates of 58 per 25,000 and 17.5 per 7000 can be expressed as 232 and 250 cases per 100,000 per year in Cities A and B, respectively. City B, despite a smaller absolute number of reported cases over a longer time period, in fact had a slightly higher frequency of occurrence of hepatitis. Thus, by providing a common time frame and unit of population, direct comparisons of disease frequencies between different populations are facilitated.

There are three general classes of mathematical parameters used to relate the number of cases of a disease or outcome to the size of the source population in which they occurred. The most basic measure is the ratio, obtained by simply dividing one quantity by another without implying any specific relationship between the numerator and denominator, such as the number of stillbirths per thousand live births. Ratio is a general term that includes a number of more specific measures, such as proportion, percentage, and rate. A proportion is a type of ratio in which those who are included in the numerator must also be included in the denominator, such as the proportion of women over the age of 50 who have had a hysterectomy, or the number of fetal deaths out of the total number of births (live births plus fetal deaths). This ratio of a part to the whole is often expressed as a percentage. A rate, strictly defined, is a ratio in which there is a distinct relationship between the numerator and denominator and, most essentially, a measure of time is an intrinsic part of the denominator. This would include the number of colds per 1000 elementary school students during a 1-month period, the number of newly diagnosed cases of breast cancer per 100,000 women during a given year, or the daily expenditure of calories per kilogram. In the medical literature, the term *rate* is often used very loosely to refer to a number of demographic and epidemiologic measures that are either true rates, proportions, or ratios. Since these terms are often used interchangeably, it is important to be aware of how any measure being reported was actually defined and calculated.

Similarly, in constructing measures of disease frequency, it is necessary to be very specific about what constitutes both the numerator and the denominator. In some circumstances, it is important to make clear whether the measure represents the number of events or the number of individuals. For example, the frequency of myopia among a population of school children could represent the number of affected eyes in relation to total eyes, or the number of children affected in one or both eyes relative to all students. Analogously, in calculating the frequency of side effects of a drug, the denominator could be either the total number of courses of treatment, in which case any individual patient could be represented more than once in the numerator, or the total number of individuals receiving the drug, in which case an individual patient could be represented in the numerator only once.

Prevalence and Incidence

The measures of disease frequency used most frequently in epidemiology fall into two broad categories: prevalence and incidence. Prevalence quantifies the proportion of individuals in a population who have the disease at a specific instant and provides an estimate of the probability (risk) that an individual will be ill at a point in time. The formula for calculating the prevalence (P) is

$$P = \frac{\text{number of existing cases of a disease}}{\text{total population}} \text{ at a given point in time}$$

For example, in a visual examination survey conducted in Framingham, Massachusetts among individuals 52 to 85 years of age [19], 310 of the 2477 persons examined had cataracts at the time of the survey. The prevalence of cataract in that age group was therefore 310 per 2477, or 12.5 percent. Thus, prevalence can be thought of as the status of the disease in a population at a point in time and as such is also referred to as point prevalence. This "point" can refer to a specific point in calendar time or to a fixed point in the course of events that varies in real time from person to person, such as the onset of menopause or puberty or the third postoperative day. The term "prevalence rate" is often used interchangeably with "prevalence," although by strict definition, prevalence is a proportion, not a rate.

In contrast to prevalence, incidence quantifies the number of new events or cases of disease that develop in a population of individuals at risk during a specified time interval. There are two specific types of incidence measures, cumulative incidence and incidence rate or density. Cumulative incidence (CI) is the proportion of people who become diseased during a specified period of time and is calculated as

$$CI = \frac{\text{number of new cases of a disease during a given period of time}}{\text{total population at risk}}$$

Cumulative incidence provides an estimate of the probability, or risk, that an individual will develop a disease during a specified period of time. For example, in a study of oral contraceptive (OC) use and bacteriuria [14], a total of 2390 women aged 16 to 49 years were identified who were free from bacteriuria. Of these, 482 were OC users at the initial survey in 1973. At a second survey in 1976, 27 of the OC users had developed bacteriuria. This results in a cumulative incidence of bacteriuria among OC users of 27 per 482 or 5.6 percent during this 3-year period. The relevant time period must be clearly specified when reporting the CI. A cumulative incidence of bacteriuria of 5.6 percent among

OC users would be viewed very differently if it referred to a 6-month period, a 3-year period, or a 10-year period.

The cumulative incidence assumes that the entire population at risk at the beginning of the study period has been followed for the specified time interval for the development of the outcome under investigation. Often, however, participants will be entered into a study over a period of a year or several years and followed to a single, common termination date. Moreover, even if all subjects enter the study at the same time, some may become lost during the follow-up period so that information is not available on these individuals at the termination of the study. In either instance, the length of follow-up, or the time during which the outcome could be observed, will not be uniform for all participants.

To account for these varying time periods of follow-up, one approach would be to restrict the calculation of the incidence to a period of time during which the entire population provided information. This would, however, necessitate disregarding the additional follow-up information available for some of the population. A more precise estimate of the impact of exposure in a population that utilizes all available information is called the incidence rate (IR), force of morbidity or mortality, or incidence density (ID). This is considered to be a measure of the instantaneous rate of development of disease in a population and is defined as:

$$ID = \frac{\text{number of new cases of a disease during given time period}}{\text{total person-time of observation}}$$

As with any measure of incidence, the numerator of the incidence density is the number of new cases in the population. The denominator, however, is now the sum of each individual's time at risk or the sum of the time that each person remained under observation and free from disease. In presenting an incidence rate, it is essential to specify the relevant time units—that is, whether the rate represents the number of cases per person-day, person-month, person-year, etc.

Figure 4-1 illustrates the calculation of person-time units, based on the experience of a hypothetical group of five subjects, two of whom developed the disease of interest during a 5-year follow-up period. The cumulative incidence of disease could thus be calculated as 2 cases per 5 individuals over a 5-year period or 8 per 100 over 1 year. However, this measure of the development of disease would be misleading, since it does not reflect the fact that only one of the five individuals (subject C) was in fact observed for the entire follow-up period. Subject A was observed for only 2 years before being lost to follow-up, while subjects B, D, and E were followed for 3.0, 4.0, and 2.5 years, respectively. Consequently, the total time at risk for this population of five subjects, ob-

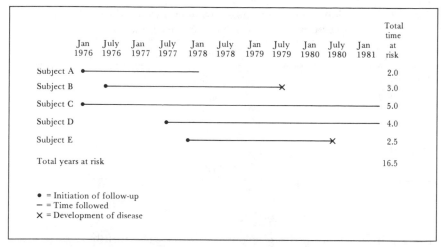

Fig. 4-1. Calculation of person-years for incidence density.

tained by adding their individual times, would be 16.5 person-years, and the incidence density (ID) would be calculated as follows:

ID = 2 cases/16.5 person-years

= 12.1/100 person-years of observation

Inherent in this calculation is the idea that a given amount of person-time can be derived from a variety of populations in different circumstances. Thus, the observation of 16 people for 1 year, of 8 people for 2 years, or of 32 people for 6 months would all result in a total of 16 person-years of observation.

To illustrate the calculation of ID, in a cohort study of postmenopausal hormone use and risk of coronary heart disease (CHD) [33], 90 cases were diagnosed among 32,317 postmenopausal women during a total of 105,786.2 person-years of follow-up. The incidence density of CHD among the participants in this study would therefore be calculated as follows:

ID = 90/105,786.2 person-years

= 85.1/10^5 person-years

In the above example, in which calculations are based on total person-years of risk experienced by the group, an assumption is made that the risk of coronary heart disease remains constant over time. However, for most diseases and death rates, the associated risk does not remain constant but rather varies for different time periods and age groups. It is therefore often useful to account for the number of person-years at risk

Table 4-2. Calculation of person-years contributed by an individual subject in a retrospective cohort study of asbestos exposure and lung cancer mortality

Time period	Person-years
1923–1934	1.5
1935–1939	5.0
1940–1944	5.0
1945–1949	5.0
1950–1954	0.5
Total	17.0

in each time period and age group. To do so, the numbers of person-years contributed by each subject to each time and age stratum are isolated, and the sums of the person-years in each stratum are then totalled to give the overall time at risk for that category. For example, in a retrospective cohort study of asbestos exposure and mortality from lung cancer in Britain [8], the period of follow-up extended from 1923 to 1954. Since overall lung cancer mortality rates in Great Britain changed over the course of the study, the observation period was divided into five strata: 1923 to 1934, 1935 to 1939, 1940 to 1944, 1945 to 1949, and 1950 to 1954. To illustrate the calculation of person-years for the different strata, consider a subject who entered the cohort in 1933 and left, because he either died or was lost to follow-up, in 1950. The distribution of this subject's total contribution of 17 person-years is outlined in Table 4-2, with the contribution of the years in which he entered and left the cohort each considered to be 0.5 person-year. A similar calculation would then be made for each individual in the study and the total person-years calculated within each time period.

Incidence density rates can be used to derive an estimate of the cumulative incidence, or an individual's risk of developing the disease during a specified period of time. If the incidence rate of the disease is low or the time period under observation short—in other words, to estimate small risks—the cumulative incidence is approximately equal to the product of the incidence rate times the length of the corresponding time period.

Issues In the Calculation of Measures of Incidence

For any measure of disease frequency, precise definition of the denominator is essential for both accuracy and clarity. This is a particular concern in the calculation of incidence. The denominator of a measure of incidence should in theory include only those who are considered "at risk" of developing the disease—that is, the total population from which the new cases could arise. Consequently, those who currently have or have already had the disease under study or persons who cannot develop the disease for reasons such as age, immunization, or prior removal of the involved organ should, in principle, be excluded from the denominator. It is often not possible to determine this information for each individual in a population, and the practical necessity for their exclusion depends on the proportion of the total population they constitute. In general, if persons not at risk are included in the denominator, the resultant measure will underestimate the true incidence of disease.

For most chronic diseases, the proportion of the general population with a history of the condition is relatively small, so that an inability to exclude these individuals from the denominator will not materially affect the incidence rate. For conditions such as endometrial cancer, however, those who are not "at risk," such as women who do not have an intact uterus, may compose a substantial proportion of the population in certain age groups. In a survey among women in New York, the proportion of women who had had a hysterectomy was over 25 percent among those aged 45 and older and approximately 35 percent for those 60 to 69 years of age [18]. These women are, of course, no longer at risk of developing endometrial cancer and should be excluded from the denominator of any incidence rate of this disease. This consideration is particularly important when comparing rates of endometrial cancer among different geographic areas or between different time periods because there are substantial regional differences and secular trends in the frequency of hysterectomy. For example, in 1979 to 1980, the rate of hysterectomy for the southern U.S. was approximately 2½ times that of women in the Northeast [31]. If women who have undergone hysterectomy are not removed from the denominator, grossly inaccurate estimates of incidence rates could result. In fact, it has been estimated that if women with a hysterectomy were excluded from the denominators, the estimates of incidence and mortality rates that have been made for uterine cancer during the period 1960 to 1973 would increase between 20 to 45 percent for each year [20].

Special Types of Incidence and Prevalence Measures

With both incidence and prevalence, either the numerator or denominator can be altered to yield specialized types of measures suitable for use in particular circumstances. These are summarized in Table 4-3.

Among the various special types of incidence rates, the two most commonly used are morbidity and mortality rates. The morbidity rate is the incidence rate of nonfatal cases in the total population at risk during a specified period of time. For example, the morbidity rate of tuberculosis (TB) in the U.S. in 1982 can be calculated by dividing the number of

Table 4-3. Special types of incidence and prevalence measures

Rate	Type	Numerator	Denominator
Morbidity rate	Incidence	New cases of nonfatal disease	Total population at risk
Mortality rate	Incidence	Number of deaths from a disease (or all causes)	Total population
Case-fatality rate	Incidence	Number of deaths from a disease	Number of cases of that disease
Attack rate	Incidence	Number of cases of a disease	Total population at risk, for a limited period of observation
Disease rate at autopsy	Prevalence	Number of cases of a disease	Number of persons autopsied
Birth defect rate	Prevalence	Number of babies with a given abnormality	Number of live births
Period prevalence	Prevalence	Number of existing cases plus new cases diagnosed during a given time period	Total population

nonfatal cases newly reported during that year by the total U.S. midyear population [3]:

$$\text{Morbidity rate of TB} = 25,520/231,534,000/\text{year}$$
$$= 11.0/10^5/\text{year}$$

Thus, in 1982, the morbidity rate or incidence rate of nonfatal TB in the United States was 11.0 per 100,000 population.

Similarly, the mortality rate expresses the incidence of death in a particular population during a period of time and is calculated by dividing the number of fatalities during that period by the total population. This can be expressed as either total mortality, which includes in the numerator deaths from all causes, or cause-specific mortality, for which the numerator is the number of deaths from a particular disease or event. For example, in the U.S. in 1982, there was a total of 1,973,000 deaths among a population of 231,534,000 individuals, giving an all-cause mortality rate of 852.1 per 100,000 per year, while there were 1807 deaths due to TB, yielding a cause-specific mortality rate of 7.8 per million per year [3]. Due to their ready availability, mortality rates are sometimes used as indices of the rate of the development of the disease in a population. Such use of death rates to represent incidence is reliable only when the disease is usually fatal and the interval between diagnosis and death is short.

In contrast to the cause-specific mortality rate, which expresses the number of deaths from a disease among all individuals in a population during a given time period, the case-fatality rate is the number of deaths from a disease divided by all cases of that illness. Thus, the case-fatality rate is a function of the severity of a disease. This measure represents the proportion of fatal cases among affected individuals and is often expressed as a percentage. For example, in the U.S. for the year 1981 to 1982, 200 cases of Reye's syndrome were reported in individuals 18 years or younger, and 70 died [29]. Thus, the case-fatality rate of Reye's syndrome for that 1-year period was 70 per 200, or 35 percent. For convenience, case-fatality rates are often constructed by dividing the number of deaths from a particular cause in a given year by the number of incident cases of the disease in that year. It should be noted that when this is done, the deaths that make up the numerator do not necessarily represent the cases that make up the denominator, as, for example, a death in 1981 might represent a case that was diagnosed a year or more previously. Therefore, a case-fatality rate derived in this manner assumes that incidence and mortality rates from the disease are relatively stable.

Another type of incidence measure that is useful in investigations of acute epidemics is the attack rate, a type of cumulative incidence which expresses the occurrence of a disease among a particular population at risk observed for a limited period of time, often due to a very specific exposure. The distinguishing feature of the attack rate is that it is useful in situations where the development of the outcome of interest rapidly follows the exposure during a time period that is fixed because of the nature of the disease process. For example, investigation of an outbreak of gastrointestinal illness in Oswego County, New York [16] revealed that 46 of the 75 people who had attended a church supper became ill within several hours, yielding an attack rate of 61 percent. Examination of the numbers of individuals who ate various foods led to the further discovery that 43 of 54 persons who ate vanilla ice cream became ill, compared with only 3 of 18 who did not. Therefore, the attack rates for those who did and did not eat vanilla ice cream were 80 and 17 percent, respectively. In such circumstances, the difference between attack rates for those exposed and nonexposed to a particular food provides important clues in the investigation of the etiology of an acute outbreak.

In addition to these special types of incidence rates, there are several types of measures of prevalence that should be mentioned, primarily because it is important to remember that they do represent prevalence despite the fact that they are often erroneously reported as measures of incidence. The first of these, the autopsy rate, is used to express the proportion of individuals who exhibit certain findings among those undergoing postmortem examinations. For example, in a case series of U.S. soldiers killed in Vietnam, the presence of atherosclerosis was reported among 105 autopsies [22]. In these data, 47 of the autopsies revealed some degree of atherosclerosis, yielding a prevalence in this young, previously healthy male population of 45 percent. While this finding is intriguing, variables such as the type of disease experienced, the circumstances under which death occurred, or standard medical practice regarding the conduct of autopsies all may influence which patients are autopsied. Such findings at autopsy may not, therefore, be representative of deaths in a general population or even of deaths among hospitalized patients.

A second type of prevalence measure often misinterpreted as an incidence rate is the frequency of birth defects. It is rarely possible to quantify the incidence or rate of development of a congenital abnormality, since the denominator for such a rate (those at risk of developing the birth defect) would have to include all products of conception, aborted fetuses and stillbirths as well as live births. Data regarding numbers of spontaneously aborted fetuses are usually not available, nor are aborted fetuses routinely examined for birth defects. Thus, a birth defect rate represents the prevalence of congenital abnormalities with the temporal reference point being birth, and the denominator being either live births or total births (live births plus stillbirths). For example, in 1981, the prevalence of ventricular septal defect in the United States was 1193 per 864,659 total births, or 138.0 per 100,000 total births [2].

One final type of prevalence rate is period prevalence, which represents the proportion of cases that exist within a population at any point during a specified period of time. The numerator thus includes cases that were present at the start of the period plus new cases that developed during this time. Period prevalence is sometimes utilized when it is particularly difficult to determine when a disease can be considered present, such as in the diagnosis of mental illness. However, this measure is not frequently used, since it combines both point prevalence (status at a single point in time) and incidence (risk of developing disease over time) in a single parameter.

Interrelationship Between Incidence and Prevalence

The proportion of the population that has a disease at a point in time (prevalence) and the rate of occurrence of new disease during a period of time (incidence) are closely related. Prevalence depends on both the incidence rate and the duration of the disease from onset to termination. If the incidence of a disease is low but those affected have the condition for a long period of time, the proportion of the population that has the disease at a particular point in time will be high relative to the incidence rate. Conversely, even if the rate of development of a disease in a population is high, if the duration is short, either through prompt recovery or death, the prevalence will be low relative to the incidence. For example, although the incidence rate of AIDS in the U.S. has been increasing at an alarming rate since the disease was first recognized [17], the prevalence has remained low because the mortality from this disease is extremely high [1]. In contrast, the yearly incidence rate of adult-onset diabetes in the U.S. is fairly low, but the prevalence is high because the disease is neither curable nor highly fatal.

Thus, a change in prevalence from one time period to another may be the result of changes in incidence rates, changes in the duration of the disease, or both. The introduction of new treatments, such as chemotherapeutic agents, that prevent death but do not produce recovery will result in an increase in the prevalence of a disease. Similarly, a decrease in the prevalence of a disease may result from a shortening of the duration of illness through more rapid recovery. For example, an observed decrease in the prevalence of hospitalization for mental illness could be due to a lowered incidence rate of psychiatric disorders in the population or merely to a decrease in the average length of stay in hospitals because of either improved treatment or the shift in medical practice to deinstitutionalization.

This interrelationship between incidence and prevalence can be expressed mathematically by saying that the prevalence (P) is proportional to the product of the incidence rate (I) and the average duration of the disease ($\bar{D}$). In particular, in the stable situation referred to as "steady state," meaning that the incidence rate of the disease has been constant over time (i.e., no epidemic or marked reduction of the disease), as has the distribution of the duration of the disease (i.e., no major change in the length of time from diagnosis to recovery or death), and assuming that the prevalence of the disease in the population is low (i.e., less than 0.1), the prevalence is approximately equal to the product of I and $\bar{D}$, as expressed by the formula:

$$P = I \times \bar{D}$$

When two of the measures are known, the third can be calculated simply by substitution. For example, in 1973 to 1977, the average annual incidence rate of lung cancer in Connecticut was 45.9 per 100,000 [37], and the average annual prevalence was 23.0 per 100,000. Therefore, the average duration of lung cancer could be calculated as follows:

$$\bar{D} = \frac{P}{I} = \frac{23.0/10^5}{45.9/10^5/\text{year}}$$
$$= 0.5 \text{ year}$$

Thus, individuals diagnosed with lung cancer during this period survived an average of 6 months from diagnosis to death. A detailed and comprehensive evaluation of the interrelationship of incidence and prevalence has been presented by Freeman and Hutchison [15].

Uses of Incidence and Prevalence Measures

Despite the close interrelationship of prevalence and incidence, each provides a somewhat different type of information with differing utility. Prevalence measures are most useful for health care providers, to assess the public health impact of a specific disease within a community and to project medical care needs for affected individuals, such as numbers of health care personnel or hospital beds that will be required. It may appear attractive to use these data to investigate etiologic relationships, since a desired sample size can often be achieved far more quickly if existing cases are used rather than waiting for new or incident cases to accumulate. However, this practical advantage must be weighed against the theoretic disadvantage that prevalent cases are determined by two sets of factors: those that affect the occurrence of disease and those that influence the duration or severity of the illness. For example, a study of prevalent cases of leukemia showed that the human leukocyte antigen HL-A2 was significantly more frequent among cases than among controls. The authors concluded that the presence of the antigen increased the risk of developing leukemia [27]. In a second study using incident cases, the data indicated that the previously observed association between the antigen and leukemia was due to improved survival of individuals with leukemia among persons with HL-A2 rather than to an increased risk of developing the disease [28]. Thus, the use of prevalent cases to study this association led to an incorrect conclusion, since those data reflected the effects of prognostic rather than etiologic factors. While the investigation of such prognostic factors is certainly important, it is not the main goal of studies designed to evaluate possible etiologic agents. Moreover, it will be more difficult to identify clearly antecedent exposures in prevalent cases since often the disease process itself will result in a conscious or unconscious change of many variables. Comparison of measures of incidence will remove the effect of survival and thus provide the clearest evidence concerning the development of the disease in relation to antecedent exposures.

Crude, Category-Specific, and Adjusted (Standardized) Rates

Rates can be presented for an entire population (crude rates) or for categories of the population defined on the basis of particular characteristics such as age, sex, or race (category-specific rates). A crude rate is a

Table 4-4. Crude and age-specific mortality rates
from cancer in the United States, 1980

Age in years	Number of cancer deaths	Population as of July 1, 1980	Mortality rate per 100,000
Under 5	686	16,348,000	4.2
5–9	777	16,700,000	4.7
10–14	720	18,242,000	3.9
15–19	1145	21,168,000	5.4
20–24	1538	21,319,000	7.2
25–29	2041	19,521,000	10.5
30–34	3040	17,561,000	17.3
35–39	4684	13,965,000	33.5
40–44	7786	11,669,000	66.7
45–49	14,230	11,090,000	128.3
50–54	26,800	11,710,000	228.9
55–59	41,600	11,615,000	358.2
60–64	53,045	10,088,000	525.8
65–74	127,430	15,581,000	817.9
75+	130,959	9,969,000	1313.7
Total	416,481	226,546,000	183.8

Source: Data from U.S. Bureau of the Census, *Statistical Abstract of the United States: 1984* (104th ed.). Washington, DC: 1983; and U.S. D.H.H.S., *Vital Statistics of the U.S., 1980.* Vol. II, Mortality, Part B. D.H.H.S. Publication No. (P.H.S.) 85–1102. Washington, DC: National Center for Health Statistics, 1985

summary measure, calculated by dividing the total number of cases of the outcome in the population by the total number of individuals in that population in a specified time period. For example, Table 4-4 presents the number of deaths from cancer in the United States in 1980 [38] as well as estimates of the midyear population [35]. As shown in the bottom line, the crude mortality rate from cancer for this year consists of the total number of cancer deaths divided by the total number of individuals in the population:

Crude 1980 cancer mortality rate $= 416,481/226,546,000/1$ year

$$= 183.8/10^5/\text{year}$$

In contrast, age-specific cancer death rates refer to the numbers of deaths due to cancer occurring among individuals in each specified age category divided by the total number of persons in that stratum. Thus, the death rate from cancer for those under 5 years of age can be calculated as follows:

$$\text{Cancer mortality rate } (< 5 \text{ years}) = 686/16,348,000/1 \text{ year}$$
$$= 4.2/10^5/\text{year}$$

One problem that arises in comparing crude rates of disease between populations is that the groups may differ with respect to certain underlying characteristics, such as age, sex, or race, that may affect the overall rate of disease. For example, the crude mortality rate from cancer in the United States in 1940 was 120.2 per 100,000 [34], as compared with 183.8 per 100,000 in 1980. These crude rates, indicating an overall 53-percent increase in cancer mortality during this 40-year period, have erroneously suggested a trend so alarming as to be considered indicative of an epidemic of cancer [13]. The problem in comparing the crude rate directly derives from that fact that in 1980, 11.3 percent of the U.S. population was aged 65 years or older [34], while in 1940 this proportion was only 6.9 percent [35]. Since cancer mortality rates rise dramatically with age, the higher crude cancer mortality rate in 1980 is attributable, at least in part, simply to the overall aging of the U.S. population.

To understand how a comparison of crude rates can be affected by differing population distributions, it must be recognized that any crude rate is actually a weighted average of the individual category-specific rates, with the weights being the proportion of the population in each category. Thus, the calculation of any crude rate can be written as:

$$\text{Crude rate } = \Sigma \text{ (category-specific rate} \times \text{ proportion of population in category)}$$

For example, as shown in Table 4-4, the crude cancer death rate in the U.S. in 1980 could be calculated by dividing the total number of deaths in that time period by the total population. As illustrated in Table 4-5, this same crude rate could also have been obtained by calculating a weighted average of the age-specific cancer mortality rates in 1980:

$$\text{Crude 1980 cancer death rate } = \frac{4.2(16,348,000) + 4.7(16,700,000) + \ldots + 817.9(15,581,000) + 1313.7(9,969,000)}{226,546,000}$$

$$= 183.8/10^5$$

As can be seen from the formula, even if two populations had identical stratum-specific rates, the crude rates for the two populations will differ if the proportions of the population within each of the various categories are different. For example, as shown in Table 4-6, if the age-specific

Table 4-5. Calculation of the crude cancer mortality rate in the U.S., 1980, as a weighted average of age-specific rates

Age in years	Mortality rate per 100,000	Population as of July 1, 1980
Under 5	4.2	16,348,000
5–9	4.7	16,700,000
10–14	3.9	18,242,000
15–19	5.4	21,168,000
20–24	7.2	21,319,000
25–29	10.5	19,521,000
30–34	17.3	17,561,000
35–39	33.5	13,965,000
40–44	66.7	11,669,000
45–49	128.3	11,090,000
50–54	228.9	11,710,000
55–59	358.2	11,615,000
60–64	525.8	10,088,000
65–74	817.9	15,581,000
75+	1313.7	9,969,000
Total		226,546,000

Crude 1980 cancer death rate =

$$\frac{4.2\,(16,348,000) + 4.7\,(16,700,000) + \ldots + 817.9\,(15,581,000) + 1313.7\,(9,969,000)}{226,546,000} = 183.8/10^5$$

cancer mortality rates are identical to those presented in Table 4-5 but the numbers of individuals in the two age groups 20 to 24 and 75+ years are reversed so that a larger proportion of the population falls in the older age group, which has a higher death rate, the crude mortality rate from cancer would increase considerably (from 183.8 to 249.2 per 100,000).

There are two ways to account for differing distributions of a characteristic between populations being compared. The first is simply to present and compare only the category-specific rates. For example, Table 4-7 presents the age-specific cancer mortality rates for 1940 and 1980 [38]. These data show that although the crude rate increased about 53 percent over this period, most of the age-specific rates tended to increase only slightly. In fact, for those under 5 years and between the ages of 25 and 49, cancer mortality rates actually decreased.

Table 4-6. Hypothetical calculation of the crude cancer mortality rate in the U.S., 1980, as a weighted average of age-specific rates, with a different age distribution of the population

Age in years	Mortality rate per 100,000	Population as of July 1, 1980
Under 5	4.2	16,348,000
5–9	4.7	16,700,000
10–14	3.9	18,242,000
15–19	5.4	21,168,000
20–24	7.2	9,969,000*
25–29	10.5	19,521,000
30–34	17.3	17,561,000
35–39	33.5	13,965,000
40–44	66.7	11,669,000
45–49	128.3	11,090,000
50–54	228.9	11,710,000
55–59	358.2	11,615,000
60–64	525.8	10,088,000
65–74	817.9	15,581,000
75 +	1313.7	21,319,000*
Total		226,546,000

Crude cancer death rate =

$$\frac{4.2\,(16{,}348{,}000) + 4.7\,(16{,}700{,}000) + \ldots + 817.9\,(15{,}581{,}000) + 1313.7\,(21{,}319{,}000)}{226{,}546{,}000} = 249.2/10^5$$

*The numbers in the two categories have been reversed from Table 4-5.

Such a consideration of category-specific rates is certainly more accurate than a comparison of the crude rates, but it requires large numbers of comparisons. In many circumstances, it is useful to have a single summary rate for each population that takes into account any differences in the structure of the populations. This is done through a procedure called adjustment, or standardization. Adjusted rates are statistically constructed summary rates that account for the difference between populations with respect to these other variables. When comparing rates adjusted for a particular factor, any remaining observed differences between the groups cannot be attributed to confounding by that variable.

The method for adjustment of rates is discussed in detail in many textbooks of biostatistics [5]. Briefly, however, the two main techniques used are referred to as the direct and indirect methods. Both methods are similar in that they consist of taking a weighted average of category-

Table 4-7. Crude and age-specific cancer mortality rates in the United States, 1940 and 1980

Age in years	Cancer mortality rates per 100,000	
	1940	1980
Under 5	4.7	4.2
5–9	3.0	4.7
10–14	2.9	3.9
15–19	4.0	5.4
20–24	6.8	7.2
25–29	11.6	10.5
30–34	23.5	17.3
35–39	43.4	33.5
40–44	80.3	66.7
45–49	133.4	128.3
50–54	209.0	228.9
55–59	309.9	358.2
60–64	443.3	525.8
65–74	695.1	817.9
75+	1183.5	1313.7
Total (crude rate)	120.2	183.8

Data from U.S. D.H.H.S., *Vital Statistics of the U.S., 1980*. Vol. II, Mortality, Part B. D.H.H.S. Publication No. (P.H.S.) 85–1102. Washington, DC: National Center for Health Statistics, 1985.

specific rates. The difference between the two lies simply in the source of the weights and the rates. The indirect method will be discussed later in this chapter, under the calculation of the standardized mortality ratio. In the direct method, adjusted rates are derived by applying the category-specific rates observed in each of the populations to a single standard population. This weighted average of the category-specific rates, with the weights taken from a standard population, provides, for each population, a single summary rate that reflects the numbers of events that would have been expected if the populations being compared had had identical distributions of the characteristic of interest. For example, as illustrated in Table 4-8, the age-adjusted cancer mortality rate for the U.S. in 1980 would be calculated by applying the 1980 age-specific cancer mortality rates to the age distribution of the population in 1940, yielding a value of 132.7 per 100,000. This standardized rate represents the hypothetical rate that would have been observed if the 1980 population had had the same age distribution as in 1940 (the standard). This means that if the age structure of the U.S. had not changed between

Table 4-8. Calculation of age-adjusted cancer mortality rates in the U.S., using the 1940 U.S. population as the standard

Age in years	1940 population (in thousands)	1980 cancer mortality rates per 100,000	Expected deaths in 1980
< 5	10,541	4.2	442.7
5–9	10,685	4.7	502.2
10–14	11,746	3.9	458.1
15–19	12,334	5.4	666.0
20–24	11,588	7.2	834.3
25–29	11,097	10.5	1165.2
30–34	10,242	17.3	1771.9
35–39	9,545	33.5	3197.6
40–44	8,788	66.7	5861.6
45–49	8,255	128.3	10591.2
50–54	7,257	228.9	16611.3
55–59	5,844	358.2	20933.2
60–64	4,728	525.8	24859.8
65–74	6,377	817.9	52157.5
75 +	2,643	1313.7	34721.1
Total	131,670		174,773.7

$$\text{Age-adjusted cancer mortality rate} = \frac{174,773.7}{131,670,000} = 132.7/10^5$$

1940 and 1980, we would have seen an overall cancer death rate of 132.7 per 100,000 during 1980. Thus, instead of the 53 percent increase observed in comparing the crude rates in 1940 and 1980, after the shift in the age structure of the U.S. population has been taken into account, cancer mortality rates have actually increased only about 10 percent during this 40-year period. Parenthetically, since this excess is virtually totally explained by increases in smoking-related cancers and more accurate diagnosis of other sites, such as prostate cancer in men, these figures provide reassuring evidence against the theory that there is currently a general epidemic of cancer in the United States [10].

In direct standardization, the standard chosen by the investigator could be the distribution of one of the populations to be compared, a distribution of the two populations combined (such as the average), or an outside standard of interest (such as the U.S. population in one of the census years). The actual values of the adjusted rates will depend on the standard population chosen. With the majority of standards, however, the magnitude of the differences for the adjusted rates will stay virtually the same.

The decision to use crude, adjusted, or category-specific rates depends on the information that an investigator is trying to obtain or impart. Crude rates represent the actual experience of the population and provide data for the allocation of health resources and public health planning. Although they are easy to calculate and widely used for international comparisons, the fact that the values may be confounded by differences between underlying population structures make any observed differences in crude rates difficult to interpret. Category-specific rates are unconfounded by that factor and provide the most detailed information about the pattern of the disease in a population. Making comparisons, however, quickly becomes cumbersome with the large number of rates that must be presented. Adjusted rates provide a summary value that removes the effect of the differences in population structure to allow for valid comparisons between groups or over time. The actual value of the adjusted rate is meaningless, however, since it has been statistically constructed based on the choice of a standard. Thus, depending on the nature of the information required, one or a combination of these measures may be chosen.

MEASURES OF ASSOCIATION

As discussed earlier, in epidemiologic research the calculation of appropriate measures of disease frequency is the basis for the comparison of populations and, therefore, the identification of disease determinants. To do this most efficiently and informatively, the two frequencies being compared can be combined into a single summary parameter that estimates the association between an exposure and the risk of developing a disease. This can be accomplished by calculating either the ratio of the measures of disease frequency for the two populations, which indicates how much more likely one group is to develop a disease than another, or the difference between the two, which indicates on an absolute scale how much greater the frequency of disease is in one group compared with the other. These measures of association, the relative risk and the attributable risk, are the two most frequently used in epidemiology.

Presentation of Data

To aid in the calculation of measures of association, epidemiologic data are often presented in the form of a two-by-two table, also called a fourfold or contingency table. The two-by-two table derives its name from the fact that it contains two rows and two columns, each representing

	Disease		
	Yes	No	Total
Exposure Yes	a	b	a + b
Exposure No	c	d	c + d
Total	a + c	b + d	a + b + c + d

Fig. 4-2. Presentation of data in a two-by-two table from a case-control or cohort study with count denominators.

the presence or absence of the exposure or disease. This creates four cells, labeled *a, b, c,* and *d,* each of which represents the number of individuals having that particular combination of exposure and disease status. Specifically, if, as illustrated in Figure 4-2, the rows represent the two levels of exposure status (exposed, nonexposed) and the columns the two levels of disease status (diseased, nondiseased), then:

a = the number of individuals who are exposed and have the disease

b = the number who are exposed and do not have the disease

c = the number who are not exposed and have the disease

d = the number who are both nonexposed and nondiseased

The margins of the table represent the total numbers of individuals in each row and column and are calculated by simply adding the relevant cells. Thus, from Figure 4-2:

$a + b$ = the total number of individuals exposed

$c + d$ = the total number nonexposed

$a + c$ = the total number with the disease

$b + d$ = the total number without the disease

The sum of all four cells $(a + b + c + d)$ is the total sample size of the study, represented by T or N.

To illustrate the construction of a two-by-two table, Table 4-9 presents the data from a case-control study of oral contraceptive (OC) use and risk of myocardial infarction (MI) [30]. Of 156 women with MI, 23 were

Table 4-9. Data from a case-control study of current oral contraceptive (OC) use and myocardial infarction in premenopausal female nurses

	Myocardial infarction		
	Yes	No	Total
Current OC use			
Yes	23	304	327
No	133	2816	2949
Total	156	3120	3276

Data from L. Rosenberg et al., Oral contraceptive use in relation to non-fatal myocardial infarction. *Am. J. Epidemiol.* 111:59, 1980.

Table 4-10. Data from a cohort study of oral contraceptive (OC) use and bacteriuria among women aged 16–49 years

	Bacteriuria		
	Yes	No	Total
OC use			
Yes	27	455	482
No	77	1831	1908
Total	104	2286	2390

Data from D. A. Evans et al., Oral contraceptives and bacteriuria in a community-based study. *N. Engl. J. Med.* 299:536, 1978.

current OC users at the time of their hospital admission. Of the 3120 control women without MI, 304 were current OC users. The number of nonexposed cases and controls can then be obtained by subtraction and the remaining margins filled in.

Similarly, Table 4-10 shows data from a cohort study of OC use in relation to the subsequent development of bacteriuria [12]. Among 2390 women aged 16 to 49 years who were free from bacteriuria, 482 were OC users at the initial survey in 1973, while 1908 were not. At a second survey in 1976, 27 of the OC users had developed bacteriuria, as had 77 of the nonusers. As before, the number of women who did not develop bacteriuria among the OC users and nonusers can then be obtained by subtraction.

In cohort studies with variable lengths of follow-up, a variation of the two-by-two table is used for data presentation, since the numbers of person-time units for exposed and nonexposed subjects are provided rather than the total numbers of individuals in each group. The usual format for presentation of such data is shown in Figure 4-3. As for tables of data with count denominators, cells *a* and *c* represent the numbers of

| | Disease | | Person-time units |
	Yes	No	
Exposure Yes	a	—	PY_1
Exposure No	c	—	PY_0
Total	$a + c$		$PY_1 + PY_0$

Fig. 4-3. Presentation of data from a cohort study with person-time denominators.

exposed and nonexposed subjects who develop the disease of interest. However, the margins now indicate the total number of person-time units (e.g., person-years) of follow-up among all exposed and nonexposed subjects, referred to as PY_1 and PY_0, respectively. However, because of the use of person-time units rather than numbers of persons in the margins, it is not possible to derive the values of cells b and d by subtraction. Moreover, since these values are not necessary to calculate the incidence rates of disease in the exposed and nonexposed groups, these two cells are usually omitted from the table.

The use of this format is illustrated by Table 4-11, which presents data on postmenopausal hormone use and coronary heart disease among postmenopausal female nurses from a prospective cohort study [33]. After a total of 54,308.7 person-years of follow-up, 30 women who reported that they had used postmenopausal hormones developed coronary heart disease. For the "never users," 60 developed coronary heart disease among 51,477.5 person-years of follow-up.

The basic two-by-two table, whether presenting count or person-time units, can also be expanded to reflect additional levels of exposure or disease status. This is generally referred to as an r-by-c table, with r representing the number of rows and c the number of columns. For example, in the case-control study of OC use and MI presented in Table 4-9, it was also of interest to determine risk of disease in relation to duration of OC use rather than simply among current users as a whole. In this circumstance, the data could be presented as a five-by-two table (Table 4-12), where the 5 rows represent four categories of current users (those who had taken OCs less than 1, 1 to 4, 5 to 9, and 10 or more years) and one category of never users.

Table 4-11. Data from a cohort study of postmenopausal
hormone use and coronary heart disease among female nurses

| | Coronary heart disease | | |
	Yes	No	Person-years
Postmenopausal hormone use			
Yes	30	—	54,308.7
No	60	—	51,477.5
Total	90		105,786.2

Data from M. J. Stampfer et al., A prospective study of postmenopausal
hormones and coronary heart disease. *N. Engl. J. Med.* 313:1044, 1985.

Table 4-12. Data from a case-control study of current oral contraceptive (OC)
use and myocardial infarction in women, by duration of use

| | Myocardial infarction | | |
	Yes	No	Total
OC use			
Current			
< 1 year	4	31	35
1–4 years	5	107	112
5–9 years	7	127	134
10+ years	7	39	46
Never	133	2816	2949
Total	156	3120	3276

Data from L. Rosenberg et al., Oral contraceptive use in relation to non-fatal
myocardial infarction. *Am. J. Epidemiol.* 111:59, 1980.

Relative Risk

The relative risk (RR) estimates the magnitude of an association between
exposure and disease and indicates the likelihood of developing the disease in the exposed group relative to those who are not exposed. It is
defined as the ratio of the incidence of disease in the exposed group
(expressed as I_e) divided by the corresponding incidence of disease in
the nonexposed group (I_0). For a cohort study with count data in the
denominator, the relative risk (or risk ratio) is calculated as the ratio of
the cumulative incidence among those exposed compared with those not
exposed. Referring to the prototype two-by-two tables presented in the

previous section, the formula for calculating the relative risk for such data is

$$RR = \frac{I_e}{I_0} = \frac{CI_e}{CI_0} = \frac{a/(a + b)}{c/(c + d)}$$

For example, in the cohort study of OC use and bacteriuria presented in Table 4-10, the relative risk would be calculated as follows:

$$RR = \frac{a/(a + b)}{c/(c + d)}$$
$$= \frac{27/482}{77/1908}$$
$$= 1.4$$

This value means that in these data, women who used OCs had 1.4 times the risk of developing bacteriuria as compared with nonusers.

For cohort studies with person-time units of follow-up, the relative risk (or rate ratio) is calculated analogously as the ratio of the incidence density in those exposed to that among those nonexposed. For example, in the cohort study of postmenopausal hormone use and coronary heart disease presented in Table 4-11, the relative risk can be calculated as:

$$RR = \frac{I_e}{I_0} = \frac{ID_e}{ID_0} = \frac{a/PY_1}{c/PY_0}$$
$$= \frac{30/54,308.7}{60/51,477.5}$$
$$= 0.5$$

A relative risk of 1.0 indicates that the incidence rates of disease in the exposed and nonexposed groups are identical and thus that there is no association observed between the exposure and the disease in the data. A value greater than 1.0 indicates a positive association, or an increased risk among those exposed to a factor. Thus, the relative risk of 1.4 calculated above indicates that OC users had 1.4 times the risk or were 40 percent (i.e., 1.4 minus the null value of 1.0) more likely to develop bacteriuria than nonusers. Analogously, a relative risk less than 1.0 means that there is an inverse association or a decreased risk among those exposed; in the above example, women who used postmenopausal hormones had 0.5 times, or only half, the risk of developing coronary heart disease compared with nonusers.

The value of the relative risk computed as the ratio of two risks or cumulative incidences depends on the time period over which the risks were calculated. This value may change depending on the length of observation; the relative risk after 10 years may be quite different from that after 1 year. This is illustrated most intuitively by considering the relative risk of all-cause mortality for an exposed and nonexposed population. Regardless of the underlying rate of death at any age, the cumulative risk of dying in the two groups will be identical over the long run (that is, 100% over an individual's lifetime), and thus the risk ratio will approach 1.0. Over a short period, cumulative incidence is approximately equal to the product of the incidence rate and time, so that the ratio of the two risks is approximately equal to the ratio of the two underlying incidence rates. Consequently, it is important that the relevant time period on which the calculation of the risk ratio was based be specified. In addition, in studies where the measure of disease frequency is prevalence, as in studies of congenital malformations, if the prevalence of disease is low and the duration is the same among those exposed and nonexposed, the relative risk based on prevalence comparisons will approximate the relative risk based on incidence. As the prevalence increases, however, the prevalence ratios will shift towards unity.

In a case-control study, where participants are selected on the basis of disease status, it is usually not possible to calculate the rate of development of disease given the presence or absence of exposure. Consequently, the formulas presented for the calculation of the relative risk in a cohort study cannot be applied to data from a case-control study. The relative risk can be estimated, however, by calculating the ratio of the odds of exposure among the cases to that among the controls. This odds ratio (OR) is expressed by the following formula:

$$OR = \frac{a/c}{b/d} = \frac{ad}{bc}$$

For example, in the case-control study of current OC use and MI presented in Table 4-9, to derive an estimate of the relative risk, the odds ratio would be calculated as follows:

$$RR = OR = \frac{ad}{bc}$$

$$= \frac{(23)\,(2816)}{(304)\,(133)}$$

$$RR = 1.6$$

Thus, these data indicate that women who were current OC users had a risk of MI 1.6 times that of nonusers.

The inability to calculate the relative risk directly in case-control studies as the ratio of incidence rates can be best illustrated by examining

Table 4-13. Calculation of the odds ratio (OR) and relative risk (RR) from a hypothetical case-control study of cigarette smoking and lung cancer among 100 cases and 100 controls

	Lung cancer		Total
	Cases	Controls	
Cigarette smoking			
Yes	70	30	100
No	30	70	100
Total	100	100	200

$$OR = \frac{ad}{bc} = \frac{(70)(70)}{(30)(30)} = 5.4$$

$$RR = \frac{a/(a+b)}{c/(c+d)} = \frac{70/100}{30/100} = 2.3$$

what happens to the estimate when the proportions of exposure in cases and controls remain the same but the number of controls is increased. Table 4-13 presents hypothetical data from a study of cigarette smoking and lung cancer among 100 cases and an equal number of controls. The proportions of smokers in these two groups are 70 and 30 percent, respectively. If we were to estimate the relative risk by calculating the odds ratio, we would conclude, as shown in the table, that smokers were 5.4 times more likely to develop lung cancer than nonsmokers. Calculating the relative risk (RR) as the ratio of cumulative incidence rates yields a value of 2.3. Table 4-14 presents the data that would result if the number of controls in the study is increased 10-fold, from 100 to 1000, but the proportions of cases and controls who smoke remain the same (70 and 30 percent). Since the proportions of exposed individuals among cases and controls remain unchanged, we would certainly want our estimate of effect also to be unaltered, regardless of the actual numbers of controls in the study. As shown in Table 4-14, estimating the relative risk as the odds ratio does indeed yield an identical estimate of 5.4. In contrast, calculating the RR as the ratio of incidence rates yields an estimate of 4.6, which is double that derived from the previous sample.

There is a firm mathematical basis for the odds ratio being not only a stable but also an unbiased estimate in case-control studies of the relative risk. Simply stated, Cornfield [6] first reasoned that when the disease is rare, that is, when the proportion of cases in the exposed and nonexposed groups is low, the total number exposed $(a + b)$ can be approximated by the number of exposed controls (b) and the total nonexposed

Table 4-14. Calculation of the odds ratio (OR) and relative risk (RR) from a hypothetical case-control study of cigarette smoking and lung cancer among 100 cases and 1000 controls

	Lung cancer		Total
	Cases	Controls	
Cigarette smoking			
Yes	70	300	370
No	30	700	730
Total	100	1000	1100

$$OR = \frac{ad}{bc} = \frac{(70)(700)}{(30)(300)} = 5.4$$

$$RR = \frac{a/(a + b)}{c/(c + d)} = \frac{70/370}{30/730} = 4.6$$

$(c + d)$ by the number of nonexposed controls (d). This is expressed mathematically as follows:

$$RR = \frac{a/(a + b)}{c/(c + d)} \cong \frac{a/b}{c/d} = \frac{ad}{bc}$$

In recent years, it has been demonstrated that this rare disease assumption is not necessary for the odds ratio to provide a valid estimate of the relative risk [23]. In fact, the odds ratio provides a valid estimate of the relative risk under conditions that prevail in most case-control studies, including that the cases of disease are newly diagnosed, that prevalent cases are not included in the control group, and that the selection of cases and controls is not based on exposure status. It should also be noted that when a case-control study is population-based—that is, when all or a known fraction of cases in a particular community are identified and a random sample of unaffected individuals are selected as controls—it is possible to calculate incidence rates of disease and the relative risk directly.

When data are presented in an expanded *r*-by-*c* table, reflecting either various exposure levels or different categories of some characteristic of the study population, the overall *r*-by-*c* table can be considered as actually comprising a number of individual two-by-two tables, in which the subjects who are serving as the comparison group, usually the nonexposed, are always entered along with those having the particular exposure level of interest. For example, in the cohort study of postmenopau-

Table 4-15. Calculation of relative risks (RRs) from a cohort study of postmenopausal hormone use and coronary heart disease with several exposure categories

	Coronary heart disease	Person-years
Postmenopausal hormone use		
Ever use	30	54,308.7
Past use	19	24,386.7
Current use	11	29,922.0
Never use	60	51,477.5

$$\text{Ever versus never use:} \quad RR = \frac{30/54308.7}{60/51477.5} = 0.5$$

$$\text{Past versus never use:} \quad RR = \frac{19/24386.7}{60/51477.5} = 0.7$$

$$\text{Current versus never use:} \quad RR = \frac{11/29922.0}{60/51477.5} = 0.3$$

Data from M. J. Stampfer et al., A prospective study of postmenopausal hormones and coronary heart disease. *N. Engl. J. Med.* 313:1044, 1985.

sal hormone use and CHD (Table 4-11), ever use of hormones can be further broken down into past use and current use. As shown in Table 4-15, the relative risks for each of these exposure levels can be calculated in comparison with never users, yielding a relative risk of 0.7 for past users of postmenopausal hormones and 0.3 for current users. Thus, past users of postmenopausal hormones had 70 percent, and current users only 30 percent, of the risk of CHD among those who had never used these preparations.

Standardized Mortality Ratios

Often in retrospective cohort studies in an occupational setting, the information that is available relates to the number of cases of disease or death that have been observed among the study population. The question is whether the number of cases in this group is unusual—that is, whether it is greater or less than one might have expected it to be. To assess this, rates from a standard population are used to calculate the number of cases that would have been expected in this group had they developed the disease at the same rate as a general population. The expected number of cases in each stratum of the study population is calculated by multiplying the stratum-specific rates in the standard population by the weights of each category, or the number of person-years of the study population in that category. The total expected number is then calculated by summing the expected numbers in each stratum. The results are presented as the standardized morbidity or mortality ratio (SMR), which is the ratio of the observed number of cases to the expected number.

$$\text{SMR} = \frac{\text{observed deaths (O)}}{\text{expected deaths (E)}} \, (\times \, 100\%)$$

The word *standardized* in the standardized morbidity or mortality ratio indicates that adjustment has been made for the effects of one or more potential confounding factors by calculating a weighted average of category-specific (and thus unconfounded) rates. This adjustment process is referred to as an indirect method of standardization, since rates from a standard population are applied to the weights (person-years of follow-up) in the exposed group to control for the effects of potential confounding factors. The standard population should be as similar as possible to the exposed group with respect to other risk factors for the outcome. Often rates from two standard populations are used: a nonexposed group (if available) from within the same occupational setting and a general population, such as U.S. white males aged 20 to 59 years.

Table 4-16 presents data from a retrospective cohort study of asbestos workers [12]. In this group, a total of 58 cancer deaths were observed between 1948 and 1963. To calculate how many cancer deaths would have been expected in this population had they died from cancer at the same rate as a general U.S. population of the same age, sex, and race, the number of person-years in each age group within the cohort is given for each follow-up interval, as well as the midpoint U.S. cancer mortality rate for white males in that age group (i.e., for the interval 1948–1952, the rate used is that for 1950). The expected number of cancer deaths in each age-time stratum is then calculated by multiplying the category-specific rate from the standard population by the person-year distribution of asbestos workers. As shown, when these expected numbers are added together, the overall number of cancer deaths expected in this cohort was 42.9. The standardized mortality ratio can then be calculated as follows:

$$\text{SMR} = \text{O/E}$$
$$= 58/42.9$$
$$= 1.35$$
$$= 135\%$$

This SMR indicates that this group of asbestos workers had a risk of cancer mortality approximately 35 percent greater than men in the gen-

Table 4-16. Indirect standardization of cancer mortality rates
for a cohort of asbestos products workers, 1948–1963

Age group	Person-years in cohort	Cancer mortality rates U.S. white males (per 100,000)	Expected cancer deaths
1948–1952:			
15–24	1250	9.9	0.1
25–34	3423	17.7	0.6
35–44	3275	44.5	1.5
45–54	2028	150.8	3.1
55–64	1144	409.4	4.7
1953–1957:			
15–24	544	11.2	0.1
25–34	3702	17.5	0.6
35–44	4382	44.2	1.9
45–54	2968	157.7	4.7
55–64	1552	432.0	6.7
1958–1963:			
15–24	4	10.3	0.0
25–34	2206	18.8	0.4
35–44	4737	46.3	2.2
45–54	4114	164.1	6.8
55–64	2098	450.9	9.5
Total			42.9

SMR = observed/expected × 100%

= 58/42.9 × 100%

= 135%

Data from P. E. Enterline, Mortality among asbestos products workers in the United States. *Ann. N.Y. Acad. Sci.* 132:156, 1965.

eral population. Note that while the standardized mortality ratio indicates an excess risk among those exposed to asbestos, the magnitude of this excess is less than what would have been estimated by a relative risk. This is because the standard (general) population consists of both exposed and nonexposed individuals. Thus, the number of cases expected on the basis of the standard population (i.e., 42.9) already reflects the effect of exposure. Because of this, a standardized mortality ratio using the general population as a standard will always underestimate any true increased or decreased risk. If available, a standardized mortality ratio using a nonexposed population as the source of the standard rates would give a more valid estimate of the true effect of the exposure.

While the interpretation of a single standardized mortality ratio is simple and straightforward, a problem arises when trying to compare a number of standardized mortality ratios from different study populations with each other. For example, if the asbestos workers were classified into two levels of exposure according to their job descriptions, an expected number of cases for each group could be calculated using age-, sex-, and race-specific rates from the general population. However, the actual number of expected cases in each group would depend on the distribution of each of the two exposed populations by age, sex, and race. Unless these are identical, which would rarely be the case, each standardized mortality ratio is in fact standardized to a different exposed population of workers despite the fact that each uses the same general population to provide the expected rates. Thus, the two standardized mortality ratios actually use different standards, are not comparable with each other, and should not be directly compared to evaluate the relative effect of the two levels of exposure. To make such a comparison validly, the direct method of standardization, in which a common standard is used for the two exposed groups, is preferred. To do this, of course, the category-specific rates in the exposed populations must be available.

Proportional Mortality Ratio

Another method of examining the impact of a disease upon an exposed population is to calculate the proportional mortality ratio (PMR). This is done when an investigator is able to ascertain the numbers and causes of deaths among the exposed group but not the structure of the population from which they arose. In the PMR, the proportion of deaths from a specified cause relative to all deaths among the cohort is compared with the corresponding proportion in the nonexposed group or general population. The PMR is therefore calculated as follows:

$$PMR = \frac{\text{proportion of deaths from specified cause (exposed)}}{\text{proportion of deaths from specified cause (comparison population)}} \ (\times \ 100\%)$$

Alternatively, the proportional mortality ratio can also be expressed in a form similar to that of the standardized mortality ratio

$$PMR = \frac{\text{observed deaths from specified cause (O)}}{\text{expected deaths from specified cause (E)}} \ (\times \ 100\%)$$

where the expected number of deaths is the number that would have occurred if the proportion of deaths from a specified cause relative to all deaths in the study population were the same as the corresponding proportion in the comparison group.

For example, in a study [26] of mortality among a cohort of nuclear shipyard workers between 1959 and 1977, a total of 146 deaths were observed, of which 56 were attributable to cancer. The proportional mortality for cancer among this cohort was therefore 56/146, or 38.4 percent. The proportional mortality for cancer in the general population of U.S. white males of comparable age in 1970 was 21.5 percent [36]. On the basis of this standard, the expected number of cancer deaths can be calculated as the total number of deaths observed in the cohort times the proportional mortality among the comparison group:

$$\text{Expected cancer deaths} = (146)\,(0.215)$$
$$= 31.4$$

The PMR can then be calculated as follows:

$$\text{PMR} = \frac{O}{E} = 56/31.4$$
$$= 1.78$$
$$= 178\%$$

Thus, the proportion of deaths attributable to cancer was almost twice as great among the nuclear shipyard workers as among a comparable U.S. population.

Like the SMR, the PMR is an estimate that is standardized to control for potential confounding effects of variables such as age, sex, race, or time. However, while the SMR requires knowledge of the structure of the exposed population in each stratum, the PMR only requires knowledge of only the proportion of cause-specific deaths observed in each stratum. Consequently, studies based on the calculation of this measure are much less time-consuming and expensive than those that require the collection of more detailed follow-up information. In addition, PMRs are frequently used in studies in which the only information available comes from the death certificates of a group of persons in a specific occupation [24]. The major problem in the interpretation of the PMR is that the relative frequency of other causes of death can affect the proportional mortality for the cause of interest. As a result, an observed excess of one cause of death in a particular exposure group may represent a true increased risk, but may also merely represent a deficit of deaths due to some other cause. Thus, while PMRs can suggest that a risk exists, an evaluation of this possibility requires that the population at risk be taken into account and that the cause-specific mortality rates be compared.

Attributable Risk

As has been discussed, the relative risk represents the likelihood of disease in exposed individuals relative to those who are nonexposed. The risk difference (RD) or attributable risk (AR) is a measure of association that provides information about the absolute effect of the exposure or the excess risk of disease in those exposed compared with those nonexposed. This measure is defined as the difference between the incidence rates in the exposed and nonexposed groups and can be calculated as follows:

$$AR = I_e - I_0$$

In a cohort study, the attributable risk is calculated as the difference of cumulative incidences (risk difference) or incidence densities (rate difference) depending on the study design. For example, in the study of OC use and bacteriuria (Table 4-10), the attributable risk would be calculated as follows:

$$
\begin{aligned}
AR = CI_e - CI_0 &= \frac{a}{(a + b)} - \frac{c}{(c + d)} \\
&= \frac{27}{482} - \frac{77}{1908} \\
&= 0.01566 = 1566/10^5
\end{aligned}
$$

Thus, the excess occurrence of bacteriuria among OC users attributable to their OC use is 1566 per 100,000. The attributable risk is used to quantify the risk of disease in the exposed group that can be considered attributable to the exposure by removing the risk of disease that would have occurred anyway due to other causes (the risk in the nonexposed). Thus, the interpretation of the attributable risk is dependent on the assumption that a cause-effect relationship exists between exposure and disease. If there is no association between exposure and disease, there will be no difference between the incidence rates in the exposed and nonexposed groups, so that AR = 0. If, however, there is a causal association between the exposure and disease and the attributable risk is greater than 0, its value indicates the number of cases of the disease among the exposed that can be attributed to the exposure itself, or alternatively, the number of cases of the disease among the exposed that could be eliminated if the exposure were eliminated. Thus, the attributable risk can be useful as a measure of the public health impact of a particular exposure.

To estimate the proportion of the disease among the exposed that is attributable to the exposure, or the proportion of the disease in that group that could be prevented by eliminating the exposure, the attributable risk is often expressed as a percentage (AR%). The attributable-risk percent, also referred to as the attributable-rate percent, attributable proportion, or etiologic fraction, is calculated as the attributable risk divided by the rate of disease among the exposed or:

$$AR\% = \frac{AR}{I_e} \times 100$$

$$= \frac{(I_e - I_0)}{I_e} \times 100$$

In the cohort study of OC use and bacteriuria, the attributable-risk percent would be calculated as follows:

$$AR\% = \frac{(AR)}{I_e} \times 100$$

$$= \frac{1566/10^5}{27/482} \times 100$$

$$= 27.96\%$$

Thus, if OC use does cause bacteriuria, about 28 percent of bacteriuria among women who use OCs can be attributed to their OC use and could therefore be eliminated if they did not use OCs.

For most case-control studies, the attributable risk cannot be calculated because the incidence rates of disease among the exposed and nonexposed groups are not available. It is, however, possible to calculate the attributable-risk percent using the following formula [4]:

$$AR\% = \frac{(RR - 1)}{RR} \times 100$$

From the data on OC use and MI presented in Table 4-9, the relative risk of MI associated with current OC use was 1.6, yielding an attributable-risk percent of:

$$AR\% = \frac{(1.6 - 1)}{1.6} \times 100$$

$$= 37.5\%$$

This study therefore suggests that if OC use causes MI, nearly 38 percent of MIs among young women who used OCs could be attributed to that exposure or could be eliminated if they were to stop using OCs.

In case-control studies in which the incidence rate in the total population of interest is known or can be estimated from other sources and the distribution of exposure among the controls is assumed to be representative of the whole population, these parameters can be used to estimate incidence rates in the exposed and nonexposed groups. Since the overall incidence rate of disease in a population (I_T) may be thought of as a weighted average of the incidence rates in various exposure categories, with the weights related to the proportions of individuals in each category, I_T can be calculated as the incidence rate among the exposed group (I_e) times the proportion of individuals in the total population who have the exposure (P_e), plus the incidence rate among the nonexposed (I_0) times the proportion of nonexposed persons (P_0). This is expressed mathematically as follows:

$$I_T = (I_e)(P_e) + (I_0)(P_0)$$

Since the relative risk is the ratio of the incidence rates among the exposed and nonexposed, the incidence rate among the exposed (I_e) members of a population is equal to the relative risk times the comparable rate in the nonexposed ($RR \times I_0$). In a case-control study, the relative risk can be estimated by the odds ratio (OR), and thus we can substitute for I_e in the formula:

$$I_T = (I_0)(OR)(P_e) + (I_0)(P_0)$$
$$= I_0[(OR)(P_e) + (P_0)]$$

To determine the incidence rate in the nonexposed, this equation is simply solved for I_0, as follows:

$$I_0 = \frac{I_T}{(OR)(P_e) + P_0}$$

Once the incidence rate among the nonexposed is determined, it can be multiplied by the odds ratio to provide an estimate of the incidence among the exposed. Given these two incidence rates (I_e and I_0), the attributable risk can then be calculated.

For example, in Doll and Hill's case-control study [9] of smoking and lung cancer, 1350 of 1357 men with the disease and 1296 of 1357 men without lung cancer had smoked cigarettes regularly for the previous 10 years, yielding a relative risk of 9.1. Using an estimate of lung cancer incidence of 480/million/year derived from other sources [7] and the proportion of smokers and nonsmokers among the controls, the incidence rates of lung cancer can be estimated, as shown in Table 4-17, as 500 per million per year among the exposed and 55 per million per year

Table 4-17. Case-control study of cigarette smoking and lung cancer, with calculation of the relative risk, estimates of the incidence rates in the exposed and nonexposed, and the attributable risk

| | Lung cancer | | Total |
	Cases	Controls	
Cigarette smoking			
Yes	1350	1296	2646
No	7	61	68
Total	1357	1357	2714

$$RR = \frac{(1350)(61)}{(1296)(7)} = 9.1$$

$$I_0 = \frac{I_T}{(RR)(P_e) + (P_0)} = \frac{480/10^6}{(9.1)(0.955) + (0.045)} = 55/10^6$$

$$I_e = (RR)(I_0) = (9.1)(55/10^6) = 500/10^6/year$$

$$AR = I_e - I_0 = 500 - 55 = 445/10^6/year$$

Data from R. Doll and A. B. Hill, A study of the aetiology of carcinoma of the lung. *Br. Med. J.* 2:1271, 1952; and R. Doll, Bronchial carcinoma: Incidence and aetiology. *Br. Med. J.* 2:521, 1953.

among the nonexposed. Thus, the excess rate of lung cancer among smokers that is attributable to smoking is

$$AR = 500/10^6/year - 55/10^6/year$$
$$= 445/10^6/year$$

If the exposure is preventive, so that I_e is less than I_0, the attributable risk is meaningless. However, an analogous measure, the preventive fraction (PF), can be defined [24]

$$PF = \frac{I_0 - I_e}{I_0}$$

Population Attributable Risk

While it is useful to estimate the proportion of cases for whom the disease is attributable to their exposure, it is also of interest to estimate the excess rate of disease in the total study population of exposed and nonexposed individuals that is attributable to the exposure. This measure, referred to as the population attributable rate or risk (PAR), helps determine which exposures have the most relevance to the health of a community [20]. The population attributable risk is calculated as the rate of disease in the population (I_T) minus the rate in the unexposed group (I_0):

$$PAR = I_T - I_0$$

Alternatively, this measure can be calculated by multiplying the attributable risk by the proportion of exposed individuals in the population (P_e):

$$PAR = (AR)\,(P_e)$$

The population attributable risk of bacteriuria associated with OC use (Table 4-10) can therefore be calculated as:

$$
\begin{aligned}
PAR &= I_T - I_0 \\
&= 104/2390 - 77/1908 \\
&= 316/10^5/\text{year}
\end{aligned}
$$

or alternatively as:

$$
\begin{aligned}
PAR &= (AR)\,(P_e) \\
&= 1566/10^5 \times (482/2390) \\
&= 316/10^5/\text{year}
\end{aligned}
$$

Thus, if OC use were stopped, the excess annual incidence rate of bacteriuria that could be eliminated among women in this study is 316 per 100,000. The attributable risk among the exposed will always be greater than the population attributable risk since the impact of removing the exposure on the number of cases of disease will always be greater for those with the exposure than for a total population, which is a combination of exposed and nonexposed individuals. To calculate the population attributable risk for a group broader than the study population, either the prevalence of exposure observed in the study population must be assumed to be an adequate reflection of the prevalence of the exposure in the total population, or another estimate must be available from an outside source. If the cohort for study has been chosen with an arbitrary distribution of exposed and nonexposed individuals (such as 200 exposed and 200 nonexposed subjects), then a population attributable risk computed for the study population would be meaningless. If an estimate of the true prevalence of the exposure were available from a source outside the study, however, the population attributable risk could be calculated.

Analogous to the attributable-risk percent among exposed individuals, the population attributable-risk percent (PAR%) expresses the proportion of disease in the study population that is attributable to the exposure and thus could be eliminated if the exposure were eliminated. The population attributable-risk percent is calculated by dividing the population attributable-risk by the rate of the disease in the population or

$$PAR\% = \frac{PAR}{I_T} \times 100$$

For example, in the cohort study of OC use and bacteriuria (Table 4-10), the incidence rate of bacteriuria in the total study population was 104 per 2390 or 4351.5 per 100,000, and the population attributable risk was 316 per 100,000. The population attributable-risk percent can then be calculated as follows:

$$PAR\% = \frac{316}{4351.5} \times 100$$

$$= 7.3\%$$

Thus, if OC use causes bacteriuria, about 7 percent of all the bacteriuria in the study population (and 28 percent of bacteriuria among women taking OCs) could be prevented if OC use were eliminated.

In a case-control study, the population attributable-risk percent can be calculated if the proportion of exposed in the control group can be used as an estimate of the proportion exposed in the population (P_e), or if the prevalence of exposure in the population is available from another source. The formula for the population attributable-risk percent can be expressed as:

$$PAR\% = \frac{(P_e)(RR - 1)}{(P_e)(RR - 1) + 1} \times 100$$

If the proportion of exposed in the control group can be used as an estimate of P_e, the population attributable-risk percent can be calculated by the equivalent formula [24]:

PAR% = AR% × (proportion of exposed cases)

For example, in the case-control study of OC use and MI presented in Table 4-9, the prevalence of OC use in the population can be estimated as the prevalence of OC use in the controls (P_e = 304/3120 = 0.0974). The population attributable-risk percent can be calculated as follows:

$$PAR\% = \frac{P_e \, (RR - 1)}{P_e \, (RR - 1) + 1} \times 100$$

$$= \frac{(0.0974) \, (1.6 - 1)}{(0.0974) \, (1.6 - 1) + 1}$$

$$= 5.5\%$$

or

$$PAR\% = AR\% \times \frac{a}{a + c}$$

$$= \frac{1.6 - 1}{1.6} \times \frac{23}{156}$$

$$= 5.5\%$$

This implies that if OC use causes MI, 5.5 percent of MIs among pre-menopausal women in the study population is attributable to OC use or could be prevented if OC use were discontinued.

As discussed earlier, in case-control studies when the incidence rate of disease in the general population is known and the rate of exposure among the controls is assumed to be representative of the population, the attributable risk can be calculated directly. In such circumstances, it is also possible to calculate the population attributable risk. For example, in the case-control study of smoking and lung cancer presented in Table 4-17, the population attributable risk can be derived as follows:

$$PAR = (AR) \, (P_e)$$

$$= (445/10^6) \, (0.955)$$

$$= 425/10^6$$

Thus, if cigarette smoking causes lung cancer, 425 cases per million men are directly attributable to this habit.

Interpretation of Measures of Association

It is important to remember that relative and attributable risks provide very different types of information. The relative risk is a measure of the strength of the association between an exposure and disease and provides information that can be used to judge whether a valid observed association is likely to be causal. In contrast, the attributable risk provides a measure of the public health impact of an exposure, assuming that the association is one of cause and effect. The magnitude of the

Table 4-18. Relative and attributable risks of mortality from lung cancer and coronary heart disease among cigarette smokers in a cohort study of British male physicians

	Annual mortality rate per 100,000	
	Lung cancer	Coronary heart disease
Cigarette smokers	140	669
Nonsmokers	10	413
Relative risk	14.0	1.6
Attributable risk	$130/10^5$/year	$256/10^5$/year

R. Doll and R. Peto, Mortality in relation to smoking: Twenty years' observations on male British doctors. *Br. Med. J.* 2:1525, 1976.

Table 4-19. Measures of disease frequency

Prevalence (P)	$\dfrac{\text{Number of persons with disease}}{\text{Number of persons in population}}$ at a point in time
Cumulative incidence (CI)	$\dfrac{\text{Number of new cases of disease in a given time period}}{\text{Total population at risk}}$
Incidence density (ID)	$\dfrac{\text{Number of new cases of disease in a given time period}}{\text{Total person-time of observation}}$

relative risk alone does not predict the magnitude of the attributable risk. This can be illustrated by examining the relationship of cigarette smoking with mortality from lung cancer and coronary heart disease in a cohort study of British male physicians [9].

As shown in Table 4-18, this investigation demonstrated a 14-fold increased death rate from lung cancer among smokers of at least one pack of cigarettes daily when compared with nonsmokers. On the other hand, the relative risk of coronary heart disease mortality among current cigarette smokers compared with nonsmokers was 1.6. Thus, cigarette smoking is a much stronger risk factor for mortality from lung cancer than for coronary heart disease. However, if smoking is causally related to both diseases, the elimination of cigarettes would prevent far more deaths among smokers from coronary heart disease than from lung cancer, as shown by the attributable risks of 256 per 100,000 and 130 per 100,000 per year, respectively. The explanation for this is that while death from lung cancer is a relatively rare occurrence, accounting for only 10 deaths per 100,000 population each year among nonsmokers, the annual death rate for coronary heart disease in that same group is 413 per 100,000. Consequently, even a 60-percent increased risk of cor-

Table 4-20. Measures of association: cohort studies

Relative risk (RR)	1. Cumulative incidence (risk) ratio =
	$$\frac{\text{Cumulative incidence in exposed }(CI_e)}{\text{Cumulative incidence in nonexposed }(CI_0)}$$
	2. Incidence density (rate) ratio =
	$$\frac{\text{Incidence rate among exposed }(I_e)}{\text{Incidence rate among nonexposed }(I_0)}$$
Attributable risk (AR)	$I_e - I_0$
Attributable-risk percent (AR%)	$\dfrac{AR}{I_e} \times 100$
Population attributable risk (PAR)	$I_T - I_0$ or $AR \times$ prevalence of exposure (P_e)
Population attributable-risk percent (PAR%)	$\dfrac{PAR}{\text{Incidence rate of disease in population }(I_T)} \times 100$

onary heart disease mortality associated with cigarette smoking will affect a much larger number of people than a 14-fold increased risk of death from lung cancer. Thus, the potential public health impact of smoking cessation on mortality will be far greater for coronary heart disease than for lung cancer.

In general, the relative risk is the measure used most commonly by those evaluating possible determinants of disease because it represents the magnitude of the association and provides information that can be used in making a judgment of causality. In contrast, once causality is assumed, from the perspective of public health administration and policy, measures of association based on absolute differences in risk between exposed and nonexposed individuals assume far greater importance. These absolute rates express either the actual incidence of a disease that is attributable to an exposure among the exposed (attributable risk) or the number of cases of disease in the total population that could be eliminated by removal of a harmful exposure (population attributable risk).

CONCLUSION

In this chapter we have considered the most commonly used measures of disease frequency (Table 4-19) and association (Tables 4-20 and 4-21)

Table 4-21. Measures of association: case-control studies

Relative risk (RR), calculated as odds ratio (OR)	$\dfrac{ad}{bc}$
Attributable-risk percent (AR%)	$\dfrac{RR - 1}{RR} \times 100$
Population attributable-risk percent (PAR%)	$\dfrac{P_e (RR - 1)}{P_e (RR - 1) + 1} \times 100$ or AR% × proportion of exposed cases
Attributable risk (AR)*	$I_e - I_0$
Population attributable risk (PAR)*	AR × proportion of exposed (P_e)

*If the study is population-based or if incidence rates can be estimated.

used in epidemiologic studies. These measures serve as the basic tools to quantify exposure-disease relationships. Part II of this textbook will discuss the various types of epidemiologic study designs that can utilize these measures to formulate and test hypotheses.

STUDY QUESTIONS

1. A case-control study was conducted to evaluate the interrelationships between several risk factors for myocardial infarction. Information on smoking status was collected from a total of 789 cases and controls. Current cigarette smoking, defined as smoking within the past three months, was reported by 157 of the 366 cases and 110 of the 423 controls.
   a. Set up the appropriate two-by-two table and calculate a measure of association between current smoking and myocardial infarction.
   b. Calculate a measure of the excess risk of myocardial infarction in cigarette smokers that is attributable to their smoking.
   State any assumptions that you make in performing these calculations and give interpretations for your results.
2. In 1985, more women in the U.S. died from lung cancer than from breast cancer [32]. During this time period, there were about 100,000 incident cases of breast cancer and 40,000 incident cases of lung cancer in this population. Comment on the prevalence, average duration, and case-fatality rates of these two diseases.

REFERENCES

1. An evaluation of the acquired immunodeficiency syndrome (AIDS) reported in health care personnel—United States. *M.M.W.R.* 32:358, 1983.
2. Centers for Disease Control. Annual summary 1982: Reported morbidity and mortality in the United States. *M.M.W.R.* 31:54, 1983.
3. Centers for Disease Control. *Tuberculosis Statistics: States and Cities, 1984.* Atlanta: Centers for Disease Control, 1985.
4. Cole, P., and MacMahon, B. Attributable risk percent in case-control studies. *Br. J. Prev. Soc. Med.* 25:242, 1971.
5. Colton, T. *Statistics in Medicine.* Boston: Little, Brown, 1974.
6. Cornfield, J. A method of estimating comparative rates from clinical data: Applications to cancer of the lung, breast, and cervix. *J.N.C.I.* 11:1269, 1951.
7. Doll, R. Bronchial carcinoma: Incidence and aetiology. *Br. Med. J.* 2:521, 1953.
8. Doll, R. Mortality from lung cancer in asbestos workers. *Br. J. Indust. Med.* 12:81, 1955.
9. Doll, R., and Hill, A. B. A study of the aetiology of carcinoma of the lung. *Br. Med. J.* 2:1271, 1952.
10. Doll, R., and Peto, R. Mortality in relation to smoking: Twenty years' observations on male British doctors. *Br. Med. J.* 2:1525, 1976.
11. Doll, R., and Peto, R. *The Causes of Cancer.* New York: Oxford University Press, 1981.
12. Enterline, P. E. Mortality among asbestos products workers in the United States. *Ann. N.Y. Acad. Sci.* 132:156, 1965.
13. Epstein, S. S. *The Politics of Cancer.* San Francisco: Sierra Club Books, 1978.
14. Evans, D. A., Hennekens, C. H., Miao, L., et al. Oral contraceptives and bacteriuria in a community-based study. *N. Engl. J. Med.* 299:536, 1978.
15. Freeman, J., and Hutchison, G. B. Prevalence, incidence and duration. *Am. J. Epidemiol.* 112:707, 1980.
16. Gross, H. Oswego County revisited. *Public Health Rep.* 91:168, 1976.
17. Hardy, A. M., Allen, J. R., Morgan, W. M., et al. The incidence rate of acquired immunodeficiency syndrome in selected populations. *J.A.M.A.* 253:215, 1985.
18. Howe, H. L. Age-specific hysterectomy and oophorectomy prevalence rates and the risks for cancer of the reproduction system. *Am. J. Public Health* 74:560, 1984.
19. Kahn, H. A., Leibowitz, H. M., Ganley, J. P., et al. The Framingham Eye Study: I. Outline and major prevalence findings. *Am. J. Epidemiol.* 106:17, 1977.
20. Lyon, J. L., and Gardner, J. W. The rising frequency of hysterectomy: its effect on uterine cancer rates. *Am. J. Epidemiol.* 105:439, 1977.
21. MacMahon, B., and Pugh, T. F. *Epidemiology: Principles and Methods.* Boston: Little, Brown, 1970.
22. McNamara, J. J., et al. Coronary artery disease in combat casualties in Vietnam. *J.A.M.A.* 216:1185, 1971.
23. Miettinen, O. S. Estimability and estimation in case-referent studies. *Am. J. Epidemiol.* 103:226, 1976.

24. Miettinen, O. S. Proportion of disease caused or prevented by a given exposure, trait or intervention. *Am. J. Epidemiol.* 99:325, 1974.
25. Monson, R. R. *Occupational Epidemiology.* Boca Raton, FL: CRC, 1980.
26. Najarian, T., and Colton, T. Mortality from leukemia and cancer in nuclear shipyard workers. *Lancet* 1:42, 1978.
27. Rogentine, G. N., Jr., Yankee, R. A., Gart, J. J., et al. HL-A antigens and disease. *J. Clin. Invest.* 51:2430, 1972.
28. Rogentine, G. N., Trapani, R. J., Yankee, R. A., et al. HL-A antigens and acute lymphocytic leukemia: The nature of the HL-A2 association. *Tissue Antigens* 3:470, 1973.
29. Rogers, M. F., Schonberger, L. B., Hurwitz, E. S., et al. Reye Syndrome surveillance, 1981–1982. *M.M.W.R.* 32:17, 1983.
30. Rosenberg, L., Hennekens, C. H., Rosner, B., et al. Oral contraceptive use in relation to non-fatal myocardial infarction. *Am. J. Epidemiol.* 111:59, 1980.
31. Sattin, R. W., Rubin, G. L., and Hughes, J. M. Hysterectomy among women of reproductive age, United States, update for 1979–80. *M.M.W.R.* 32:1, 1983.
32. Silverberg, E., and Lubera, J. Cancer statistics, 1986. *CA* 36:9, 1986.
33. Stampfer, M. J., Willett, W. C., Colditz, G. A., et al. A prospective study of postmenopausal hormones and coronary heart disease. *N. Engl. J. Med.* 313:1044, 1985.
34. U.S. Bureau of the Census. *Sixteenth Census of the U.S., 1940.* Characteristics of the Population, Part I, United States Summary. Washington, DC: 1942.
35. U.S. Bureau of the Census. *Statistical Abstract of the United States: 1984* (104th ed.). Washington, DC: U.S. Govt. Printing Office, 1983.
36. U.S. D.H.E.W. *Vital Statistics of the United States 1973.* Vol. II, Mortality. Rockville, MD: National Center for Health Statistics, 1975.
37. U.S. D.H.H.S. *Surveillance, Epidemiology, and End Results: Incidence and Mortality Data, 1973–77.* N.I.H. Publication No. 81-2330. Bethesda, MD: National Cancer Institute, 1981.
38. U.S. D.H.H.S. *Vital Statistics of the U.S., 1980.* Vol. II, Mortality, Part B. D.H.H.S. Publication No. (P.H.S.) 85-1102. Washington, DC: National Center for Health Statistics, 1985.

II. TYPES OF EPIDEMIOLOGIC STUDIES

5

Descriptive Studies

Descriptive studies describe patterns of disease occurrence in relation to variables such as person, place, and time. The data provided by descriptive studies are essential for public health administrators as well as epidemiologists. Specifically, for public health administrators, knowledge of which populations or subgroups are most or least affected by disease allows the most efficient allocation of resources and the targeting of particular segments of the population for education and/or prevention programs. For epidemiologists, the identification of descriptive characteristics frequently constitutes an important first step in the search for determinants or risk factors that can be altered or eliminated to reduce or prevent disease.

Descriptive studies use information from such diverse sources as census data, vital statistics records, employment health examinations, clinical records from hospitals or private practices, as well as national figures on consumption of foods, medications, or other products. Since this information is often routinely collected and readily available, descriptive studies are generally far less expensive and time-consuming than analytic studies. While features inherent in their design usually preclude the ability to test epidemiologic hypotheses, descriptive studies are very useful to describe patterns of disease occurrence as well as to formulate research questions. Indeed, they may well be the most frequently encountered epidemiologic design strategy in the medical literature [23].

In this chapter, we review each of the specific types of descriptive studies, including their particular strengths and limitations. We also illustrate the use of descriptive data in the formulation of epidemiologic hypotheses.

TYPES OF DESCRIPTIVE STUDIES

There are three main types of descriptive studies: correlational studies, which consider patterns of disease among populations; case reports or

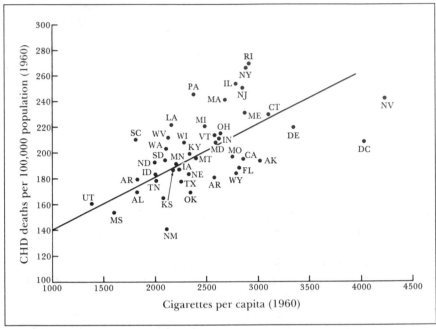

Fig. 5-1. Coronary heart disease mortality rates in the United States by per capita cigarette sales in 1960, by state. (From G. D. Friedman, Cigarette smoking and geographic variation in coronary heart disease mortality in the United States. *J. Chronic Dis.* 20:769, 1967.)

case series; and cross-sectional surveys of individuals. Each of these descriptive study designs provides information on various characteristics of person, place, or time, and each has unique strengths and limitations.

Correlational Studies

In correlational studies, measures that represent characteristics of entire populations are used to describe disease in relation to some factor of interest such as age, calendar time, utilization of health services, or consumption of a food, medication, or other product. For example, to describe patterns of mortality from coronary heart disease (CHD) in 1960, death rates from 44 states were correlated with per capita cigarette sales (Figure 5-1). Death rates were highest in states with the most cigarette sales, lowest in those with the least sales, and intermediate in the remainder [24]. This early observation contributed to the formulation of the hypothesis that cigarette smoking causes fatal CHD, which has been substantiated in a large number of subsequent analytic epidemiologic studies [71].

The correlation coefficient, denoted by r, is the descriptive measure of association in correlational studies. This coefficient quantifies the extent to which there is a linear relationship between exposure and disease—that is, whether for every unit of change in level of exposure, the disease frequency increases or decreases proportionately. The value of the correlation coefficient can vary between $+1$ and -1.

A chief strength of correlational studies, which contributes to their frequent use as a first step in investigating a possible exposure-disease relationship, is that they can be done quickly and inexpensively, often using already available information. Governmental and private health agencies routinely collect demographic and product consumption data that can be correlated with disease incidence, mortality, or utilization of health resources. Similarly, the availability of data from surveillance programs or national and international disease registries can permit comparisons of disease rates in different geographic regions. There are, however, features inherent in the design of correlational studies that limit their interpretability.

The chief limitation of correlational studies is the inability to link exposure with disease in particular individuals. For example, to evaluate whether Papanicolaou smears were correlated with mortality from cancer of the cervix, the percentage decrease in cervical cancer mortality between the two periods 1950 to 1954 and 1965 to 1969 as well as the percentage of women undergoing Papanicolaou smear screening annually was examined [16]. These two periods were chosen because the mid-1950s marked the widespread adoption of this screening procedure as well as the beginning of a decline in mortality from cervical cancer. There is a fairly strong and statistically significant positive correlation, with the states reporting the highest percentage of women screened exhibiting the largest decline in cervical cancer mortality and, conversely, those with the lowest screening rates having the smallest percent decreases. These data raise the question that screening programs may result in a decrease in mortality from cervical cancer. This hypothesis, however, cannot be tested from such data, since it is not possible to determine whether in fact it was the women who had been screened for the disease who actually experienced the lower mortality rates.

A second major limitation of correlational studies is the lack of ability to control for the effects of potential confounding factors. For example, in a study of average per capita daily intake of pork in relation to breast cancer mortality rates in 28 countries in 1964 to 1965 [35], there was a very strong positive correlation between these two variables, suggesting a possible association between pork intake and death from breast cancer. Increased pork consumption, however, may merely be a marker for a number of other factors that are related to elevated risk of breast cancer, such as increased intake of dietary fat, decreased intake of vegetables, or higher socioeconomic status. It is not possible to separate the effects of such potential confounding factors using correlational data. This lim-

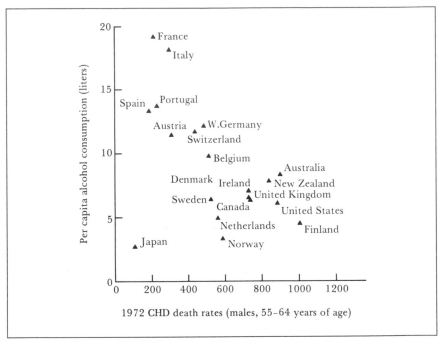

Fig. 5-2. Per capita alcohol consumption and coronary heart disease mortality rates in 20 countries in 1972. (From R. E. LaPorte, J. L. Cresanta, and L. H. Kuller, The relation of alcohol to CHD and mortality: Implication for public health policy. *J. Public Health Policy* 1:198, 1980.)

itation is further illustrated by noting that a very strong positive correlation can be demonstrated between per capita number of color television sets and CHD mortality rates in various countries. Of course, per capita number of color televisions is certainly related to other life-style variables that are known to increase risk of CHD, such as blood pressure, blood cholesterol level, cigarette smoking, and physical inactivity. Thus, the presence of a correlation does not necessarily imply the presence of a valid statistical association. Conversely, the lack of a correlation in such studies does not necessarily imply the absence of a valid statistical association. For example, during the early 1970s, the use of oral contraceptives (OCs) in the United States increased, while at the same time mortality rates from CHD among all women of childbearing age declined about 30 percent [63]. Thus, these correlational data do not support the suggestion of a positive association between use of OCs and risk of fatal CHD. However, a large number of analytic studies, both case-control [51] and cohort [4, 30, 31, 74] have consistently shown that women who use OCs experience, on average, a twofold increase in risk of fatal CHD compared with nonusers. Careful consideration of this apparent discrepancy indicates that this association would have been difficult to de-

Table 5-1. Dose-response relationship of alcohol intake with CHD mortality from the Chicago Western Electric Company Study

Average daily consumption of alcohol (number of drinks)	Age-adjusted CHD mortality rate (per 1000)
< 1	80
1	77
2–3	73
4–5	55
6+	155

Source: A. R. Dyer, et al., Alcohol consumption and 17-year mortality in the Chicago Western Electric Company Study. *Prev. Med.* 9:78, 1980.

tect in correlational data. Specifically, there are roughly 800,000 deaths due to CHD in the United States each year, of which about 18,000 occur among women of childbearing age. As regards OCs, even with a doubling of risk, the number of deaths from CHD that are attributable to their use each year is only about 100. Consequently, in the experience of all women of childbearing age in the U.S., an increase of a few hundred cases of fatal CHD among users would be impossible to detect from correlational data given the concurrent decrease of several thousands of CHD deaths among the millions of women of childbearing age who did not use OCs.

Finally, correlational data represent average exposure levels rather than actual individual values. Thus, while it may appear from correlational data that there is an overall positive or negative linear association, this might actually be masking a more complicated relationship between the exposure and disease. For example, Figure 5-2 shows a striking inverse correlation between per capita alcohol consumption and CHD mortality [39]. These data indicate that those with the highest levels of alcohol consumption are at the lowest risk of CHD mortality, and that those with the lowest consumption levels have the highest risks. In fact, the data from analytic studies among individuals show that the relationship between alcohol and CHD mortality is not a simple inverse linear one. In fact, the association is best represented by a J-shaped curve, where individuals consuming the largest amounts of alcohol have the highest risks, and those drinking small to moderate amounts daily have risks of fatal CHD even lower than those of both heavy drinkers and nondrinkers [29]. For example, as shown in Table 5-1, in the Chicago Western Electric Company Study [20], a prospective cohort study of 1832 white males followed between 1957 and 1975, the CHD mortality rate for those drinking less than one drink daily was 80 per 1000. For those consuming one or two to three drinks daily, the rates were 77 and 73 per 1000, respectively, while for those whose daily intake was four to five drinks, the CHD death rate was only 55 per 1000. Those consuming six or more drinks daily experienced a dramatically higher CHD mortality rate of 155 per 1000, which is nearly double that of nondrinkers and over three times that of more moderate drinkers. Such a nonlinear relationship can rarely be identified from correlational studies, in which the exposure represents an average consumption for a population rather than the actual consumption patterns of the individuals.

Case Reports and Case Series

While correlational studies consider whole populations, case reports and case series describe the experience of a single patient or a group of patients with a similar diagnosis. These types of studies, in which typically an astute clinician identifies an unusual feature of a disease or a patient's history, may lead to formulation of a new hypothesis. In this way, case reports and case series represent an important interface between clinical medicine and epidemiology.

Case reports are among the most common types of studies published in medical journals, accounting for over a third of all articles in one systematic review [23]. Case reports document unusual medical occurrences and can represent the first clues in the identification of new diseases or adverse effects of exposures. For example, in recent years, case reports have raised the question of new health hazards related to a number of currently popular physical activities, including "Frisbee finger" [22], "jogger's whiplash" [64], "Space-Invaders wrist" [44], and "breakdancing neck" [43]. Similarly, as mentioned in Chapter 2, it was a single case report that led to the formulation of the hypothesis that OC use increases risk of venous thromboembolism [36].

Case series are collections of individual case reports, which may occur within a fairly short period of time. This design has historical importance in epidemiology, as it was often used as an early means to identify the beginning or presence of an epidemic. Even at present, the routine surveillance of accumulating case reports often suggests the emergence of a new disease or epidemic [38]. Investigation of the activities of the affected individuals in the case series can then lead to formulation of a hypothesis. At that time, an analytic study, most frequently using a case-control approach, can be done to compare the experiences of the case series with that of a group of individuals who did not develop the disease to identify possible causal factors.

The collection of a case series rather than reliance on a single case report can mean the difference between formulating a useful hypothesis and merely documenting an interesting medical oddity. For example, in 1974, Creech and Johnson [17] reported a case series of three men with angiosarcoma of the liver among workers at a vinyl chloride plant. This number in such a small population during the time period studied was clearly in excess of what was expected and led to the formulation of the hypothesis that occupational exposure to vinyl chloride caused hepatic angiosarcoma. Later the same year, this hypothesis was substantiated by data from two analytic studies [57, 69]. A single case report from that plant might not have been sufficient to allow formulation and subsequent testing of this hypothesis.

The usefulness of case reports and case series in the recognition of new diseases and the formulation of hypotheses concerning possible risk factors can be illustrated by the early epidemiology of acquired immunodeficiency syndrome (AIDS) [61]. Between October 1980 and May 1981, 5 cases of *Pneumocystis carinii* pneumonia were reported among young, previously healthy, homosexual men in Los Angeles [10]. This case series was unusual in that this type of pneumonia had previously occurred only in older cancer patients whose immune systems were suppressed, usually as a result of chemotherapy [75]. Similarly, in early 1981, an unprecedented number of cases of Kaposi's sarcoma were diagnosed in young homosexual men. Again, this was noteworthy because previously this malignancy had been seen almost exclusively in the elderly and affected men and women equally [11]. As a result of these case series, the Centers for Disease Control immediately initiated a surveillance program to quantitate the magnitude of this problem and to develop diagnostic criteria for what appeared to be a new disease. This program quickly identified that homosexual men were at high risk of developing this syndrome. Subsequent case reports and case series suggested that AIDS also resulted from blood-borne transmission among intravenous drug abusers as well as recipients of transfusions [2] and hemophiliacs receiving blood products [12]. These descriptive data provided clues used in the design and conduct of analytic studies, which subsequently led to the identification of a number of specific risk factors for the development of AIDS. The availability of sera from these cases and comparable controls also has contributed to the identification of human immunodeficiency virus (HIV) as the transmissible agent [61].

While case reports and case series are very useful for hypothesis formulation, they cannot be used to test for the presence of a valid statistical association. One fundamental limitation of the case report is that it is based on the experience of only one person. The presence of any risk factor, however suggestive, may simply be coincidental. Although case series are frequently sufficiently large to permit quantification of frequency of an exposure, the interpretability of such information is severely limited by the lack of an appropriate comparison group. This lack can either obscure a relationship or suggest an association where none actually exists. For example, in an attempt to explore the possible association between the use of OCs and hepatocellular carcinoma in women,

Table 5-2. Case series of oral contraceptive use and hepatocellular carcinoma

	All cases		Age in years					
			16–25		26–35		36–45	
	No.	%	No.	%	No.	%	No.	%
OC users	39	31.0	11	28.2	17	43.6	11	28.2
OC nonusers	26	20.6	7	26.9	4	15.4	15	57.7
OC use unknown	61	48.4	17	27.9	19	31.1	25	41.0
Total	126		35		40		51	

Source: J. Vana and G. P. Murphy, Primary malignant liver tumors: Association with oral contraceptives. *N.Y. State J. Med.* 79:321, 1979.

data were collected on 126 cases identified between 1970 and 1975 as part of a national survey [73]. As shown in Table 5-2, the percentages of users and nonusers of OCs were calculated for the total group of cases and for three subgroups by age. Among the 126 cases of liver cancer, 39, or 31 percent, were users of OCs, while in the age group 26 to 35 years, this figure rose to 43.6 percent. Because there was no comparison group, however, it is not possible to determine whether that rate of OC use was different from that among all healthy women in that age category. The authors themselves cite estimates of 25- to 37-percent use nationwide during the mid-1970s, suggesting that the rates observed in their case series may have been no different from the national average. (Parenthetically, in this case series, such a high proportion of women were categorized as unknown with respect to OC use that it is not possible to draw any firm conclusions concerning the actual pattern of use among these women.) While this hypothesis certainly seems biologically plausible, information from a case series can merely raise the question.

Cross-Sectional Surveys

A third type of descriptive study is the cross-sectional or prevalence survey, in which exposure and disease status are assessed simultaneously among individuals in a well-defined population. There can be a specific time window, such as a given calendar year during which a community-wide survey is conducted, or a fixed point in the course of events that varies in real time from person to person, such as a preemployment physical examination, entrance into high school or college, or retirement. Thus, cross-sectional surveys provide information about the frequency and characteristics of a disease by furnishing a "snapshot" of the health experience of the population at a specified time. Such data can be of great value to public health administrators in assessing the health status and health care needs of a population. For example, in 1956, the U.S. Congress passed the National Health Survey Act, which established periodic surveys to obtain data on the prevalence of acute and chronic diseases, disabilities, utilization of health care resources, and relevant demographic and personal characteristics for the purposes of effective health care planning and administration. Under the overall administration of the National Center for Health Statistics, this program includes the Health Interview Survey, which collects data through personal household interviews from a random sample of the population, and the Health Examination Survey, which utilizes standardized physical examinations and laboratory tests [72]. In 1971, a nutritional component was added and the name changed to the Health and Nutrition Examination Survey. In each of these cross-sectional surveys, the subjects provide information at a single interview or examination. These data are used to assess the prevalence of certain acute and chronic conditions, ranging from upper respiratory infections to cardiovascular diseases and disabling conditions; the distribution of physiologic or biochemical measurements such as height, weight, blood cholesterol, or visual acuity; and the impact of these health experiences as measured by the number of days of hospitalization, days lost from work, frequency of visits to a doctor or dentist, and health insurance coverage.

Cross-sectional surveys can also be used to provide information on the prevalence of disease or other health outcomes in certain occupations. For example, detailed questionnaires were sent to all 2856 production workers at a rubber tire manufacturing plant in the eastern United States [50]. These forms included information on chronic bronchitis, persistent cough and phlegm, and a variety of other symptoms suggestive of the development of obstructive lung disease. Subjects also completed a detailed work history that provided information on employment in specific areas of the plant with different presumed levels of exposure to potentially hazardous conditions. Analysis of these cross-sectional data revealed four particular work areas with high prevalence of respiratory symptoms, which persisted after age and cigarette smoking were taken into account: milling, calendaring, tube curing, and tube inspection. This survey led to the formulation of hypotheses tested in a subsequent analytic study, which documented the role of working with heated rubber in the development of respiratory symptoms [41].

Since exposure and disease status are assessed at a single point in time, in many cases, it is not possible to determine whether the exposure preceded or resulted from the disease. Figure 5-3 illustrates this interrelationship in the context of a hypothetical occupational exposure. Suppose there are 100 workers in each of two jobs in a particular industry, one of which (job A) involves a known hazardous exposure and the other of

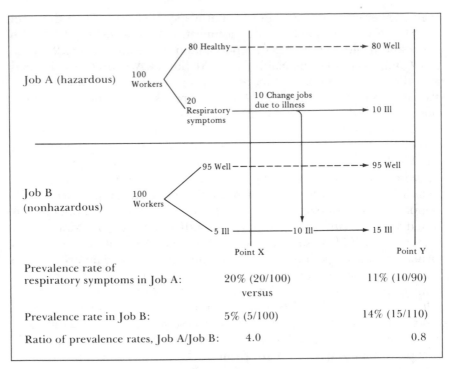

Fig. 5-3. Hypothetical illustration of the interrelationship between an occupational exposure and prevalence of disease, as measured by a cross-sectional survey. (Adapted from A. J. McMichael et al., Chronic respiratory symptoms and job type within the rubber industry. *J. Occup. Med.* 18:611, 1976.)

which (job B) clearly does not. If we were to conduct a cross-sectional survey at point X, we might find that four times as many workers in job A had chronic respiratory symptoms than in job B (20/100 versus 5/100). In contrast, if we surveyed this population at point Y, we would in fact find a greater prevalence rate of respiratory symptoms among workers in job B, not because that job assignment had become more hazardous, but because 10 of the affected workers who were in the job with known hazardous exposure (job A) chose to change to the job assignment with no known exposure because of their illness. Thus, being in job B at point Y for those with respiratory symptoms would in fact be the effect of those symptoms, not their cause.

This type of "chicken or egg" dilemma is common to virtually all cross-sectional data. For example, a survey was conducted in Evans County, Georgia from 1960 to 1962 among all residents over the age of 40 as well as a 50-percent random sample of residents aged 15 to 39 years [45].

Table 5-3. Cross-sectional survey of coronary heart disease (CHD) among
white male farm owners, aged 40–74 years, by occupational physical activity

	Number examined	Number with CHD	Prevalence rate	Age-adjusted prevalence rate
Not physically active	89	14	157.2/1000	126/1000
Physically active	90	3	33.3/1000	36/1000
Total	179	17	95.0/1000	87/1000

Source: J. R. McDonough et al., Coronary heart disease among Negroes and
Whites in Evans County, Georgia. *J. Chronic Dis.* 18:443, 1965.

The 3102 participants were given comprehensive medical examinations,
and extensive information was collected on demographic, occupational
and medical history variables. To explore a possible relationship with
physical activity, the investigators compared the prevalence rates of
CHD among white farm owners who did and did not do their own labor.
As shown in Table 5-3, the prevalence rate of CHD among those who
were not physically active in their work was nearly five times higher than
that among those who engaged in farm labor (157.2 versus 33.3/1000).
When the possibility of differing age distributions of men in the two
groups was controlled by calculation of age-adjusted rates, a marked difference between the two groups persisted. Nevertheless, it is impossible
to determine from these cross-sectional data whether physical activity is
truly protective or whether farmers with symptoms of CHD are simply
more likely to decrease their physical labor.

Since cross-sectional surveys must consider prevalent rather than incident cases, the data obtained will always reflect determinants of survival as well as etiology. For example, data from the Evans County study
[45] showed a lower prevalence of CHD among blacks than whites. Since
this only reflects the status of the population at the time of the survey,
it in no way implies that the development of CHD is lower among blacks
and whites. In fact, if blacks both develop and die from CHD at higher
rates than whites this would be compatible with the observed lower prevalence of CHD among blacks at any point in time. Cross-sectional data
cannot distinguish between these alternative explanations.

In one special circumstance, a cross-sectional survey can be considered
as a type of analytic study and used to test epidemiologic hypotheses.
This can occur only when the current values of the exposure variables
are unalterable over time, thus representing the value present at the
initiation of the disease. Such variables include factors present at birth,
such as eye color or blood group. However, in most cross-sectional sur-

veys, the risk factors may be subject to alteration subsequent (or even consequent) to the development of disease. In these instances, the data can be used to describe characteristics of individuals with the disease and to formulate hypotheses, but not to test them.

HYPOTHESIS FORMULATION FROM DESCRIPTIVE STUDIES

For any public health problem, the first step in the search for possible solutions is to formulate a reasonable and testable hypothesis. There are three methods of hypothesis formulation about disease etiology that have been derived from the five canons of inductive reasoning proposed by John Stuart Mill [55]. The first, referred to as the "method of difference," involves recognizing that if the frequency is markedly different in two sets of circumstances, the disease may be caused by some particular factor that differs between them. Studies comparing disease frequencies in different countries can provide data for this method of hypothesis formulation. For example, the observation that certain cancers are very rare in one country but very common in another became part of the basis for the current belief in the avoidability of a large proportion of human cancers by manipulation of environmental or life-style variables [19]. A second, common process in hypotheses formulation is the "method of agreement." This refers to the observation that a single factor is common to a number of circumstances in which a disease occurs with high frequency. For example, in AIDS, the unusually high frequency among intravenous drug abusers, recipients of transfusions, and hemophiliacs raised the possibility that one mode of transmission involved introduction of the virus into the bloodstream [61]. Finally, the "method of concomitant variation" refers to circumstances in which the frequency of a factor varies in proportion to the frequency of disease. Correlational studies are particularly useful sources of data for this type of hypothesis formulation, as illustrated in Figure 5-1, where CHD mortality rates rise with per capita cigarette consumption, and Figure 5-2, where CHD mortality decreases with increasing per capita consumption of alcohol.

Whatever the method, hypothesis formulation begins with a general consideration of the descriptive characteristics of a disease. This process has been likened to the parlor game "20 Questions," in which an imagined object must be identified on the basis of answers to a limited number of queries [49]. Thus, a determination of the basic descriptive characteristics of a disease in relation to person, place, and time is roughly the epidemiologic equivalent of learning the answers to the standard opening question, "Is it animal, vegetable, or mineral?"

Table 5-4. Death rates per 100,000 population from
coronary disease in the United States, 1981, by age and sex

Age	White men	White women
< 1	2.0	1.8
1–4	2.2	2.0
5–14	0.9	0.8
15–24	2.6	1.6
25–34	9.4	4.2
35–44	60.6	16.2
45–54	265.6	71.2
55–64	708.7	243.7
65–74	1669.9	769.4
75–84	3751.5	2359.0
85 +	8596.0	7215.1

Source: U.S. D.H.H.S., *Health United States 1984.* D.H.H.S. Publication No.
(P.H.S.) 85–1232. Hyattsville, MD: National Center for Health Statistics, 1984.

Person

Descriptive data on person address the question, "Who is getting the
disease?" The characteristics of person must include the unalterable but
essential descriptors of age and sex. In addition, variables as varied as
religion, marital status, personality type, and race, as well as socioeconomic factors such as education, income, or occupation, can be considered. Each variable can furnish a different type of clue about the pattern
and possible etiology of the disease. A classic example of a contribution
of this type of descriptive epidemiology is the research of Joseph Goldberger on pellagra in the early twentieth century [26]. By observing that
the disease was very common among the inmates of an asylum and virtually nonexistent among the nurses and attendants, all of whom shared
a common physical environment, he speculated that the development of
pellagra was less likely to be infectious and more likely to be a consequence of factors such as diet, which did differ between the two groups.
He then tested this hypothesis in an analytic study and showed that pellagra resulted from a dietary deficiency of nicotinic acid, part of the
vitamin B complex [27].

Age and sex are such fundamental characteristics of person that they
should always be routinely considered in any epidemiologic study. For
example, Table 5-4 shows CHD death rates by age and sex in the United
States in 1981 [72]. At every age over 15 years, there is a striking difference between the rates for men and women. Since the gap begins to
narrow after age 54, the average age at menopause [76], these descrip-

tive data have suggested a possible protective effect of endogenous estrogen levels. If this were true, women who experience an early menopause, either naturally or through surgery or irradiation, should have increased risks of CHD compared with women having a late age at menopause. While the descriptive data alone are insufficient to permit an assessment of whether age at menopause is related to risk of CHD in women, the results of analytic studies have supported this hypothesis [14]. The observed differences between the sexes in risk of CHD might also merely reflect differences in levels of risk factors such as cigarette smoking, blood cholesterol, blood pressure, or physical activity. Similarly, differences in social class, access to health care, or dietary patterns may be responsible for the patterns seen. This possibility of confounding limits the ability to interpret all descriptive data. Nevertheless, as shown by the above example, descriptive studies of differences between disease rates among subgroups of a single population classified by these variables can provide valuable leads for further epidemiologic investigation.

With respect to age, as seen in Table 5-4, CHD is rare among young adults, and has an ever increasing frequency among the middle-aged and elderly. This pattern is quite different for other diseases such as multiple sclerosis, which occurs most frequently between the ages of 20 and 35 years [42], and measles, which is most common under the age of 15 years [13]; both these diseases virtually never develop in individuals over age 60. The relation of age with disease can frequently provide important clues about etiology. For example, Figure 5-4 shows the incidence rates of Hodgkin's disease in Brooklyn, New York from 1943 to 1952, according to age at onset [46]. There are two distinct peaks in frequency, one in early adulthood at about age 29, and the other at about age 73. This unusual age-incidence pattern led to formulation of the hypothesis that Hodgkin's disease comprises two entities, each with somewhat different etiologies and clinical features [15, 47]. Specifically, younger patients manifest characteristics suggestive of an inflammatory and infectious disease process, including a high frequency of fever and the similarity in time (not age) of onset of cases occurring within a single family. On the other hand, individuals over age 50 exhibit features of neoplastic disease, such as pathologic evidence of sarcoma and a high case-fatality rate. This hypothesis, which was formulated from descriptive data, has been supported by findings from analytic studies evaluating differences in histology of Hodgkin's disease in younger versus older patients [58].

The interpretation of observations concerning the age distribution of disease is not always simple or straightforward. A change in the age distribution of a disease from one time period to another could be due to a number of factors, such as improvements in the technology for diagnosing the disease or the discovery of a new and effective therapy. It could also result from a common, general exposure during a specific

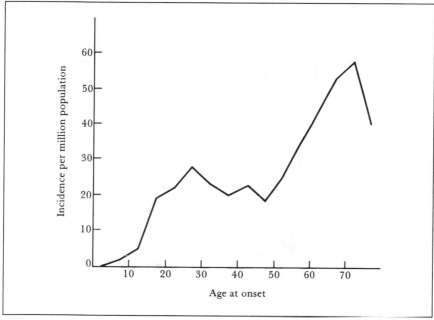

Fig. 5-4. Incidence rates of Hodgkin's disease by age in Brooklyn, 1943–1952. (From B. MacMahon. Epidemiologic evidence on the nature of Hodgkin's disease. *Cancer* 10:1045, 1957.)

period, such as an infectious agent or ionizing radiation, that results in increased risk of disease decades later. Thus, it is difficult to interpret differences in disease rates between 60-year-old men in 1900 and 60-year-old men in 1960. It is possible, however, to differentiate between various effects by performing birth cohort analyses, which consider incidence rates of a disease not by age at onset, but by date of birth.

Birth cohort analysis of mortality data was first described by Farr in 1870, and one classic example, reported by Frost [25] in 1939, involves the comparison of death rates from tuberculosis. Figure 5-5 shows mortality rates among men from this disease in Massachusetts by age at death in the years 1880, 1910, and 1930. While it is clear that there was a marked decline in mortality from tuberculosis between 1880 and 1930, the pattern of risk seemed to be changing, with the highest mortality in 1930 among middle-aged men aged 50 to 60 years rather than among young adults, as had been previously noted. When a birth cohort analysis was performed (Fig. 5-6), which plots the distribution of age at death from tuberculosis by year of birth rather than year of death, a very different pattern emerged. The curves of mortality with age are actually very similar for all the groups, with each having a peak between ages 20 and 30 and declining steadily thereafter. It thus became clear that the

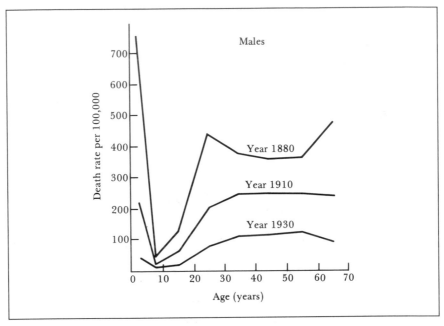

Fig. 5-5. Death rates from tuberculosis in Massachusetts men by age, 1880, 1910, and 1930. (From W. H. Frost, The age selection of mortality from tuberculosis in successive decades. *Am. J. Hyg.* 30:91, 1939.)

1930 age-specific mortality pattern resulted from the fact that men in their fifties at that time belonged to the 1880 birth cohort, who had experienced a much greater exposure to tuberculosis than men in the subsequent groups, who were born after major preventive and therapeutic advances had materially reduced both incidence and mortality.

Place

The second basic question addressed by descriptive studies is, "Where are the rates of disease highest and lowest?" Descriptive characteristics related to place can provide major insights into disease etiology. For example, mortality rates for specific cancers vary widely in different countries [19]. Table 5-5 shows, for a number of cancer sites, the geographic areas reporting the highest and lowest incidence rates and the ratio of those rates. The range of variation is great, from a low of 6 : 1 for bladder and ovarian cancers to a high of 300 : 1 for esophageal malignancy. It is also striking that some countries that have the highest incidence rate for one cancer site have the lowest for another. England has very high rates of lung cancer but the lowest rates of liver cancer; Japan has the highest frequency of stomach cancer but the lowest incidence rates for bladder, prostate, ovarian, and uterine malignancies. Moreover, Japan

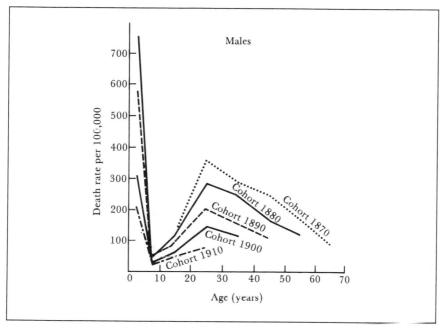

Fig. 5-6. Death rates from tuberculosis in Massachusetts men by age, according to year of birth. (From W. H. Frost, The age selection of mortality from tuberculosis in successive decades. *Am. J. Hyg.* 30:91, 1939.)

and Nigeria both have the lowest incidence rates of sites for which the United States experiences the highest rates, namely bladder, colon, prostate, and uterine cancers. The patterns noted from these descriptive data have contributed to the belief that most human cancers are potentially avoidable and to the formulation of research questions concerning a large number of specific etiologic exposures [19].

Geographic comparisons of disease frequency can be made between countries or between regions within a single country. With respect to the former, studies of migrants provide epidemiologists with a unique opportunity to distinguish between possible roles of genetics and environment. For example, mortality from colon cancer is much lower in Japan than in the U.S. [19]. This difference could, in theory, be due to genetic differences between Orientals and whites, but might also result from one or more dietary or other life-style factors that are dissimilar between the two cultures. Studies of migrants from Japan to the United States can help distinguish between effects of "nature" and "nurture." For example, Table 5-6 shows relative risks for stomach, liver, and colon cancer among Japanese men living in Japan, Japanese immigrants to California, and sons of Japanese immigrants, compared with white men in California [9]. These data exhibit a consistent pattern. For stomach and liver

Table 5-5. Geographic areas of highest and lowest
incidence of selected cancer sites, with ratios of incidence rates

	Cancer site	High incidence area	Low incidence area	Ratio high-low
Men	Bladder	United States	Japan	6 : 1
	Colon	United States	Nigeria	10 : 1
	Esophagus	Iran	Nigeria	300 : 1
	Liver	Mozambique	England	100 : 1
	Lung	England	Nigeria	35 : 1
	Pancreas	New Zealand (Maori)	India	8 : 1
	Prostate	United States (blacks)	Japan	40 : 1
	Stomach	Japan	Uganda	25 : 1
Women	Breast	British Columbia	Israel (non-Jewish)	7 : 1
	Cervix	Colombia	Israel (Jewish)	15 : 1
	Ovary	Denmark	Japan	6 : 1
	Uterus	United States	Japan	30 : 1

Source: R. Doll and R. Peto, *The Causes of Cancer.* New York: Oxford University
Press, 1981.

Table 5-6. Relative risks of mortality from cancer of the stomach, liver, and
colon among Japanese men in Japan, Japanese immigrants to California, and
sons of Japanese immigrants compared with white men in California, aged
45–64 years

Cancer sites	Relative risk (compared with California whites)		
	Japanese in Japan	Japanese immigrants to California	Sons of Japanese immigrants
Stomach	8.4	3.8	2.8
Liver	4.1	2.7	2.2
Colon	0.2	0.4	0.9

Source: P. Buell and J. E. Dunn, Cancer mortality among Japanese Issei and
Nisei of California. *Cancer* 18:656, 1965.

cancer, both of which are much more common in Japan than among whites in the United States, men who were born in Japan but migrated to California have considerably lower risks of death than men of the same age in Japan. Risks of mortality from these two cancers among the sons of Japanese immigrants are still lower. In contrast, the risk of colon cancer, which is extremely common in California but rare in Japan, approaches that of white men in California with migration, from 0.2 among Japanese in Japan, to 0.4 among immigrants to California and 0.9 among sons of immigrants.

These patterns raise several important issues. First, in all three instances, migration is associated with changes in cancer mortality rates from those of the native land toward those of the new country. This finding that the death rates among Japanese so clearly and consistently move toward the experience in the U.S., even within a single generation, strongly suggests that the occurrence of these cancers is largely determined by environmental rather than genetic factors. On the other hand, for each cancer there remains a residual difference between the mortality rates. For stomach and liver cancer, the sons of Japanese immigrants have lower risks than the Japanese immigrants themselves and far lower risks than the Japanese in Japan, but still higher risks than California whites. These data are compatible with each of two plausible interpretations. First, they may reflect differences in genetic susceptibility to these malignancies. Second, it is also possible that migrants retain certain environmental determinants of their current risk that are correlated with their ethnic origins. In this regard, diet, and specifically the consumption of smoked or cured foods [34], has been raised as an important etiologic factor in stomach cancer.

Genetic hypotheses can be tested in investigations designed specifically to quantitate heritability. Of available design options, twin studies provide the most powerful tool of epidemiologists to quantify the relative roles of genetics and environment [48]. There is, however, an increased awareness that even clearly inherited disorders such as phenylketonuria have important environmental determinants, specifically phenylalanine in the diet. Such considerations have focused primary attention on the identification of specific and alterable environmental causes rather than concentrating on determining relative roles of nature and nurture.

In addition to international comparisons, disease frequency can be compared between various regions within a larger population. For example, throughout the world, mortality from multiple sclerosis is much higher in northern latitudes than in southern regions [1, 42]. Such data have contributed to the formulation of a number of hypotheses concerning risk factors for this disease. In a large number of analytic studies testing various hypotheses during the past 20 years, an association be-

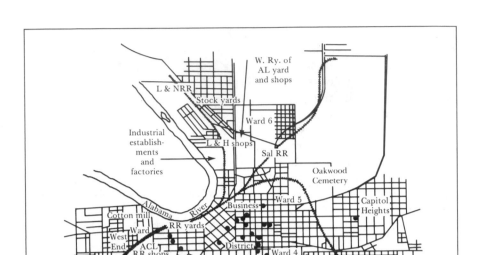

Fig. 5-7. A. Cases of mild typhus in Montgomery, Alabama, 1922–1925, plotted according to residence. B. Cases of mild typhus in Montgomery, Alabama, 1922–1925, plotted according to place of employment (or residence, if unemployed). (From K. F. Maxcy, An epidemiological study of endemic typhus [Brill's disease] in the Southeastern United States with special reference to its mode of transmission. *Public Health Rep.* 41:2967, 1926.)

tween latitude and multiple sclerosis has persisted. While the range of possible etiologic factors has constantly been expanded, no more specific environmental factor has been reliably identified [21]. Any future etiologic hypothesis, however, must be consistent with this descriptive feature of a north-south gradient.

Similarly, in 1975, the U.S. Department of Health, Education and Welfare published an atlas of maps of cancer mortality rates by county [52], which showed that deaths from lung cancer among white men were elevated in some geographic regions, particularly in large metropolitan areas. It also revealed high rates in a cluster of adjacent counties along the southeast Atlantic coast. This intriguing geographic variation led to a search for further clues from descriptive data on lung cancer death rates by demographic, socioeconomic, racial, and occupational charac-

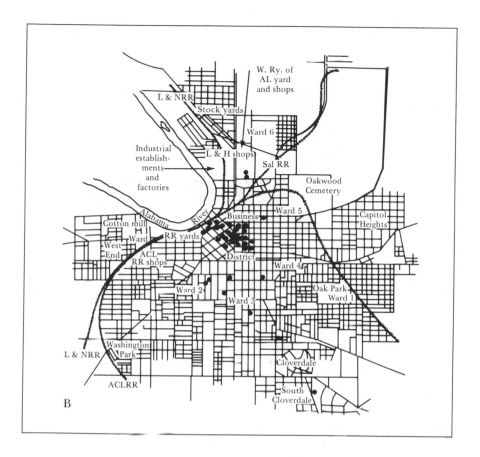

B

teristics by county [5]. These data showed that after taking into account the degree of urbanization and other demographic features of the counties, lung cancer mortality was significantly higher in counties where paper, chemical, petroleum, and transportation industries were located. Concurrent analyses of descriptive data from the state of Florida indicated excess lung cancer mortality in the northern region of the state, particularly in Duval County [32]. All these descriptive findings contributed to the formulation of the hypothesis that employment in a particular industry accounted for the observed excess of lung cancer. Results of two case-control studies from Georgia [6] and Florida [7] indicated that employment in shipbuilding during World War II in these coastal regions was associated with the increased lung cancer mortality in white men, possibly due to exposure to asbestos.

Descriptive data on place can be presented very efficiently in a pictorial manner, with a map indicating either the location of actual cases of disease or areas of varying frequencies. An example of the former, also referred to as a spot map, is illustrated in Figure 5-7, which plots cases

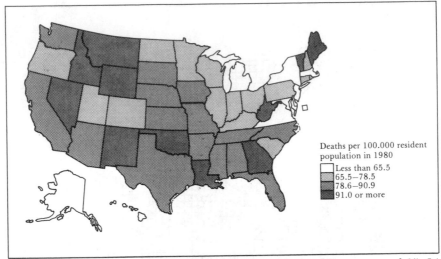

Fig. 5-8. Death rates for motor vehicle accidents among white men, aged 15–24 years, in the United States, 1979–1980. (From U.S. D.H.H.S. *Health United States 1984.* D.H.H.S. Publication No. (P.H.S.) 85–1232. Hyattsville, MD: National Center for Health Statistics, 1984.)

of mild typhus in Montgomery, Alabama during 1922 to 1925, in relation to residence (Fig. 5-7A) and place of employment (Fig. 5-7B) [53]. As shown in Figure 5-7A, there did not appear to be any marked clustering of cases. When the cases were plotted by place of employment (or by residence for those who were unemployed), the vast majority were grouped in the business district adjacent to the railroad yards, which encompassed feed stores and food depots. This observation led to the hypothesis that endemic typhus in the southern United States was not being transmitted by lice, but rather by flea-infested rats or mice. This important etiologic hypothesis was subsequently corroborated in analytic studies [53, 77].

A map of different regions within a larger population can be similarly informative. Figure 5-8 depicts U.S. death rates for motor vehicle accidents among white males, 15 to 24 years of age, in 1979 to 1980 [72]. Most of the high-mortality states are located in the western U.S., while most of those with the lowest rates are on the east coast. This raises the question that differences in rates may be related to factors such as number of miles driven, average speeds, highway versus city driving, the availability of alternate forms of transportation, as well as minimum driving and drinking ages, all of which may differ between the urban, densely populated east coast and the rural, more sparsely populated west. All these hypotheses require analytic studies designed to test the role of specific factors [33].

Time

Descriptive data on time address such questions as "When does the disease occur commonly or rarely?" and "Is the frequency of the disease at present different from the corresponding frequency in the past?" In some respects, changes in disease rates over time correspond to the classic concept of an epidemic, which involves a marked increase in disease frequency during a relatively short interval. For diseases or outcomes with a short latency period, such time clustering suggested from descriptive data can sometimes be traced, through analytic studies, to the introduction of a specific causal agent. For example, in Germany in late 1959, there was a single case report of an extremely unusual congenital malformation affecting the limbs and digits. Cases continued to accumulate, and by September 1961, there appeared to be a marked increase over the previous year in the number of cases of these malformations. These descriptive data led to the hypothesis that these malformations were due to to a recently introduced new drug. In mid-November 1961, the specific hypothesis was formulated that thalidomide, a sleeping pill first introduced in Germany in 1956, was responsible. Review of all reported cases between 1957 and 1961 indicated a 200-fold increase in the frequency of these birth defects during that period. In addition, in analytic studies, mothers of affected infants were compared with those of healthy children, and an extremely high proportion of those with affected infants had indeed taken thalidomide, compared with virtually none of the controls. On the basis of these observations, thalidomide was taken off the market in Germany at the end of November 1961 [54].

More recently, a similar time-clustering of reports of toxic shock syndrome (TSS) led to the formulation of important etiologic hypotheses. Figure 5-9 shows the number of confirmed cases of TSS in the United States by month from January 1977 to October 1981 [62]. This striking increase occurred primarily in menstruating women who used tampons, in particular the superabsorbent tampon Rely. This tampon had been introduced to the market in August 1978, the point at which the number of cases of TSS began to rise steadily. This hypothesis was tested in analytic studies [18, 40, 66, 67], and the product was removed from the market by the Proctor and Gamble Company in September 1980. As shown in Figure 5-9, after the removal of the Rely tampon from the market, there was an almost immediate drop in the number of cases of TSS. Although this action was temporally associated with the abrupt termination of the epidemic of this disease, it was not yet clear what aspect of the use of superabsorbent tampons increased risk of developing TSS. Several mechanisms were proposed, including abrasion of the vaginal wall by the tampon or its applicator, or chemical changes due to the composition of the tampons themselves. Recent studies have implicated

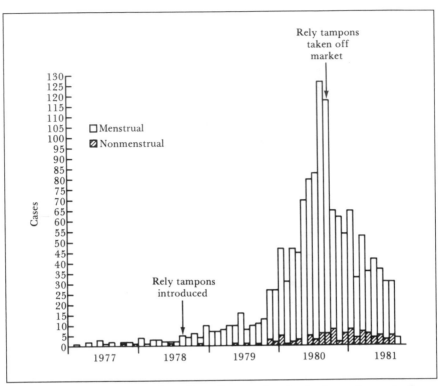

Fig. 5-9. Monthly number of confirmed cases of toxic shock syndrome in the United States, 1977–1981, in relation to the introduction and removal of the Rely tampon from the market. (From A. L. Reingold et al., Toxic shock syndrome surveillance in the United States, 1980 to 1981. *Ann. Intern. Med.* 96:875, 1982.)

the fiber of the tampon itself in creating an environment favorable for the production of the toxin that causes TSS [56].

There are two other types of time patterns that can suggest possible etiologic hypotheses. Cyclic changes, such as seasonal patterns, have proved particularly valuable in the investigation of acute diseases or those with a short latent period. For example, in the 1920s, comparison of the seasonal patterns of endemic typhus in the southern United States and epidemic typhus in Europe (Fig. 5-10) led to the hypothesis that these were two different disease entities with different modes of transmission [53]. Specifically, the distribution of typhus in the U.S. peaked in the late summer and early autumn, which was the reverse of the pattern of epidemic typhus in Europe, which was most frequent in the winter and spring. Since the disease in Europe was known to be louse-borne and the seasonal pattern of onset was consistent with that of other louse-

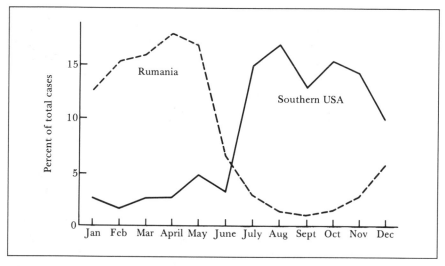

Fig. 5-10. Seasonal distribution of epidemic typhus in Rumania and endemic typhus in the southern United States, 1922–1925. (From K. F. Maxcy, An epidemiological study of endemic typhus [Brill's disease] in the southeastern United States with special reference to its mode of transmission. *Public Health Rep.* 41:2967, 1926.)

borne diseases, a different mode of transmission was suggested for endemic typhus. Subsequent analytic studies implicated flea-infested rats as the mode of transmission for endemic typhus in the U.S. [77].

To evaluate the epidemiology of chronic diseases, examining the secular trend, or changes in frequency that take place over years or decades, can be particularly useful. Secular trends can be due to one or more of a number of different factors, including

1. Changes in diagnostic techniques, leading to increased reporting of a particular diagnosis even though the disease may not actually be more common
2. Changes in the accuracy of enumerating the population at risk of developing the disease, leading to changes in rates, which again may not reflect alteration in actual frequency
3. Changes in the age distribution of the population, which could result in an alteration in crude rates of disease even though age-specific rates remain constant
4. Changes in survival from a disease due to improved treatments or greater effects of usual therapy following earlier diagnosis
5. Changes in actual incidence of the disease due to alterations in environmental or life-style factors.

For example, in the 1960s there began an approximate 30-percent decline in mortality from CHD in the United States [63]. During this same period, a large number of other factors have also changed in the U.S. population. Descriptive data reveal that between 1963 and 1983, consumption of eggs, whole milk, butter, and cream have decreased, while per capita intake of vegetable oils, margarine, poultry, and fish have increased [59]. Current cigarette smoking among men has decreased from 53 percent in 1955 [71] to 35 percent in 1983 [72], and the proportion of individuals with high blood pressure receiving adequate treatment has markedly increased [8]. While all these primary prevention measures are temporally related to the decline in mortality, improvements in treatment of CHD have also occurred. For example, coronary care units have been reported to decrease in-hospital mortality from about 35 percent to 15 to 20 percent [37]. Further, a number of new surgical techniques, such as coronary artery bypass grafting [65], as well as thrombolytic therapy, such as streptokinase [68], tissue plasminogen activator [70], and aspirin [3], all have been proposed to decrease mortality following myocardial infarction. These data raise the question that the decline in CHD mortality may be related to changes in both the prevention and treatment of CHD. Although it has been suggested that the majority of this decline is due to decreases in incidence rates [28, 60] because of primary prevention, such a hypothesis requires testing using analytic epidemiologic designs.

CONCLUSION

Data from descriptive epidemiologic studies are useful to public health administrators planning for health care utilization and resource allocation. They are also valuable to epidemiologists in describing patterns of disease as well as contributing important information to the formulation of etiologic hypotheses. There are a number of descriptive epidemiologic study design options, including correlational studies of populations as well as case reports, case series, and cross-sectional surveys among individuals. Each type of study provides valuable information on who is getting the disease (person), where it is more and less common (place), and when it is occurring (time). Since descriptive studies provide data on populations rather than individuals (correlational studies), lack an adequate comparison group (case reports and case series), or cannot usually discern the temporal relationship between an exposure and disease (cross-sectional surveys), they generally cannot test etiologic hypotheses. To do so requires utilization of the analytic design strategies to be detailed in the next several chapters.

STUDY QUESTIONS

1. In which special circumstances can cross-sectional surveys be used to test hypotheses?
2. Why can the presence or absence of correlations from correlational studies be misleading in assessing the presence of a valid statistical association?
3. These data relate to an unusual episode that actually occurred.

SOCIO-ECONOMIC CLASS	Adult Males		Adult Females		Children		Total	
	N	DEATH RATE (%)	N	DEATH RATE (%)	N	DEATH RATE (%)	N	DEATH RATE (%)
High	173	66.5	144	3.5	5	0.0	322	37.3
Middle	160	91.9	93	16.1	24	0.0	277	58.5
Low	454	87.9	179	45.3	76	71.1	709	75.3
Unknown	875	78.4	23	8.7	0	—	898	76.6
Total	1662	81.0	439	23.5	105	51.4	2206	68.2

a. Describe the epidemiologic features of this episode.
b. Based on the descriptive characteristics, formulate a hypothesis concerning the etiology of this episode.

REFERENCES

1. Alter, M. Etiologic considerations based on the epidemiology of multiple sclerosis. *Am. J. Epidemiol.* 88:318, 1968.
2. Ammann, A. J., Cowan, M. J., Wara, D. W., et al. Acquired immunodeficiency in an infant: Possible transmission by means of blood products. *Lancet* 1:956, 1983.
3. Aspirin for heart patients. *F.D.A. Drug Bull.* 15:34, 1985.
4. Beral, V., and Kay, C. R. Royal College of General Practitioners Oral Contraception Study: Mortality among oral contraceptive users. *Lancet* 2:727, 1977.
5. Blot, W. J., and Fraumeni, J. F., Jr. Geographic patterns of lung cancer: Industrial correlations. *Am. J. Epidemiol.* 103:539, 1976.
6. Blot, W. J., Harrington, J. M., Toledo, A., et al. Lung cancer after employment in shipyards during World War II. *N. Engl. J. Med.* 299:620, 1978.
7. Blot, W. J., Davies, J. E., Brown, L. M., et al. Occupation and the high risk of lung cancer in northeast Florida. *Cancer* 50:364, 1982.
8. Borhani, N. O. Mortality Trends in Hypertension, United States, 1950–1976. In R. J. Havlik and M. Feinleib (eds.), *Proceedings of the Conference on the Decline in Coronary Heart Disease Mortality.* U.S. D.H.E.W., N.I.H. Publication No. 79-1610, 1979. Pp. 218–233.

9. Buell, P., and Dunn, J. E. Cancer mortality among Japanese Issei and Nisei of California. *Cancer* 18:656, 1965.
10. Centers for Disease Control. *Pneumocystis* pneumonia—Los Angeles. *M.M.W.R.* 30:250, 1981.
11. Centers for Disease Control. Kaposi's sarcoma and *Pneumocystis* pneumonia among homosexual men—New York City and California. *M.M.W.R.* 30:305, 1981.
12. Centers for Disease Control. *Pneumocystis carinii* pneumonia among persons with hemophilia A. *M.M.W.R.* 31:365, 1982.
13. Centers for Disease Control. Annual summary 1982: Reported morbidity and mortality in the United States. *M.M.W.R.* 31(54), 1983.
14. Colditz, G. A., Willett, W. C., Stampfer, M. J., et al. Menopause and risk of coronary heart disease in women. *N. Engl. J. Med.* 316:1105, 1987.
15. Cole, P., MacMahon, B., and Aisenberg, A. Mortality from Hodgkin's disease in the United States: Evidence for the multiple-aetiology hypothesis. *Lancet* 2:1371, 1968.
16. Cramer, D. W. The role of cervical cytology in the declining morbidity and mortality of cervical cancer. *Cancer* 34:2018, 1974.
17. Creech, J. L., Jr., and Johnson, M. N. Angiosarcoma of liver in the manufacture of polyvinyl chloride. *J. Occup. Med.* 16:151, 1974.
18. Davis, J. P., Chesney P. J., Wand, P. J., et al. Toxic shock syndrome: Epidemiologic features, recurrence, risk factors, and prevention. *N. Engl. J. Med.* 303:1429, 1980.
19. Doll, R., and Peto, R. *The Causes of Cancer.* New York: Oxford University Press, 1981.
20. Dyer, A. R., Stamler, J., Paul, O., et al. Alcohol consumption and 17-year mortality in the Chicago Western Electric Company Study. *Prev. Med.* 9:78, 1980.
21. Ellison, G. W. (moderator). Multiple sclerosis. *Ann. Intern. Med.* 101:514, 1984.
22. Faust, H. S., and Dembert, M. L. Frisbee finger. *N. Engl. J. Med.* 295:304, 1975.
23. Fletcher, R. H., and Fletcher, S. W. Clinical research in general medical journals: A 30-year perspective. *N. Engl. J. Med.* 301:180, 1979.
24. Friedman, G. D. Cigarette smoking and geographic variation in coronary heart disease mortality in the United States. *J. Chronic Dis.* 20:769, 1967.
25. Frost, W. H. The age selection of mortality from tuberculosis in successive decades. *Am. J. Hyg.* 30:91, 1939.
26. Goldberger, J. The etiology of pellagra: The significance of certain epidemiological observations with respect thereto. *Public Health Rep.* 29:1683, 1914.
27. Goldberger, J., and Wheeler, G. A. The experimental production of pellagra in human subjects by means of diet. *Hyg. Lab. Bull.* 120:7, 1920.
28. Goldman, L., and Cook, E. F. The decline in ischemic heart disease mortality rates: An analysis of the comparative effects of medical interventions and changes in lifestyle. *Ann. Intern. Med.* 101:825, 1984.
29. Hennekens, C. H. Alcohol. In N. Kaplan and J. Stamler (eds.), *Prevention of Coronary Heart Disease.* Philadelphia: Saunders, 1983. Pp. 130–138.

30. Hennekens, C. H., Evans, D., and Peto, R. Oral contraceptive use, cigarette smoking and myocardial infarction. *Br. J. Fam. Planning* 5:66, 1979.
31. Hennekens, C. H., and MacMahon, B. Oral contraceptives and myocardial infarction. *N. Engl. J. Med.* 20:1166, 1977.
32. Hennekens, C. H., Davies, J. E., Levine, R. S., et al. Trends of lung cancer in northern Florida. *South. Med. J.* 74:566, 1981.
33. Hingson, R. W., Scotch, N., Mangione, T., et al. Impact of legislation raising the legal drinking age in Massachusetts from 18 to 20. *Am. J. Public Health* 73:163, 1983.
34. Hirayama, T. The Epidemiology of Cancer of the Stomach in Japan with Special Reference to the Role of Diet. In R. Harris (ed.), *Proceedings of the 9th International Cancer Congress.* U.I.C.C. Monograph Series, vol. 10. Berlin: Springer-Verlag, 1967. Pp. 37–49.
35. Hirayama, T. Epidemiology of breast cancer with special reference to the role of diet. *Prev. Med.* 7:173, 1978.
36. Jordan, W. M. Pulmonary embolism. *Lancet* 2:1146, 1961.
37. Killip, T. Impact of Coronary Care on Mortality from Ischemic Heart Disease. In R. J. Havlik and M. Feinleib (eds.), *Proceedings of the Conference on the Decline in Coronary Heart Disease Mortality.* U.S. D.H.E.W., N.I.H. Publication No. 79-1610, 1979. Pp. 135–46.
38. Langmuir, A. D. The surveillance of communicable diseases of national importance. *N. Engl. J. Med.* 268:182, 1963.
39. LaPorte, R. E., Cresanta, J. L., and Kuller, L. H. The relation of alcohol to CHD and mortality: Implication for public health policy. *J. Public Health Policy* 1:198, 1980.
40. Latham, R. H., Kehrberg, M. W., Jacobson, J. A., et al. Toxic shock syndrome in Utah: A review of a case-control study and surveillance. *Ann. Intern. Med.* 96:906, 1982.
41. Lednar, W. M., Tyroler, H. A., McMichael, A. J., et al. The occupational determinants of chronic disabling pulmonary disease in rubber workers. *J. Occup. Med.* 19:263, 1977.
42. Limburg, C. C. The geographic distribution of multiple sclerosis and its estimated prevalence in the U.S. *Assoc. Res. Nerv. Dis. Proc.* 28:15, 1950.
43. McBride, D. O., Lehman, L. P., and Mangiardi, J. R. Break-dancing neck. *N. Engl. J. Med.* 312:186, 1985.
44. McCowan, T. C. Space-Invaders wrist. *N. Engl. J. Med.* 304:1368, 1981.
45. McDonough, J. R., Hames, C. G., Stulb, S. C., et al. Coronary heart disease among Negroes and Whites in Evans County, Georgia. *J. Chronic Dis.* 18:443, 1965.
46. MacMahon, B. Epidemiologic evidence on the nature of Hodgkin's disease. *Cancer* 10:1045, 1957.
47. MacMahon, B. Epidemiology of Hodgkin's disease. *Cancer Res.* 26:1189, 1966.
48. MacMahon, B. Gene-environment interaction in human disease. *J. Psychiatr. Res.* 6(Suppl. 1):393, 1968.
49. MacMahon, B., and Pugh, T. F. *Epidemiology: Principles and Methods.* Boston: Little, Brown, 1970.
50. McMichael, A. J., Gerber, W. S., Gamble, J. F., et al. Chronic respiratory

symptoms and job type within the rubber industry. *J. Occup. Med.* 18:611, 1976.

51. Mann, J. I., and Inman, W. H. W. Oral contraceptives and death from myocardial infarction. *Br. Med. J.* 2:245, 1976.

52. Mason, T. J., McKay, F. W., Hoover, R., et al. *Atlas of Cancer Mortality in U.S. Counties: 1950–1969.* D.H.E.W. Publication No. (N.I.H.) 75-780. Washington, DC: Government Printing Office, 1975.

53. Maxcy, K. F. An epidemiological study of endemic typhus (Brill's disease) in the Southeastern United States with special reference to its mode of transmission. *Public Health Rep.* 41:2967, 1926.

54. Mellin, G. W., and Katzenstein, M. The saga of thalidomide. *N. Engl. J. Med.* 267:1184, 1962.

55. Mill, J. S. *A System of Logic, Ratiocinative and Inductive* (5th ed.). London: Parker, Son and Bowin, 1862.

56. Mills, J. T., Parsonnet, J., Tsai, Y-C., et al. Control of production of Toxic-Shock-Syndrome Toxin-1 (TSST-1) by magnesium ion. *J. Infect. Dis.* 151:1158, 1985.

57. Monson, R. R., Peters, J. M., and Johnson, M. N. Proportional mortality among vinyl chloride workers. *Lancet* 2:397, 1974.

58. Newell, G. R., Cole, P., Miettinen, O. S., et al. Age differences in the histology of Hodgkin's disease. *J.N.C.I.* 45:311, 1970.

59. Page, L., and Marston, R. M. Food Consumption Patterns, U.S. Diet. In R. J. Havlik and M. Feinleib, (eds.), *Proceedings of the Conference on the Decline in Coronary Heart Disease Mortality.* U.S. D.H.E.W., N.I.H. Publication No. 79-1610, 1979. Pp. 236–243.

60. Pell, S., and Fayerweather, W. E. Trends in the incidence of myocardial infarction and in associated mortality and morbidity in a large employed population, 1957–1983. *N. Engl. J. Med.* 312:1005, 1985.

61. Peterman, T. A., Drotman, D. P., and Curran, J. W. Epidemiology of the acquired immunodeficiency syndrome (AIDS). *Epidemiol. Rev.* 7:1, 1985.

62. Reingold, A. L., Hargrett, N. T., Shands, K. N., et al. Toxic shock syndrome surveillance in the United States, 1980 to 1981. *Ann. Intern. Med.* 96:875, 1982.

63. Rosenberg, H. M., and Klebba, A. J. Trends in Cardiovascular Mortality with a Focus on Ischemic Heart Disease: United States, 1950–1976. In R. J. Havlik and M. Feinleib (eds.), *Proceedings of the Conference on the Decline in Coronary Heart Disease Mortality.* U.S. D.H.E.W., N.I.H. Publication No. 79-1610, 1979. Pp. 11–39.

64. Rosier, R. P., and Lefer, L. G. Jogger's whiplash. *J.A.M.A.* 239:2114, 1978.

65. Sabiston, D. C., Jr. Effect of Coronary Artery Bypass Grafts in CHD. In R. J. Havlik and M. Feinleib (eds.), *Proceedings of the Conference on the Decline in Coronary Heart Disease Mortality.* U.S. D.H.E.W., N.I.H. Publication No. 79-1610, 1979. Pp. 172–188.

66. Shands, K. N., Schmid, G. P., Dan, B. B., et al. Toxic shock syndrome in menstruating women: Association with tampon use and *Staphylococcus aureus* and the clinical features in 52 cases. *N. Engl. J. Med.* 303:1436, 1980.

67. Shands, K. N., Schleck, W. F. III, Hargrett, N. T., et al. Toxic shock syndrome: Case-control studies at the Centers for Disease Control. *Ann. Intern. Med.* 96:895, 1982.

68. Stampfer, M. J., Goldhaber, S. Z., Yusuf, S., et al. Effect of intravenous strep-tokinase on acute myocardial infarction. *N. Engl. J. Med.* 307:1180, 1982.
69. Tabershaw, I. R., and Gaffey, W. R. Mortality study of workers in the man-ufacture of vinyl chloride and its polymers. *J. Occup. Med.* 16:509, 1974.
70. T.I.M.I. Study Group. The thrombolysis in myocardial infarction (TIMI) trial: Phase I findings. *N. Engl. J. Med.* 312:932, 1985.
71. U.S. D.H.E.W. *Smoking and Health: A Report of the Surgeon General.* D.H.E.W. Publication No. (P.H.S.) 7-50066. Rockville, MD: U.S. D.H.E.W., 1979.
72. U.S. D.H.H.S. *Health United States 1984.* D.H.H.S. Publication No. (P.H.S.) 85-1232. Hyattsville, MD: National Center for Health Statistics, 1984.
73. Vana, J., and Murphy, G. P. Primary malignant liver tumors: Association with oral contraceptives. *N.Y. State J. Med.* 79:321, 1979.
74. Vessey, M. P., McPherson, K., and Johnson, B. Mortality among women partici-pating in the Oxford/Family Planning Association Contraceptive Study. *Lancet* 2:731, 1977.
75. Walzer, P. D., Perl, D. P., Krogstad, D. J., et al. *Pneumocystis carinii* pneumonia in the United States: Epidemiologic, diagnostic, and clinical features. *Ann. Intern. Med.* 80:83, 1974.
76. Willett, W. C., Stampfer, M. J., Bain, C., et al. Cigarette smoking, relative weight and menopause. *Am. J. Epidemiol.* 117:651, 1983.
77. Woodward, T. E. President's address: Typhus verdict in American industry. *Trans. Am. Clin. Climatol. Assoc.* 82:7, 1970.

6

Case-Control Studies

A case-control study is a type of observational analytic epidemiologic investigation in which subjects are selected on the basis of whether they do (cases) or do not (controls) have a particular disease under study. The groups are then compared with respect to the proportion having a history of an exposure or characteristic of interest. Because of this design, case-control studies offer a number of advantages for evaluating the association between an exposure and a disease. This approach was begun in developed countries in the twentieth century, in part as a response to needs that accompanied the shift from acute to chronic diseases as major public health problems [8]. Specifically, the case-control design offered a solution to the difficulties of studying diseases with very long latency periods, since investigators could identify affected and unaffected individuals and then look backward in time to assess their antecedent exposures rather than having to wait a number of years for the disease to develop. Thus, case-control studies are particularly efficient, in terms of both time and costs, relative to the other analytic approaches. Moreover, since case-control studies select participants on the basis of their disease status, this design allows investigators to identify adequate numbers of diseased and nondiseased individuals. Consequently, this strategy is particularly well suited to the evaluation of rare diseases, which would otherwise need to follow tremendously large numbers of individuals in order to accumulate a sufficient number who develop a particular outcome. Finally, case-control studies allow for the evaluation of a wide range of potential etiologic exposures that might relate to a specific disease as well as the interrelationships among these factors. Such studies can, therefore, be used to test specific hypotheses or, in the absence of an a priori hypothesis, to explore a range of exposures among affected and nonaffected individuals. This type of study design is especially useful in the early stages of the development of knowledge about a particular disease or outcome of interest.

The major potential problem in a case-control study relates to the fact that both the exposure and disease have already occurred at the time the participants enter into the study. As a result, this design is particularly susceptible to bias from the differential selection of either the cases or controls into the study on the basis of their exposure status as well as from differential reporting or recording of exposure information between study groups based on their disease status. This potential for bias, as well as the fact that some consider the logic of an investigation progressing temporally from effect (disease) to cause (antecedent exposure) as inherently flawed, has led to a degree of skepticism in the past concerning the value of case-control investigations [16]. While this potential for bias cannot be ignored, it is not a reason to avoid case-control studies. Rather, it merely requires that careful consideration be made of the sources from which the bias may arise in any particular investigation in order to minimize or, preferably, to avoid, its occurrence [29]. Moreover, the logic of elucidating a potential cause from observing an effect is an approach used often in everyday life. Well designed and conducted case-control studies can provide valuable information on the association between an exposure and disease. In fact, because of their advantage in being able to evaluate diseases that occur many years following relevant exposures in a timely and cost-effective manner, case-control studies have become the most common analytic epidemiologic study design encountered in the medical literature today [8].

It should be noted that some investigators use the term *retrospective studies* as synonymous with *case-control studies* because such designs look backward from the effect to ascertain the possible cause. As discussed in Chapter 2, we believe it to be more informative to reserve the term *retrospective* to refer to the timing of the relevant events with respect to the initiation of the study. In this context, the terms *retrospective* and *prospective* are most commonly used to differentiate the two types of cohort studies. While in either type of cohort study the participants are selected on the basis of their exposure status, in a retrospective cohort study all relevant events, both exposure and disease, have already occurred at the time the study has begun. In a prospective cohort design, while the exposure may or may not yet have occurred at the beginning of the study, the outcomes of interest have certainly not yet developed. When the word *retrospective* is used to denote the timing of the study, a case-control study can clearly also be termed either *retrospective* or *prospective*. Specifically, if all the cases of the disease have been diagnosed at the time the investigator initiates the study, it is a retrospective case-control study. On the other hand, if the study is begun and all new cases that are diagnosed within the next period of time (such as a number of years) are included in the investigation, the study is a prospective case-control design. Thus, in the context of these definitions the use of the term *retrospective* to refer to all case-control studies is inappropriate. In general, however, the distinction between a retrospective and prospective case-control study is not made.

ISSUES IN THE DESIGN AND CONDUCT OF CASE-CONTROL STUDIES

For a case-control study to provide sound evidence of whether there is a valid statistical association between an exposure and disease, comparability of cases and controls is essential. The aspects of comparability that must be considered include factors such as their baseline risk of developing the disease other than from the exposure(s) under study, as well as the accuracy and completeness of data. Consequently, the major issues to be considered in designing and conducting a case-control study are the selection of the study groups and the sources of information about exposure and disease.

Definition and Selection of Cases

One of the first issues to be considered in the design of a case-control study is the definition of the disease or outcome of interest. It is important that this represent as homogeneous a disease entity as possible since very often similar manifestational entities of disease have very different etiologies. For example, until 1940, the designation "uterine cancer" on death certificates encompassed malignancies of both the corpus uteri and the uterine cervix [21], thus hampering epidemiologic studies. Since that time, etiologic investigations have found that these two diseases have very different risk factors, low number of sexual partners and high socioeconomic status for uterine cancer, contrasted with high number of sexual partners and low socioeconomic status for cervical malignancy [11]. Similarly, many investigations of drug exposure in relation to the development of specific congenital malformations have considered all congenital malformations as a group due to the inadequate sample size for any single entity. However, since no single teratogen increases risk uniformly for all malformations, such a strategy may mask any true increased risks associated with use of a particular drug.

To help ensure that cases selected for study represent a homogeneous entity, one of the first tasks in any study is to establish strict diagnostic criteria for the disease. For example, in the investigation of toxic shock syndrome, one of the first priorities of the Centers for Disease Control was to develop specific criteria for the disease, listed in Table 6-1 [27]. Similarly, case-control studies of myocardial infarction often use diagnostic criteria formulated by the World Health Organization, including documented electrocardiographic abnormalities, enzyme changes, and

Table 6-1. Diagnostic criteria for toxic shock syndrome

---

1. Fever: temperature greater than 38.9°C (102°F)
2. Rash (diffuse macular erythroderma)
3. Desquamation, particularly of palms and soles, 1–2 weeks after onset of illness
4. Hypotension (systolic blood pressure less than 90 mm Hg for adults, or less than 5th percentile by age for children under 16 years of age, or orthostatic syncope)
5. Involvement of 3 or more of the following organ systems:
   a. Gastrointestinal tract (vomiting or diarrhea at onset of illness)
   b. Muscular system (severe myalgia or creatinine kinase level at least twice the upper limits of normal [ULN])
   c. Mucous membranes (vaginal, oropharyngeal, or conjunctival hyperemia)
   d. Renal tract (blood urea nitrogen or creatinine level at least twice the ULN; or 5 + leukocytes per high power field—in the absence of a urinary tract infection)
   e. Hepatic system (total bilirubin, aspartate transaminase or alanine transaminase at least twice the ULN)
   f. Hematologic system (platelets ≤ 100,000/mm³)
   g. Central nervous system (disorientation or alterations in consciousness without focal neurologic signs when fever and hypotension are absent)
6. Negative results on the following tests, if obtained:
   a. Blood, throat, or cerebrospinal fluid cultures
   b. Seriologic tests for Rocky Mountain spotted fever, leptospirosis, and measles

---

Source: A. L. Reingold, et al. Toxic shock syndrome surveillance in the United States, 1980 to 1981. *Ann. Intern. Med.* 96:875, 1982.

characteristic chest pain [38]. Depending on the certainty of the diagnosis, and the amount of information available, it is often useful to perform analyses separately for cases classified as definite, probable, or possible.

Once the diagnostic criteria and definition of the disease have been clearly established, the individuals with this condition can be selected from a number of sources. These include identifying persons with the disease who have been treated at a particular hospital or medical care facility during a specified period of time or selecting all persons with the disease in a defined general population at a single point or during a given period of time. The first approach, referred to as a hospital-based case-control study, is more common because it is relatively easy and inexpensive to conduct. The second, the population-based case-control study, involves locating and obtaining data from all affected individuals or a random sample from a defined population. The scientific advantage of a population-based design is that it avoids bias arising from whatever selection factors lead an affected individual to utilize a particular health care facility or physician. Moreover, the population-based approach allows the description of the entire picture of the disease in that population and the direct computation of rates of disease in exposed and nonexposed individuals [7]. Because the logistic and cost considerations are often prohibitively large, however, population-based case-control studies are not routinely done.

Regardless of the source, the affected individuals can represent either incident (newly diagnosed) or prevalent (existing at a point in time) cases of the disease. Certainly, the inclusion of prevalent cases, especially of a rare condition, will greatly increase the sample size available for study in a given time period. Since prevalent cases reflect determinants of duration as well as the development of the disease, however, the interpretation of the findings from such a study may be complicated. Unless the effect of the exposure on the duration of illness is known, it will not be possible to determine the extent to which a particular characteristic is related to the prognosis of the disease once it develops rather than to its cause. Moreover, it is much more difficult to ensure that reported events relate to a time before the development of the disease rather than to a consequence of the disease process itself. For example, in a case-control study of coffee consumption and risk of peptic ulcer, it may be unclear whether the pattern of coffee drinking reported by the cases reflects the period before the development of the disease, when it could be causally related, or is merely a response to the first preclinical symptoms of the condition. While clarification of the temporal sequence between exposure and disease is always an issue in case-control studies, it is a more serious problem when prevalent rather than incident cases are used. Certainly, as discussed in Chapter 4, there are certain situations in which the use of prevalent cases is unavoidable, such as in a study of congenital malformations. Whenever possible, however, it is preferable to limit cases to those newly diagnosed within a specified period.

One issue that has often been raised is whether the cases in a case-control study should be selected to be representative of all persons with the disease. In other words, for a study of myocardial infarction (MI) among men, some believe that a random sample of all cases of MI in a community would be preferable to choosing cases of MI among white males ages 45 to 74 admitted to one of five area hospitals. The proposed rationale for selecting a random sample derives from the fact that findings from a study that utilized representative cases would be more readily generalizable to the broader population of all men. However, as stated in Chapter 3, the primary concern in the design of any study must be validity, not generalizability. A case-control study can be restricted to a particular type of case on whom complete and reliable information on exposure and disease can be obtained. If the cases selected for study do differ from others with the disease by age, sex, race, or severity of illness, the frequency of exposure among those cases will also be likely to differ from that among other cases of the disease. The control subjects should be selected to be comparable to the cases, and as a consequence will represent not the population of all nondiseased persons but the population of nondiseased persons who would have been included as cases had they developed the disease. Such a case-control study will, therefore, provide a valid estimate of the association between the exposure and the disease, and a judgment concerning the generalizability of the findings can then safely be made. Validity should not be compromised in an attempt to achieve generalizability, since a lack of confidence in the validity of findings from a study will preclude any ability to generalize the results.

Selection of Controls

The selection of an appropriate comparison group is perhaps the most difficult and critical issue in the design of a case-control study. Controls are necessary to allow the evaluation of whether the frequency of an exposure or specified characteristic observed in the case group is different from that which would have been expected based on the experience of a series of comparable individuals who do not have the disease. There is no control group that is optimal for all situations. The selection of a control group is made for a particular group of cases and involves consideration of a number of issues including the characteristics and source of the cases, the need to obtain comparable information from cases and controls, as well as practical and economic considerations. Depending on the source from which the cases were chosen—whether the cases were those seen in the office of a single medical practitioner or all those developing the disease throughout the entire state, for example—the controls must be selected to represent not the entire nondiseased population but the population of individuals who would have been identified and included as cases had they also developed the disease. Thus, in a manner analogous to selection of cases, the controls included may well differ from the general population with respect to a number of characteristics and, as a result, with regard to exposure. The crucial requirement is that they be comparable to the source population of the cases and that any exclusions or restrictions made in the identification of cases apply equally to the controls and vice versa.

Among the specific issues to be considered in selecting controls is the source of subjects. There are several possible sources commonly used, including hospital controls, general population controls, and special control series such as friends, neighbors, or relatives of cases. Each offers particular advantages and disadvantages that must be considered for any particular study in view of the nature of the cases, their source, and the type of information to be obtained.

One of the most frequently utilized sources of controls for investigations in which cases have been identified at one or more hospitals consists of patients at the same hospitals who have been admitted for conditions other than the disease being studied. For example, in a case-control study evaluating the association of cigarette smoking with myocardial infarction among women [31], cases were identified from admissions to coronary care units at 152 participating hospitals. Controls were drawn from among admissions to the surgical, orthopedic, and medical services of the same institutions and included patients with muskuloskeletal and abdominal diseases, trauma, and a variety of other noncoronary conditions.

There are a number of important practical and scientific advantages to using hospitalized controls. The first is that they are easily identified and readily available in sufficient numbers, thus minimizing the costs and effort involved in their assembly. Second, because they are hospitalized, they are more likely than healthy individuals to be aware of antecedent exposures or events. In this respect, their comparability to cases in their accuracy of reporting information will reduce the potential for recall bias. Third, using patients hospitalized with other diseases as controls means that they are likely to have been subject to the same intangible selection factors that influenced the cases to come to this particular physician or hospital. Finally, hospital controls, like cases, are more likely to be willing to cooperate than healthy individuals, thus minimizing bias due to nonresponse.

The chief disadvantage of using hospitalized controls is that they are, by definition, ill and therefore differ from healthy individuals in a number of ways that may be associated with illness or hospitalization in general. Thus, the experience of these other patients may not accurately represent the exposure distribution in the population from which the cases derived. Studies using both hospitalized and nonhospitalized controls have demonstrated that as a group, hospitalized patients are more likely to smoke cigarettes [1, 37], use oral contraceptives [37], and be heavy drinkers of alcohol [23] than nonhospitalized individuals. The result of using hospital controls for a study of any of these risk factors could be a biased estimate of effect. For example, a hospital-based investigation of smoking and bladder cancer might fail to find a difference in exposure frequencies among cases and controls, not because there truly is no association, but simply due to the high frequency of smoking among hospitalized controls. Similarly, a hospital-based case-control study of coffee and bladder cancer could find positive associations that were spurious if the control group was selected from those hospitalized for chronic conditions, since such patients tend to drink less coffee than healthy people in the community [28].

Although an advantage of using hospitalized patients as a source of controls is that in general they share the same selective processes by which the cases were identified, it is important to realize that this is not equally true for all diseases. For example, if a hospital is known to be a referral center for the treatment of a particular condition, it will certainly be a good source of cases for a case-control study, but those patients may not be comparable with individuals having other diseases in the same hospital since the referral patients are likely to be drawn from a wider geographic area and perhaps from a generally higher socioeconomic group than those with other illnesses.

The question of which category or categories of diseases should be included in a hospitalized control group is an important one. The concern is that the diseases for which the controls were hospitalized may also be associated with the risk factors under study. Thus, in practical terms, patients with diseases known to be associated, either positively or negatively, with the exposure of interest should be excluded from the control series. For example, cigarette smoking is an important risk factor for many respiratory diseases, such as bronchitis and pneumonia [36]. Including patients with such diseases in the comparison group for a case-control study of smoking and lung cancer would result in an observed proportion of smokers among the controls that would be unrepresentative of the healthy population with respect to smoking. The use of controls with bronchitis and pneumonia would therefore result in an underestimate of the true risk associated with smoking, since the two groups would be artificially more alike in terms of proportions of smokers. In the same way, in a case-control study of oral contraceptive use and cervical cancer, including in the control series women who had used barrier methods of contraception would result in a biased estimate of any true risk associated with oral contraceptive use, since barrier methods of contraception are associated with decreased risk of cervical cancer. Similarly, persons with conditions that might have resulted in a change in exposure levels should be excluded from the control group. For example, in studying effects of coffee consumption, the comparison group should not include patients with peptic ulcer, who may have been advised to reduce their coffee drinking as a result of their condition. The problem, however, is that for many exposures, especially those related to lifestyle, it is not always possible to be confident that the diagnostic group(s) chosen is truly unrelated to the factor under study.

When the cases have been chosen from a hospitalized population but the use of hospitalized controls is not scientifically desirable or feasible, the comparison group may be selected from the general population. This is also the source that should be utilized when the cases have been selected to represent affected individuals in a defined general population. In this circumstance, the use of general population controls assures the greatest level of comparability, since they come from the same source population that gave rise to the cases.

Selecting controls from the general population can be accomplished in a number of different ways, including canvassing households in targeted neighborhoods, random-digit telephone dialing, or the identification of individuals from population registers or voting lists [30]. The selection of healthy participants from the community does involve a number of difficulties, however. Identifying and interviewing controls from the general population is usually more costly and time-consuming than for hospital controls. Population lists are not always available, and it is frequently difficult to contact healthy people with busy work and leisure activity schedules. Moreover, the quality of the information may differ between cases and controls because those in the general population may not recall exposures with the same level of accuracy as those who have developed the disease. Finally, individuals who have not recently experienced an adverse health outcome tend to be less motivated to participate, so that the frequency of individuals who refuse to participate among community controls is nearly always substantially greater than that seen among both cases and hospitalized controls. Since individuals who agree to participate may differ systematically from those who either refuse or can never be contacted in ways that may be related to the risk of developing the disease of interest, this can be a serious threat to the validity of the study results. For example, in studying physical activity as a risk factor for coronary disease, the use of community controls identified through a systematic household survey might result in a comparison group with a higher proportion of less active individuals simply because such persons are more likely to be at home when the interviewer calls. Thus, as with hospital controls, the use of population controls must be carefully considered in the context of the particular hypothesis under study.

A third source of controls consists of special groups such as friends, relatives, spouses, or neighbors of the cases. Such groups share the advantage of general population controls in that they are healthy but are also more likely to be cooperative than members of the general population because of their interest in the case. They may also offer a degree of control of important confounding factors related to ethnic background, socioeconomic status, or environment that is not otherwise easily achieved. On the other hand, if the study factor itself is one for which family members and friends are likely to be similar to the cases, an underestimate of the true effect of the exposure of interest may result. This is a particular concern in studies of factors such as diet or smoking history, where individuals who are closely associated are likely to have similar exposures. In such circumstances, these groups would not constitute an adequate control series.

Once the source of the control series has been determined, the next question to consider is whether to use one, two, or more control groups. Ideally, there should be a single control group most comparable to the cases and therefore best suited for the study. As mentioned earlier, however, it is often difficult, especially with hospitalized controls, to be confident that the comparison group is appropriate and that the conditions for which the controls are hospitalized are not also in some way related to the exposure under study. In this circumstance it may be useful to use several control groups drawn from patients with different diagnoses and compare the observed results. For example, patients with cancer of the breast may be compared with controls having gynecologic cancers, noncancerous elective gynecologic surgery, or emergency surgery such as appendectomy, or those injured in accidents. Similarly, in a pilot case-control study of medication use and Reye's syndrome [17], four sources of controls—emergency room, hospitalized, school, and community controls—were identified. If the experience of the cases consistently differs from all the other groups with respect to the exposure of interest, the credibility of the conclusion that it is the experience of the cases themselves that is unusual is strengthened. On the other hand, if different effects are observed when the various control groups are utilized, this may provide useful information as to the nature of the association under study as well as the possible biases that could be present.

The use of multiple control groups is also indicated when there is concern that one selected group has a specific deficiency that could be overcome by the inclusion of another control group. For example, in a case-control study of coffee and pancreatic cancer, the cases could be compared with a group of controls hospitalized for a variety of other conditions. While the use of a hospitalized control series is very attractive from the standpoint of cost, convenience, willingness to participate, and minimization of recall bias, there would be serious concern that hospitalized patients as a group had coffee consumption patterns that were different from a nonhospitalized population regardless of the admission diagnosis. To address this, a second control series could be added consisting of individuals selected from the general population. A comparison of the observed association between coffee and pancreatic cancer for each of these control series would provide information concerning the true effect as well as the adequacy of the use of a hospitalized control group to study such a hypothesis.

After the source and number of control groups for a study have been determined, it is necessary to decide how many and the manner in which individual subjects will be selected. With respect to the size of the series, when the number of available cases and controls is large and the cost of obtaining information from both groups is comparable, the optimal control-to-case ratio is 1 : 1. When the sample size of cases is limited, with only a small number being available for study, or when the cost of obtaining information is greater for cases or controls, the control-to-case ratio can be altered to achieve the desired sample size. As the number of controls per case increases, the power of the study also increases. It is not generally recommended that this ratio increase beyond 4 : 1, however, unless the data are available at very little extra cost, because there is only a small increase in statistical power with each additional control beyond this point [9].

When the entire population of potentially eligible controls is known, a random sample of the required size can be chosen. Similarly, the group from which the sample will be drawn can be assembled in some sort of order and individuals selected systematically—that is, every tenth, hundredth, or thousandth person listed. As long as the order of the group of potential controls is not determined by some variable likely to be important to the study, such as socioeconomic or educational status, the difference between these two methods is minimal, and the choice of which to use is generally based on practical considerations.

When the total population of potential controls cannot easily be enumerated, such as when hospital controls are to be used and it is not desirable to have to wait for the total number of patients hospitalized during a certain period to be known before beginning data collection, paired sampling can be used. In this method, one or more controls are selected for each case on the basis of some previously defined temporal or geographic relationship with the case. For example, in a hospital-based study, the control for each case might be the next consecutive admission of the same age and sex, or perhaps even the next admission from the same neighborhood as the case. For investigations using community controls, the basis for selection might be proximity of residence or the position of a name on a voting list. Regardless of the specific method of selection employed, it is important to follow clearly defined, objective, and reproducible procedures. Haphazard selection could easily lead to systematic biases. For example, exclusion of individuals who are more difficult to contact may bias the result if noncooperation is related to the exposure under study. Similarly, if selection of records is influenced by the ease of reading the patient's name or thickness of the files, a systematic bias could result related to ethnicity or severity of illness and length of hospitalization.

Ascertainment of Disease and Exposure Status

After the case and control series have been defined in terms of characteristics and sources, the information on the disease and exposure must be obtained. In this regard, it is important to recall that any potential source of information must be carefully considered in terms of its ability to provide accurate as well as comparable information for all study groups.

Information about disease status can be obtained from many sources, including review of death certificates, case registries that maintain on-going surveillance, office records of physicians, hospital admission or discharge records, and pathology department log books. For example, in a case-control study of oral contraceptives and nonfatal myocardial infarction [19], all women under age 46 who were hospitalized for myo-cardial infarction during the first 6 months of 1975 were identified through reviews of hospital discharge diagnoses compiled by the Com-mission on Professional and Hospital Activities, an organization that ob-tains data from approximately 40 percent of all acute-care hospitals in the United States. This review identified 954 women meeting the crite-ria, representing 621 hospitals, from which the study population of 107 cases was selected. If the catchment area for cases is smaller and con-fined to a single geographic location, it is possible for the investigators to identify cases through ongoing surveillance of hospital admissions. This was done in a case-control study of alcohol, diet, and other risk factors for myocardial infarction [4] in which cases were selected through twice weekly on-site reviews of special study logs filled out by the nurses in the coronary and intensive care units of each participating hospital. This log contained all eligibility information and permitted im-mediate identification of potential cases.

Information about exposure can be obtained from the study subjects themselves, by either interview or mail questionnaire [13]; from a sur-rogate, such as spouses of participants [12] or mothers of children [35]; or from information recorded in medical records [3]. Procedures used to obtain information must be as similar as possible for cases and con-trols. For example, it is preferable that the place and circumstances of interviews be the same to avoid a situation in which, for example, cases are interviewed in the hospital and the population controls at home. In some situations it may be possible for the interviewers or medical records abstractors to be blinded to the case or control status of subjects. More-over, those obtaining the information should remain, insofar as possible, unaware of the specific hypotheses being tested. These latter measures serve to minimize the possibility of observation bias introduced when an interviewer subconsciously probes or scans records more intensively for a history of exposure among the cases.

In this regard, the ability to obtain exposure information from records completed before the occurrence of outcome events is especially valu-able, since it is unlikely that the accuracy or completeness of the data would be dependent on whether the subject later developed the disease. For example, in a case-control study of risk factors for neuroblastoma [20], birth certificates of cases and controls were reviewed to determine birth weight, gestational age, and a number of other medical and demo-graphic variables. Similarly, in a study of the association between pre-natal x-ray exposure and childhood malignancies [24], medical records of mothers of both cases and controls were searched to determine whether abdominal or other x-rays had been done. In these examples, it is unlikely that the subsequent development of disease would have affected the accuracy or completeness of the available exposure information, since the data had been recorded before the development of the outcome events.

One of the central issues in the ascertainment of exposure in a case-control study concerns the basis on which a given individual should be considered exposed. This decision involves defining the part of a person's exposure history that should be considered relevant to the etiology of the disease under study and will depend on some understanding of the mechanisms of the disease process as well as the limits of the possible induction period. To evaluate an association between smoking and lung cancer, it is less the amount currently smoked than the total duration of smoking that is etiologically important. On the other hand, to evaluate smoking and MI, the current habit is the most relevant exposure. In many circumstances, however, the most appropriate time window for the evaluation of the possible harmful effects of an exposure is not clear. The problem is that if a case-control study utilizes information spanning too wide a period (such as "ever use," which includes any history of exposure from birth to diagnosis), some period of exposure that cannot be causally related to the disease will be included. This will result in a type of misclassification that will dilute or underestimate the effect of the relevant exposure. One approach is to evaluate the data from differing time windows of exposure and in this way gain information about the period that appears most relevant to risk of disease.

ISSUES IN ANALYSIS

The analysis of a case-control study is basically a comparison between cases and controls with respect to the frequency of an exposure whose potential etiologic role is being evaluated. In the vast majority of case-control studies, this comparison is made primarily by estimating the relative risk as computed by the odds ratio, as discussed in Chapter 4. If the case-control study is population-based, or if estimates of disease incidence are available from an outside source, rates of disease for those exposed and nonexposed can be computed and compared directly. By testing the significance of this measure of association and calculating confidence intervals, as presented in Chapter 10, the role of chance can be evaluated. Cases and controls must, of course, also be compared to ensure similarity with respect to other baseline differences that could be associated with the risk of developing the outcome under study.

ISSUES IN INTERPRETATION

In all analytic epidemiologic studies, an evaluation of the validity of the findings requires consideration of the roles of chance, bias, and confounding as possible alternative explanations. There are, however, a number of issues of particular importance in the interpretation of the results of case-control studies. The major issue in interpretation relates to the potential for a number of types of bias. Many of the biases are certainly not unique to case-control studies, but they are more of a possibility because of the inherent nature of this type of investigation. A second issue relates to the interpretation of data-derived hypotheses.

The Role of Bias

Selection bias can occur whenever the inclusion of cases or controls into the study depends in some way on the exposure of interest. Selection bias is a particular problem in case-control studies, since exposure and disease have both occurred at the time subjects are selected for study. There are a number of situations that can result in this bias. In all of these, however, the common element is that the relationship between the exposure and disease observed among those who participate in the study is different from that for individuals who would have been eligible to participate but were unwilling or not selected by the investigator. For example, concerns about the existence of selection bias are always raised when response rates are either low or unequal for cases and controls, since it is known that those who agree to participate are different from those who do not in ways that may be related to the exposure and outcome under investigation. Similarly, if alternate controls are selected to replace those who were originally chosen but could not be contacted or refused to participate, biased estimates could also result. For example, in a case-control study [6] investigating the efficacy of Papanicolaou (Pap) smears in reducing mortality from cervical cancer, controls were identified through a household survey. For each of 1060 controls who participated, an average of 12 households had to be approached before a control for the study could be located. The usual reason for failure to obtain a control from the originally designated house was that no one was home at the time the neighborhood was canvassed. If availability at home were related to the likelihood of having had a Pap smear within the last 5 years, then the estimate of relative risk from this study would be biased. Suppose that women who were not home tended to be employed and employed women were more likely to have had a Pap smear than those unemployed. In this case, having unemployed women constitute the control series would underestimate the magnitude of any protective effect of Pap smears on cervical cancer mortality. Although this potential for bias in selection of the controls was a major concern, the investigators were able to demonstrate that the exposure frequencies were similar for those controls identified initially and a sample of those who had to be excluded due to initial unavailability.

Another example of the potential for selection bias resulted from the great deal of media attention given to early case-control studies linking toxic shock syndrome to tampon use. As a result, when later case-control studies of this disease were conducted, there was concern that the widespread publicity and knowledge of this possible association might have influenced the selection of cases in two ways. First, women using tampons at the time of the onset of their disease might have been more likely to see a physician than those with similar symptoms who were not tampon users, resulting in an artificially high proportion of reported cases among women who use tampons. In addition, there was concern that physicians examining patients with such symptoms might be more likely to diagnose toxic shock syndrome among tampon users [33]. In fact, later case-control studies reported relative risks similar to those from studies conducted before the tampon use hypothesis became widely publicized.

The possible role of selection bias as an alternative explanation for an observed association between postmenopausal hormone use and risk of uterine cancer led to a controversy during the 1970s. Several earlier case-control studies had reported an extremely strong, approximately seven-fold association [32, 39], but one group of investigators argued that almost the entire effect was due to a form of selection or diagnostic bias [15]. Specifically, these investigators proposed that women who use estrogens are more likely to experience uterine bleeding as a consequence of the medication and then see a physician for evaluation. In this way, estrogen users may be more likely to be diagnosed with an early "pseudocancer" than women who do not use such agents. Thus, the use of estrogens may result in a diagnostic evaluation that identifies a condition that otherwise might not have been detected. In a subsequent review of this criticism [18], it was concluded that although the proposed selection bias was certainly possible, it was unlikely to be sufficiently strong to account for the increased risk observed. Moreover, the fact that the association persisted when the cases were restricted to those with invasive disease added support to this latter interpretation [10].

Observation bias, or errors in obtaining information from subjects once they have been entered into the study, may also be a particular problem in a case-control design. This type of bias may arise because information on exposure is often provided by the participant after the onset of disease. Knowledge of the disease status may, therefore, influence the reporting of information by the subject or the recording or interpretation of this information by the investigator. Of particular concern is the potential for recall bias and misclassification.

Recall bias relates to differences in the ways exposure information is remembered or reported by cases, who have experienced an adverse health outcome, and by controls, who have not. A common method of collecting information in a case-control investigation is by interviewing either the study subjects themselves or some surrogate, such as spouses of participants or mothers of affected children. Individuals who have experienced a disease or other adverse health outcome tend to think about the possible "causes" of their illness and thus are likely to remember their exposure histories differently from those who are unaffected by the disease. This bias may also affect the recall of families of affected individuals. For example, in a study of maternal x-ray exposure and childhood cancer [34], children who had died from malignancies were identified through death certificate review, and controls of the same age, sex, and geographic location were selected at random from local birth registries. Information about exposure to prenatal x-rays was obtained by interviewing the mothers of both cases and controls. The investigators found that mothers exposed to abdominal x-rays had a 90-percent greater risk of having a child who died of malignancy than mothers who did not have this exposure. The concern was that this observed increased risk could be due, totally or in part, to the fact that mothers of cases might be more likely to remember or report prenatal x-rays than mothers of healthy controls. To address this issue, a subsequent study was conducted [24] in which exposure to x-rays was ascertained solely through medical records rather than any questioning of the mothers themselves. Since these records were compiled prior to the birth of the child, they could not be influenced by the subsequent diagnosis of the disease. Although the magnitude of effect was lessened after recall bias was taken into account, there was still a statistically significant 40-percent increased risk of childhood malignancy associated with x-ray exposure [25]. Since the potential for recall bias exists in every case-control study that relies on information obtained from the participants themselves, it is important that this issue be considered carefully in the design as well as in the interpretation of published results.

Misclassification refers to errors in the categorization of either exposure or disease status. Such errors are inevitable in any study, but the consequences of this type of bias depend on whether the misclassification with respect to one axis (either exposure or disease) is or is not independent of the classification of the other axis. When the misclassification of one axis is independent of the other, that is, when the exposure or disease classification is incorrect for the same proportions of subjects in the groups compared, then the misclassification is random or nondifferential. For example, if in a case-control study of prior history of hypertension and risk of stroke, 80 percent of cases and controls who had such a history accurately reported it and 90 percent of cases and controls who had no such history reported that information correctly, then misclassification of exposure had occurred but is totally indepen-dent of disease status. On the other hand, if these proportions differ, for example, if 90 percent of the cases who had a history of hypertension accurately reported their history as compared with 60 percent of con-trols, then the misclassification of exposure is not independent of disease status and is termed nonrandom or differential. The potential for non-random misclassification is often a concern when the fact of either hav-ing experienced or not having experienced the outcome event is likely to affect the accuracy with which subjects recall relevant exposures (as in recall bias). In contrast, misclassification is more likely to be random in other situations, such as when exposure information is obtained from records maintained prior to the occurrence of outcome events. In this case, it is quite possible that proportion of the records would be either incomplete or inaccurate. However, it is unlikely that the accuracy or completeness of these records would differ between the cases and con-trols.

Random misclassification always results in an underestimate of the true relative risk; consequently, any association that is observed could not be a spurious one. In contrast, when there is differential misclassi-fication, the result could be either an exaggeration or an underestimate of effect, depending on the particular situation. Nondifferential mis-classification is often believed to be a less serious problem with respect to the validity of the findings since the bias introduced is always towards the null. However, if substantial random misclassification exists, which is always a potential problem because of the inherent difficulties in ac-curately ascertaining exposure alluded to earlier in this chapter, then a study can report a finding of little or no effect when in fact an associa-tion truly exists.

Interpretation of Data-Derived Hypotheses

While most case-control studies test the specific hypothesis that the dis-ease of interest is caused by a particular etiologic exposure, investigators often collect information on a number of additional risk factors that they also wish to explore. In other case-control studies, especially those of diseases about which little is known, no hypotheses are specified a priori and data pertaining to a multitude of potential risk factors are obtained. In such circumstances, it is important to distinguish between tests of a hypothesis that has been specified in advance and those "fishing expe-ditions" in which one or more associations emerge when the data are analyzed. The latter are referred to as data-derived hypotheses and must be interpreted with the same caution afforded the results of descriptive epidemiologic investigations. While such data can be used to formulate a hypothesis, testing of that association must be done in a study designed to address that specific question.

CONCLUSION

Like every epidemiologic study design, the case-control study has unique strengths and limitations that must be considered when selecting this particular strategy for the evaluation of a hypothesis or when interpreting published results. As summarized in Table 6-2, from a practical standpoint, one of the chief advantages of case-control studies is that they can be conducted far more rapidly and less expensively than investigations requiring an extended period of follow-up. Thus, they are uniquely well suited to the evaluation of diseases with long latent periods. A second practical and scientific advantage is that since participants are selected on the basis of disease status, case-control studies are optimal for the investigation of rare diseases. Finally, case-control studies offer the opportunity to investigate multiple etiologic factors simultaneously. This is particularly advantageous as an initial attempt to identify causal or preventive factors for a disease about which very little is known.

With respect to disadvantages, a case-control study is not an efficient design for the evaluation of a rare exposure unless the study is very large or the exposure is common among those with the disease (i.e., the attributable-risk percent is high). This has been the case in a number of investigations that have utilized the case-control approach to evaluate the effect of a rare exposure on a rare disease, such as vinyl chloride and angiosarcoma of the liver [2], asbestos and mesothelioma [5, 22, 26], and prenatal diethylstilbestrol (DES) exposure and cancer of the vagina [14].

Table 6-2. Strengths and limitations of the case-control study design

Strengths

    Is relatively quick and inexpensive compared with other analytic designs

    Is particularly well-suited to the evaluation of diseases with long latent periods

    Is optimal for the evaluation of rare diseases

    Can examine multiple etiologic factors for a single disease

Limitations

    Is inefficient for the evaluation of rare exposures, unless the attributable-risk percent is high

    Cannot directly compute incidence rates of disease in exposed and nonexposed individuals, unless study is population based

    In some situations, the temporal relationship between exposure and disease may be difficult to establish

    Is particularly prone to bias compared with other analytic designs, in particular selection and recall bias

Second, unless the case-control study is population-based, direct calculation of the incidence of disease in exposed and nonexposed groups is not possible. As shown in Chapter 4, however, estimates of these incidence rates can sometimes be made and a valid estimate of the relative measure of association between exposure and disease can always be calculated. Third, the temporal relationship between exposure and disease may be difficult to establish. Finally, probably the greatest limitation of case-control studies is that they are more susceptible to bias than other analytic study designs. It is particularly important that potential sources of such biases be recognized in the design phase of a study so that precautions can be taken to avoid or minimize their effects. When possible, it is optimal to quantify the effects of such biases and to take them into account in analyzing the data.

Case-control studies have particular utility in investigating both rare diseases and the potential roles of multiple risk factors. Because of lower costs and greater efficiency, the conduct of case-control studies is often a useful first step in the identification of risk factors for a disease. If properly designed and conducted, the case-control study is a valuable research tool that can provide reliable tests of particular epidemiologic hypotheses.

STUDY QUESTIONS

1. Discuss the strengths and limitations of case-control studies.
2. Compare and contrast the utility of hospital and neighborhood controls.
3. Why is the potential for bias a particular problem in case-control studies as opposed to other analytic designs?
4. What types of bias are of most concern in case-control studies?

REFERENCES

1. Bonham, G. S. *Use Habits of Cigarettes, Coffee, Aspirin and Sleeping Pills, United States, 1976.* Vital and Health Statistics, Series 10. Data from the National Health Survey, no. 131. *D.H.E.W.* Publication No. (P.H.S.) 80-1559, 1979.
2. Brady, J. S., Liberatore, F., Harper, P., et al. Angiosarcoma of the liver: An epidemiologic study. *J.N.C.I.* 59:1383, 1977.
3. Buring, J. E., Bain, C. J., and Ehrmann, R. L. Conjugated estrogen use and risk of endometrial cancer. *Am. J. Epidemiol.* 124:434, 1986.
4. Buring, J. E., Willett, W., Goldhaber, S. Z., et al. Alcohol and HDL in nonfatal myocardial infarction: Preliminary results from a case-control study. *Circulation* 68:227, 1983.
5. Churg, A., Wiggs, B., Depaoli, L., et al. Lung asbestos content in chrysotile workers with mesothelioma. *Am. Rev. Respir. Dis.* 130:1042, 1984.

6. Clark, E. A., and Anderson, T. W. Does screening by "Pap" smears help prevent cervical cancer? A case-control study. Lancet 2:1, 1979.
7. Cole, P. A population-based study of bladder cancer. In R. Doll and I. Vodopija (eds.), *Host Environment Interactions in the Etiology of Cancer in Man.* Lyon, France: International Agency for Research on Cancer, IARC Scientific Publications No. 7, 1973. Pp. 83–87.
8. Cole, P. The evolving case-control study. *J. Chronic Dis.* 32:15, 1979.
9. Gail, M., Williams, R., Byar, D. P., et al. How many controls? *J. Chron. Dis.* 29:723, 1976.
10. Gordon, J., Reagan, J. W., Finkle, W. D., et al. Estrogen and endometrial carcinoma. An independent pathology review supporting original risk estimate. *N. Engl. J. Med.* 297:570, 1977.
11. Henderson, B. E., Gerkins, V. R., and Pike, M. C. Sexual Factors and Pregnancy. In J. R. Fraumeni, Jr. (ed.), *Persons at High Risk of Cancer: An Approach to Cancer Etiology and Control.* New York: Academic, 1975. Pp. 267–283.
12. Hennekens, C. H., Drollette, M. E., Jesse, M. J., et al. Coffee drinking and death due to coronary heart disease. *N. Engl. J. Med.* 294:633, 1976.
13. Hennekens, C. H., Speizer, F. E., Rosner, B., et al. Use of permanent hair dyes and cancer among registered nurses. *Lancet* 1:1390, 1979.
14. Herbst, A. L., Ulfelder, H., and Poskanzer, D. C. Adenocarcinoma of the vagina: Association of maternal stilbestrol therapy with tumor appearance in young women. *N. Engl. J. Med.* 284:878, 1974.
15. Horwitz, R. I., and Feinstein, A. R. Alternative analytic methods for case-control studies of estrogens and endometrial cancer. *N. Engl. J. Med.* 299:1089, 1978.
16. Horwitz, R. I., and Feinstein, A. R. Methodologic standards and contradictory results in case-control research. *Am. J. Med.* 66:556, 1979.
17. Hurwitz, E. S., Barrett, M. J., Bregman, D., et al. Public Health Service study on Reye's syndrome and medications: Report of the pilot phase. *N. Engl. J. Med.* 313:849, 1985.
18. Hutchison, G. B., and Rothman, K. J. Correcting a bias? *N. Engl. J. Med.* 299:1129, 1978.
19. Jick, H., Dinan, B., and Rothman, K. J. Oral contraceptives and nonfatal myocardial infarction. *J.A.M.A.* 239:1403, 1978.
20. Johnson, C. C., and Spitz, M. R. Neuroblastoma: Case-control analysis of birth characteristics. *J.N.C.I.* 74:789, 1985.
21. Kessler, I. I. Cervical cancer epidemiology in historical perspective. *J. Reprod. Med.* 12:173, 1974.
22. McDonald, A. D., and McDonald, J. C. Malignant mesotheliomas in North America. *Cancer* 46:1650, 1980.
23. McIntosh, I. D. Alcohol-related disabilities in general hospital patients: A critical assessment of the evidence. *Int. J. Addict.* 17:609, 1982.
24. MacMahon, B. Prenatal x-ray exposure and childhood cancer. *J.N.C.I.* 28:1173, 1962.
25. MacMahon, B., and Hutchison, G. B. Prenatal x-ray and childhood cancer: A review. *Acta Un. Int. Cancer* 20:1172, 1964.
26. Newhouse, M. L., Berry, G., and Skidmore, J. W. A mortality study of workers manufacturing friction materials with chrysotile asbestos. *Ann. Occup. Hyg.* 26:899, 1982.

27. Reingold, A. L., Hargrett, N. T., Shands, K. N., et al. Toxic shock syndrome surveillance in the United States, 1980 to 1981. *Ann. Intern. Med.* 96:875, 1982.
28. Rosenberg, L., Slone, D., Shapiro, S., et al. Case-control studies on the acute effects of coffee upon the risk of myocardial infarction: Problems in the selection of a hospital control series. *Am. J. Epidemiol.* 113:646, 1981.
29. Sackett, D. L. Bias in analytic research. *J. Chron. Dis.* 32:51, 1979.
30. Schlesselman, J. J. *Case-Control Studies: Design, Conduct, Analysis.* New York: Oxford University Press, 1982.
31. Slone, D., Shapiro, S., Rosenberg, L., et al. Relation of cigarette smoking to myocardial infarction in young women. *N. Engl. J. Med.* 298:1273, 1978.
32. Smith, D. C., Prentice, R., Thompson, D. J., et al. Association of exogenous estrogens and endometrial cancer. *N. Engl. J. Med.* 293:1164, 1975.
33. Stallones, R. A. A review of the epidemiologic studies of toxic shock syndrome. *Ann. Intern. Med.* 96:917, 1982.
34. Stewart, A., Webb, J., and Hewitt, D. A survey of childhood malignancies. *Br. Med. J.* 1:1495, 1958.
35. Stewart, A., Webb, J., Giles, D., et al. Malignant disease in childhood and diagnostic irradiation in utero; preliminary communication. *Lancet* 2:447, 1956.
36. U.S. D.H.E.W. *Smoking and Health: A Report of the Surgeon General.* D.H.E.W. Publication No. (P.H.S.) 7-50066. Rockville, MD: U.S. D.H.E.W., 1979.
37. West, D. W., Schuman, K. L., Lyon, J. L., et al. Differences in risk estimations from a hospital and a population-based case-control study. *Int. J. Epidemiol.* 13:235, 1984.
38. World Health Organization. *IHD Registers: Report of the Fifth Working Group.* Copenhagen: World Health Organization, 1971.
39. Ziel, H. K., and Finkle, W. D. Increased risk of endometrial cancer among users of conjugated estrogens. *N. Engl. J. Med.* 293:1167, 1975.

7

Cohort Studies

The second major type of observational analytic design is the cohort or follow-up study, in which a group or groups of individuals are defined on the basis of presence or absence of exposure to a suspected risk factor for a disease. At the time exposure status is defined, all potential subjects must be free from the disease under investigation, and eligible participants are then followed over a period of time to assess the occurrence of that outcome.

As a consequence of this design, cohort studies offer a number of advantages for evaluating the relationship between exposure and disease. First, because participants are free from the disease at the time their exposure status is defined, the temporal sequence between exposure and disease can be more clearly established. Second, cohort studies are particularly well suited for assessing the effects of rare exposures. For many exposures, especially those that arise in occupational settings, the proportions of exposed persons among a group of individuals with the disease would be far too small to permit meaningful comparisons of risk. Because cohort studies enroll participants on the basis of their exposure status, this design allows the investigators to identify adequate numbers of exposed and nonexposed subjects. Finally, cohort studies allow for the examination of multiple effects of a single exposure. For example, the Nurses' Health Study, an ongoing cohort study of over 120,000 female nurses in the U.S., has examined the relationship of oral contraceptive use with breast [27] and ovarian [48] cancer, malignant melanoma [1], as well as myocardial infarction [43]. Thus, a cohort design can provide information on the full range of health effects of a single exposure.

Since cohort studies often involve following large numbers of individuals for many years, they are generally very time-consuming and expensive. Consequently, cohort studies are often conducted after a hypothesized relationship has been explored and evaluated in a case-control design. While some investigators tend to regard cohort studies as more logical and direct, and thus as inherently superior, it is important to keep in mind that both the case-control and cohort designs have unique strengths and limitations. As will be discussed more fully later, cohort studies tend to minimize the potential for selection bias, which is a particular concern in case-control studies. On the other hand, cohort studies have an equally serious potential for bias associated with the losses to follow-up that are likely to occur when participants must be followed for months, years, or even decades. While the potential for such problems must certainly be carefully considered in the design and interpretation of a particular case-control or cohort study, the selection of one observational design over another in a given circumstance should be made on the basis of the particular hypothesis being tested, the resources available, and the current state of knowledge rather than on any a priori belief in the inherent worth of any particular option. The goal is to choose the specific design option that will yield the most valid and informative result.

TYPES OF COHORT STUDIES

Cohort studies may be classified as either prospective or retrospective, depending on the temporal relationship between the initiation of the study and the occurrence of the disease. By definition, both prospective and retrospective cohort study designs classify subjects in the study on the basis of presence or absence of exposure. In retrospective cohort studies, however, all the relevant events (both the exposures and outcomes of interest) have already occurred when the study is initiated. In prospective studies, the relevant exposures may or may not have occurred at the time the study is begun, but the outcomes have certainly not yet occurred. Thus, after the selection of the cohort, participants must be followed into the future to assess incidence rates of disease.

For example, in 1965, Enterline [14] conducted a retrospective cohort study of asbestos exposure and lung cancer mortality. A group of asbestos workers was identified from social security tax returns filed with the United States Bureau of Internal Revenue during 1948 to 1951. All deaths that occurred among this group between 1948 and 1963 were identified from claims filed with the Social Security Administration, and the corresponding certificates were obtained from the various state health departments. Mortality from lung cancer among the asbestos workers was compared with that of a group of cotton textile workers as well as with the experience of the general population of white males of the same age in the U.S. The results of these comparisons indicated excess lung cancer mortality among asbestos workers. A subsequent investigation was then initiated using a prospective cohort design that included all 17,800 male members of the Asbestos Insulation Workers union in the United States and Canada as of January 1, 1967 [46]. These subjects were followed until 1975 to determine their mortality rates from lung cancer, for comparison with the general population of white males of the same age. This prospective study corroborated the positive association between asbestos exposure and mortality from lung cancer that had been first identified using the retrospective cohort design.

In some instances, a cohort study is ambidirectional; data are collected both retrospectively and prospectively on the same cohort. This type of design is most useful for exposures having both short-term and long-term effects, such as a chemical that may increase the risk of birth defects within a few years of exposure as well as cancer risk after one or two decades. For example, to study the possible deleterious consequences of exposure to dioxin (Agent Orange), the U.S. Air Force School of Aerospace Medicine conducted a cohort study of Air Force personnel. The study population included an exposed group of 1264 participants in the "Ranch Hand" project, who were involved in defoliant spraying in Vietnam between 1962 and 1971, as well as a group of 1264 nonexposed men who flew a variety of cargo missions in Southeast Asia during the same time period [25]. These data were analyzed retrospectively to compare the experiences of exposed and nonexposed subjects on a variety of health outcomes that could be assessed within a relatively short period after exposure, such as dermatologic conditions, infertility, birth defects, liver abnormalities, and psychological disorders. Since another serious concern was the possibility of increased cancer risk, the cohort is also being followed prospectively to allow for the long latency period between exposure and the subsequent development of malignancy [18].

The choice of a retrospective or prospective cohort design for the evaluation of a particular hypothesis is based on a number of scientific and logistic considerations. Retrospective cohort studies can usually be conducted much more quickly and cheaply than their prospective counterparts because all relevant events have already occurred at the time the study is initiated. Thus, the retrospective design is particularly efficient for a cohort investigation of diseases with long latency periods requiring many years to accrue sufficient end points. However, since retrospective cohort studies usually evaluate exposures that occurred many years previously, they depend on the routine availability of relevant exposure data in adequate detail from pre-existing records. Since these data were often recorded for purposes other than investigation of the hypothesis of interest, this can result in incomplete and possibly noncomparable information for all study subjects. Moreover, often information on potential confounding factors such as diet, smoking, or other lifestyle characteristics is not available from such records. In a prospective investigation, the investigator can often use more recent records or even assess the exposure directly or through questioning the participants themselves, and information on potential confounders can also be obtained from study subjects. Thus, the gain in efficiency and cost inherent in a retrospective cohort design must be considered in the context of the adequacy of the data available. If the sample size is large and follow-up is complete, data from prospective cohort studies can be regarded as particularly reliable and informative.

An additional modification of the basic cohort design that is often utilized in epidemiologic research involves inserting a case-control study into either a retrospective or prospective cohort study. For example, to evaluate whether serum levels of a number of micronutrients are associated with subsequent cancer risk, blood samples could be collected at baseline from all participants in a cohort study. In a traditional cohort study, the cohort would then be followed for the next 10 to 20 years to compare the incidence of cancer among those with differing levels of each micronutrient. In a case-control within a cohort, or nested case-control design, however, the blood samples taken at baseline would simply be frozen and stored, and all participants would be followed for development of the disease. When a sufficient number of cancer cases had accrued, the blood samples for these individuals would then be analyzed, as would those for a comparison group of individuals without cancer selected from within the cohort, as in a case-control study. By performing the blood analyses on a subgroup of the study population rather than on every member, nested case-control studies can often be conducted at a fraction of the usual cost for a cohort study. Such an approach is a particularly efficient way to deal with expensive test that would otherwise have to be made on tens of thousands of individuals.

ISSUES IN THE DESIGN OF COHORT STUDIES

Selection of the Exposed Population

The group of individuals selected to comprise the exposed population in a cohort study can come from a variety of sources. The choice of a particular group will depend on a variety of scientific and feasibility considerations, including the frequency of the exposures under study, the need to obtain complete and accurate exposure and follow-up information on all study participants, and the nature of the particular research questions being evaluated.

For relatively common exposures, such as cigarette smoking or coffee drinking, a sufficiently large number of exposed individuals could probably be identified from a number of possible populations. For rare exposures, however, such as those related to particular occupations or environmental factors in specific geographic locations, it is more efficient to choose a group specifically because they have undergone some unusual exposure or experience, the effects of which are to be evaluated. Such special exposure groups would include individuals in certain occupations, such as rubber processing, uranium mining, or shipbuilding; those who have undergone a particular medical therapy, such as x-ray treatment for ankylosing spondylitis or repeated fluoroscopic examinations for tuberculosis; individuals living near a suspected environmental hazard, such as a nuclear testing ground or toxic waste dump site; groups with unusual dietary or lifestyle practices, such as Seventh Day Adventists or Mormons; or those who were exposed by being present at a given event, such as the dropping of the atomic bomb at Hiroshima or a major industrial accident. The advantage of selecting a special exposure population is that it allows the accrual of sufficient exposed individuals in a reasonable period of time.

The use of these cohorts can lead to the identification of etiologic agents in the special circumstances being investigated. In addition, they can provide an efficient means of identifying risk factors operating in the general population. Since these groups have been exposed to higher levels of the exposure than the general population, if the exposure did have an effect on the incidence of a particular disease, these would be reasonable cohorts in which to see the first evidence of such a relationship. Thus, to evaluate the relationship between physical activity and risk of coronary heart disease, a number of cohort studies have been conducted among special exposure groups such as longshoremen [38] or busmen in London [36]. The information obtained from these investigations, with their clear advantages in terms of reduced sample size as well as the ability to ascertain exposure accurately and follow the participants to determine outcomes of interest, can then be generalized to assess the role of physical activity in the etiology of coronary heart disease for the general population.

In addition, the use of a special exposure cohort permits the evaluation of rare outcomes that would otherwise require a prohibitively large number of individuals to test with assurance. Even though an outcome may be extremely rare in a general population, it may be sufficiently common in a special exposure group to allow for an adequate number of cases to be collected. For example, the annual incidence rate of mesothelioma among the general population of males in the U.S. is approximately 8.24 per million [40]. Therefore, a cohort study that included 20,000 men would be unlikely to identify any cases of this disease even after 5 years of follow-up. Since mesothelioma is relatively common among people exposed to asbestos, however, a cohort study of 20,000 such workers might yield a sufficient number of cases to explore various exposure-disease relationships. Thus, while cohort studies are in general not optimal for the evaluation of rare diseases, if the outcome is not rare among those exposed—that is, if the attributable-risk percent is high— a cohort design can be used efficiently.

Since a primary requirement for the validity of a cohort study is the ability to obtain complete and accurate information on all participants, particularly with respect to the ascertainment of data on the exposures and outcomes of interest, cohort studies are often conducted among groups specifically chosen not for their exposure status, but for their ability to facilitate the collection of relevant information. Among the different groups targeted for cohort studies are members of certain professions, such as doctors [12] or nurses [3]; workers in various occupations [35, 41] or entire companies [13]; union members [46]; participants in prepaid medical care plans [24]; veterans [42]; students or alumni of particular colleges [37]; and residents of well-defined communities [10]. Each of these groups offers some logistic advantage to the investigator, ranging from the availability of annually updated addresses, to a mechanism for periodic follow-up, to the provision of complete medical and employment records. Since the groups were not selected because of unusually high levels of specific exposures, these populations are most usefully studied when the exposures of interest are common or the groups are very large.

Thus, the choice of a particular group to serve as the study population for any given cohort study is related to both the hypotheses under investigation and specific features of the design. For example, to evaluate the possible relationship of exposure to an industrial solvent with risk of cancer, a retrospective cohort design could be used to identify a number of specific individual plants that used that solvent and also had available extensive personnel records about specific work assignments within the factory. This was in fact the design chosen under a contractual agreement between the United Rubber, Cork, Linoleum and Plastic Workers of America and the six major rubber manufacturers in the United States to initiate studies of industrial exposures and cancer risk [30, 34]. These funds supported five retrospective cohort studies among workers at plants in Akron, Ohio, using information from employment records and death certificate reviews. In contrast, to allow for the investigation of a number of common risk factors for relatively common chronic diseases, the best choice of study population might be a general cohort, drawn from a geographically and demographically well-defined area, who can be surveyed to establish baseline exposure status with respect to a number of factors and then examined periodically to ascertain future outcomes. One classic design of this type is the Framingham Heart Study, a prospective cohort study that has followed approximately 5100 residents of this Massachusetts community for over 30 years. The town of Framingham was chosen as the site for this study not because the population was believed to have any unique characteristics related to the exposures or outcomes that were to be investigated, but because of a number of factors that would allow investigators to identify and follow participants for many years. The fact that it was a stable population, had a number of occupations and industries represented, had a single, major hospital that was utilized by the vast majority of the population, and prepared annually updated population lists that would facilitate follow-up, all contributed to the success of this undertaking. Specifically, the use of a general population cohort has permitted assessment of the effects of a wide variety of factors on the risk of numerous diseases, including coronary heart disease [10], rheumatic heart disease [47], congestive heart failure [29], angina pectoris [20], intermittent claudication [21], stroke [22], gout [19], gallbladder disease [16], and a number of eye conditions [26].

Selection of the Comparison Group

Once the source of exposed subjects has been determined, the next consideration is the selection of an appropriate comparison group of non-exposed individuals. The choice of this group for a cohort study is as important and difficult as the selection of controls in a case-control study. The major principle underlying this decision is that the groups being compared should be as similar as possible with respect to all other factors that may be related to the disease except the determinant under investigation, so that if there is really no association between the exposure and the disease, the disease rates in the populations being compared will be essentially the same. Moreover, it is important to ensure that the information that can be obtained from the nonexposed group is adequate for comparison with the exposed population.

In cohort studies in which a single, general cohort is entered and its members then classified into exposure categories, an internal comparison group can be utilized. That is, the experience of those cohort members classified as having a particular exposure is compared with that of members of the same cohort who are either nonexposed or exposed to a different degree. For example, in the cohort study of British physicians begun by Doll and Hill [12] in 1950, mortality from lung cancer among those who never smoked was compared with that among all smokers as well as with the experience of those who smoked differing numbers of cigarettes. The investigators found increased death rates from lung cancer among those who smoked compared with those who did not, as well as marked and steady rises in lung cancer mortality with increasing levels of cigarette smoking. Similarly, in the Framingham Heart Study [10], baseline levels of blood cholesterol as well as systolic and diastolic blood pressure were determined and the participants divided into quintiles of exposure based on these values. The rates of coronary heart disease within each level were then calculated and compared. It is important to note that when several risk factors are being considered simultaneously, the nonexposed group should be defined as those with none of the risk factors under evaluation. Thus, the comparison group should consist of a single, well-defined reference population rather than one whose composition shifts according to the specific factor being analyzed at that time.

For cohort studies that involve the use of a special exposure group, such as in an occupational setting or for a particular environment, it is often not possible to identify a portion of the cohort that can safely be assumed to be nonexposed for comparison. In this instance, an external comparison group is used, such as the general population of the area in which the exposed individuals reside. The disease experience observed in the study group is compared with that expected on the basis of the frequency of disease in the general population at the time the cohort is being followed. For example, to evaluate potential risks associated with occupation in the rubber industry, the mortality experience of a group of rubber workers at a tire manufacturing plant in Akron, Ohio, was compared with mortality rates for the U.S. population of the same age and sex [32]. The investigators found that the all-cause mortality rate for the rubber workers was only 82 percent of that seen in the general population.

Comparisons with population rates are, of course, possible only for outcomes for which population rates are available, such as mortality, cancer incidence, or other situations where special data can be obtained. Moreover, the use of the experience of the general population as a valid indicator of the experience of a nonexposed group assumes that only a small proportion of that population is actually exposed through any source to the risk factor under investigation. To the extent that a part of the general population is, in fact, exposed, such a comparison will underestimate the true association between exposure and disease.

The major disadvantage of using the general population as a comparison group is that its members may not be directly comparable to those of the study cohort. First, people who are employed are, on average, healthier than those who are not. Since the general population includes people who are unable to work due to illness as well as those who are employed, rates of disease and death among the general population are almost always higher than they are for members of the work force [23, 31]. This was observed in the study of rubber workers cited above [32], in which all-cause mortality for rubber workers was only 82 percent of that among U.S. males as a whole. The effect of this phenomenon, termed the "healthy worker" effect is that any excess risk associated with a particular occupation will again tend to be underestimated by a comparison with the general population. Moreover, even if the population from which the expected rates are taken is chosen to be as generally similar as possible to that from which the exposed cohort derived, including basic demographic and geographic characteristics, it may well be different with respect to other risk factors for the disease, such as smoking or consumption of particular foods or alcoholic beverages. Since this information is not available on individuals in a general population, any observed differences may in fact be due to the effects of confounding that cannot be controlled.

To address these issues, one alternative to using rates of disease in the general population as the comparison group is to compare the experience of the special exposure cohort with that of another cohort similar in demographic characteristics but considered nonexposed. In studies of occupational exposures, one such group would consist of workers with different types of jobs performed at different locations within a single facility. For example, disease rates of presumably nonexposed office workers at a factory could be compared with those of exposed production workers within the same industrial setting. In the study of a tire manufacturing plant in Ohio [32], the cohort of rubber workers was subdivided into a number of occupational groups according to usual area of employment, such as curing, tire building, inspection, and so on. Mortality rates in these different groups were calculated and compared with those for all subjects in the study [33]. Another potential source of a comparison group is identification of a cohort of similar workers who are involved in another occupation that does not expose them to the factor of interest. For example, in the Ranch Hand study [25], where the exposed group included pilots flying defoliation missions, a comparison group was chosen from Air Force personnel flying a variety of cargo missions in the same area of Vietnam during the same period. Similarly, to evaluate the potential risk to radiologists of long-term exposure to low-dose ionizing radiation, radiologists have been compared with internists and other medical specialists [28], since these groups would likely be comparable with respect to demographic characteristics, health awareness, and utilization of medical care. In a study of asbestos processing and lung cancer [14], the experience of the cohort of exposed workers employed in the asbestos textile industry was compared with that of a cohort of workers in the cotton textile industry because workers in this industry engage in the same kinds of tasks and share many socioeconomic characteristics but are occupationally nonexposed to asbestos. The advantage of using a comparison cohort is that the group can be selected to be more comparable with the exposed cohort than the general population would be. Moreover, information on potential confounding factors can be obtained on individuals in the study and residual differences controlled in the analysis.

In many cohort studies, it may be useful to have multiple comparison groups, especially when no single group appears sufficiently similar to those who are exposed to provide assurance about the validity of the comparison. In such circumstances, the study results may be more convincing if a similar association were observed for a number of different comparison groups. For example, in the asbestos study described above [14], in addition to comparison with the group of cotton textile workers, mortality rates were also compared with those of the general U.S. white male population. Asbestos workers had excess mortality from all causes, from lung cancer and other respiratory diseases, and from hypertensive heart disease relative to both cotton textile workers and the general population. Thus, the mortality experience of asbestos workers was not only greater than that of the general population, but also substantially higher than that of a group of men doing similar work but without asbestos in their environment. The consistency of the results of these two comparisons enhanced the belief in the existence of true increased disease risks associated with the manufacture of asbestos products. Similarly, in evaluating potential adverse health outcomes associated with the use of oral contraceptives, choice of an appropriate comparison group has been a crucial consideration. Some studies have used for comparison a group of women not using oral contraceptives, while others have selected a group using some form of contraception other than the oral contraceptive pill. Women using no method of contraception may differ substantially from users of any type of contraception in terms of ability or desire to become pregnant or the nature of their sexual practices. On the other hand, women using various forms of contraception are likely to differ from oral contraceptive users with respect to religion, socioeconomic status, ethnic group, and a number of health and other lifestyle factors. Thus, it may be that no one comparison group is clearly superior, and information on the role of oral contraceptives and disease can best be elucidated by comparing the results from cohort studies using these various designs.

Sources of Data

When any cohort study is being designed, a major consideration is the availability of accurate and complete information that will allow the classification of all cohort members according to whether they have been exposed to the factor(s) under investigation or developed any of the outcomes of interest. Information concerning the exposure may be obtained from a number of sources, including records collected independently of the study, such as medical or employment records; information supplied by the study subjects themselves, through interviews or questionnaires; data obtained by medical examination or other testing of the participants; or direct measurements of the environment in which cohort members have lived or worked. Outcome information may also be ascertained from existing records, including death certificates or medical records, from questionnaires, or from physical examinations. Each of these sources offers particular advantages and disadvantages that must be considered in designing or interpreting a specific study.

Sources of Exposure Information

The methods or techniques used to ascertain exposure in a cohort study will vary from one investigation to another and from one risk factor to another. In many cohort studies, preexisting records, such as those kept by hospitals or employers, may contain sufficient data to classify individuals according to exposure status as well as provide demographic and other necessary information. Moreover, in some circumstances, this may in fact be the only way to obtain such data accurately. For example, a possible association between irradiation and subsequent development of leukemia was evaluated by following a cohort of 13,352 patients treated with x-ray therapy between 1934 and 1954 for ankylosing spondylitis [8]. While patients would undoubtedly know whether they had received x-ray therapy or not, they would probably not be aware of the dose of radiation received. This information would be available only through the medical record.

The use of preexisting records offers a number of advantages. First, such information is usually available for a high proportion of the cohort and is relatively inexpensive to obtain. To ensure that sufficient data on the relevant exposures are obtained, it is, therefore, often desirable to collect routinely whatever information is available from the records even if additional sources will also be needed. In addition, since the data were recorded prior to any knowledge of an individual's development of the outcome under study, and, in most cases, for reasons totally unrelated to the investigation, the use of such information will allow objective and unbiased classification of exposure status.

For many exposures, the level of detail present in preexisting records concerning an exposure may be insufficient to address specific research questions adequately. In addition, such records frequently do not contain data on potential confounding variables such as food consumption patterns, smoking, exercise, and other lifestyle factors. Such information can only be provided by the individuals themselves. Thus, interviews and questionnaires completed by study subjects are particularly useful for collecting information on exposures that are not routinely recorded. A potential for bias always exists in the use of such data, however, since it cannot be obtained as objectively as from preexisting records. Individuals who are ill or who have preconceived notions concerning the association under investigation may be more likely to give responses they believe to be desired by the investigator. Similarly, stigma associated with certain exposures, such as alcohol or drug use, may influence a respondent's answer. It is therefore especially important in studies that cannot use objective sources for the ascertainment of exposure to ensure that information is obtained in a comparable manner for all participants.

For some exposures or characteristics of interest, such as blood pressure or cholesterol level, a medical history may not provide adequate information, so that a direct physical examination and/or blood testing may be necessary. If obtained in a comparable manner for all participants, these data can provide an objective and unbiased means of classifying study subjects with respect to exposure.

Typically, individuals do not know their specific levels of exposure to pollutants or industrial chemicals, and many of the commonly used proxy measurements, such as job title or distance from the source, are at best only approximate. For certain occupational and environmental exposures, adequate information cannot be obtained from any of the sources mentioned above. In these cases, direct measurement of the air or water in a particular location may be required. For example, in the Harvard Six Cities air pollution study [15], the air in each of the study communities was measured repeatedly for levels of sulphur dioxide, mass respirable particles, sulfates, nitrogen dioxide, and ozone. Monitoring was carried out by continuous fixed station sampling in representative locations in each city, indoor/outdoor monitoring every 6 days in at least 10 cities per community, and periodic 24-hour personal monitoring of selected subjects, who also kept a daily log of their activities. However, while direct measurement may be possible for the evaluation of current or future exposures, it may be problematic in situations where the exposure of interest occurred prior to the initiation of the study. In such circumstances, current levels of the exposure are likely to be lower than previous levels due to changes in the working environment, such as the institution of safeguards. For example, in order to assess possible health risks associated with employment in the rubber industry in the U.S. today, data have been examined from a number of retrospective cohort studies. The evaluation of a possible excess risk of bladder cancer has been complicated by the fact that beta-naphthylamine, a known bladder carcinogen, was removed from the work environment as of 1949 [6]. Thus, since many of these cohorts included men who were employed in the industry some time prior to 1949 and therefore may have been exposed to this carcinogen during some or all of their employment, it has been difficult to assess whether an excess mortality from bladder cancer exists in current industrial settings.

To obtain adequate information on exposure in a given cohort study may require the use of a number of sources of data. For example, a retrospective cohort study [5] was conducted to evaluate the risk of breast cancer among women receiving repeated fluoroscopic examinations of the chest in the course of air-collapse therapy for tuberculosis. Data were collected from medical records, interviews with physicians, and patient contacts concerning the number of pneumotherapy treatments, the duration of each fluoroscopic examination, the use of filtration, and the orientation of the patient during therapy. These data were supplemented by physical measurements taken from fluoroscopic machines representing the type used when the patients were treated to estimate the total radiation dose to the breast received by each woman in the cohort. Similarly, data on various risk factors in the Framingham Heart Study [10] have been obtained from questionnaires (for factors such as age, smoking, and family history), laboratory determinations (serum cholesterol, glucose, and triglycerides), physical examination (blood pressure, body mass index, and height), and special diagnostic procedures (electrocardiogram and x-rays).

In many cohort studies, a single classification of exposure is made for each individual at the time of his or her entry into the study. Frequently, however, changes in exposure levels for the factors of interest will occur during the course of long-term follow-up. Individuals may cut down on their smoking habits, change jobs, or begin to eat a diet lower in saturated fats. Similarly, the introduction into the workplace of a new piece of standard equipment may affect the level of exposure experienced by all workers in a single plant or entire industry. Such changes will tend to result in an underestimate of the true strength of the association between an exposure and disease. Consequently, many cohort studies are designed to allow for periodic reexamination or resurvey of the members of the cohort to allow for revision of exposure categories according to the new information. The analysis can then take into account the total length of exposure, any changes in exposure status, and the reasons for these changes. The periodic requestioning of cohort members will also allow data to be collected on exposures or risk factors that were not recognized to be of interest at the initiation of the study. For example, in the Framingham Heart Study [10], growing interest in the possibility that level of physical activity might be related to risk of cardiovascular disease led to the inclusion of questions on energy expenditure at the fourth biennial examination.

Sources of Outcome Data

The sources of outcome data for a cohort study will necessarily depend on the specific resources available as well as the particular disease under evaluation. The goal is to obtain complete, comparable, and unbiased information on the subsequent health experience of every study subject. The approach used to obtain outcome information may range from routine surveillance of obituaries and death certificates to periodic health examinations of members of the cohort. Combinations of the various sources of outcome data may be necessary to obtain complete follow-up information.

For diseases that are frequently fatal, outcome information for all members of a cohort may be obtained solely from death certificates. While these are readily available, the reliability of such information depends on the specific outcome of interest. Death certificates are completely acceptable when total mortality is the end point of interest, since the occurrence of death can be established with virtual certainty. For cause-specific mortality, however, death certificate information is far less reliable, since the cause of death recorded may be subject to interpretation. The adequacy of death certificates for the determination of cause-specific mortality depends on the particular disease under investigation. Criteria for the postmortem diagnosis of conditions such as coronary heart disease are less straightforward than for others, such as cancer. Moreover, there is a potential for bias in collecting or interpreting study data from such records, especially when the records are vague or incomplete, if the abstractor is also aware of a participant's exposure status. Therefore, additional confirmatory information is often obtained from autopsies, physician and hospital records, or next of kin.

For nonfatal end points, outcome data can be obtained from physicians' records, hospital discharge logs, population-based disease registries, or prepaid health plans. Data can also be obtained directly from the participants, a procedure that offers similar advantages and disadvantages as for collecting exposure information. To overcome the possibility of bias due to a subject's awareness of the hypothesis under investigation, questionnaires are often used to identify those who report an event of interest, and additional information, such as hospital records or pathology reports, is then obtained to confirm the diagnosis. The adequacy of self-reported diagnoses depends on the particular disease of interest. An assessment of the validity of self-reports in the Nurses' Health Study [7], for example, indicated that for conditions with clear diagnostic criteria such as fractures, hypertension, or cancers of the breast, skin, large bowel, and thyroid, over 90 percent of self-reports were confirmed by relevant medical records. For other conditions, such as cancers of the lung, ovary, and uterus, myocardial infarction, and stroke, a much lower level of confirmation was observed. Thus, for many outcomes of interest, additional documentation may be required.

For certain diseases, accurate and reliable outcome information can only be obtained from periodic direct medical examinations of members of the cohort. While more expensive and time-consuming than other sources of outcome data, this approach allows for the collection of objective information using standardized diagnostic procedures for all subjects. Many studies of cardiovascular disease, including the Framingham Heart Study [10], rely on periodic health examinations. Since a complete physical examination also includes a medical history, it is important to ensure that the individual performing the examination remains unaware of the participant's exposure status.

Whatever the procedures for identifying the outcomes of interest, it is crucial for the validity of the study that they are equally applied to all exposed and nonexposed individuals. If, for example, the exposed group in an occupational setting has periodic health examinations provided by the industry and the experience of this group is compared with that of the general population, a biased estimate of the rate of occurrence of the outcome among the exposed could result simply because of their greater opportunity to have the disease diagnosed. Consequently, if the only information available on a general population comparison group is cause of death as recorded on the death certificate, then cause of death from the death certificate must also be used as the mechanism to ascertain outcomes for the special exposure cohort, even if additional information could be obtained for that group.

Approaches to Follow-Up

In any cohort study, whether retrospective or prospective, the ascertainment of outcome data involves tracing or following all study participants from the point of exposure into the future, to determine whether they develop the disease of interest. Failure to obtain such information on every subject, or collecting it on a greater proportion of individuals in either the exposed or nonexposed group, is the major source of potential bias in cohort investigations and could render the results of a study uninterpretable. Consequently, collecting follow-up data on every person enrolled represents the major challenge of a cohort study, as well as the major cost in terms of time, fiscal resources, and ingenuity.

The length of the required period of follow-up, or the interval that elapses between definition of exposure status and ascertainment of outcome, will be related to the length of the latency period for the outcome(s) of interest. Outcomes that have a latency period of days to weeks, such as acute illnesses, or months, such as congenital malformations or spontaneous abortions, require far shorter periods of observation than chronic diseases with latency periods lasting many years or even decades, such as cancer and coronary heart disease. In general, the longer the observation period required, the more difficult it will be to achieve complete follow-up, because people are more likely to move, change jobs, change their names, or, in prospective studies, lose touch with the study organization. There are, however, a variety of resources available that, if used creatively, can greatly diminish the numbers of individuals on whom follow-up information is unavailable. For example, in the study of breast cancer after repeated fluoroscopy [5], the sources of outcome data included the outpatient records of the sanitorium from which subjects had been identified; the Massachusetts Department of Vital Statistics; town residents' lists; telephone directories; relatives and friends of the subjects, identified in various ways; records of state tuberculosis agencies; divorce records; town election boards; Motor Vehicle Bureau records; the Internal Revenue Service; military records; employment records; as well as physicians and other individuals mentioned in the subject's medical records. These procedures resulted in the location of 93.6 percent of the 1764 study subjects. The remaining small percentage of women who were lost to follow-up were divided equally between the exposed and nonexposed groups, offering reassuring evidence that the study results were not biased with respect to losses to follow-up.

ISSUES IN ANALYSIS

The basic analysis of data from a cohort study involves the calculation of rates of the incidence of a specified outcome among the cohorts under investigation. These rates can be compared for those exposed and nonexposed, as well as for those exposed to various levels of the factor or to a combination of factors. The specific calculations of disease incidence in a given study will depend on whether the denominator includes numbers of individuals or person-time units of observation. Using these rates, both relative and absolute measures of association can be calculated, as presented in Chapter 4, and tested, as will be discussed in Chapter 10. The groups must also be compared to ensure similarity with respect to other baseline differences that could be associated with risk of developing the outcomes under study.

ISSUES IN INTERPRETATION

As with any epidemiologic investigation, an evaluation of the validity of a cohort study requires consideration of the roles of chance, bias, and confounding as alternative explanations for the study findings. There are, however, a number of issues of particular importance in the interpretation of the results of a cohort study that arise as a result of its inherent design or because of the types of research questions that are most usually being addressed.

The Role of Bias

In general, the potential for selection bias is less of a concern in cohort than in case-control studies. In prospective cohort studies, since exposure is assessed prior to the occurrence of disease, it is unlikely that the outcome could influence the classification of exposure. In retrospective cohort studies, however, as in case-control studies, both the exposure and outcome have occurred at the start of the investigation. If knowledge of the disease affects the selection or classification of exposed and nonexposed individuals to be included in the study, selection bias may result.

One major source of error in cohort studies arises from the degree of accuracy with which subjects have been classified with respect to their exposure and disease status. Any observational study is unlikely to categorize all individuals correctly. In cohort studies, a number of those exposed will be considered nonexposed, and a number of those who are truly nonexposed will be classified as exposed. Similarly, errors will be made with respect to ascertainment of the outcomes of interest. The validity of the study data will be affected not only by the accuracy and completeness of the information on which the classifications were based, but also by the degree to which the errors were made differentially among the study groups. Thus, while misclassification (of exposure or outcome) is a problem in every cohort study, its effect will depend on whether the misclassification was independent of the other study axis (outcome or exposure).

Nondifferential or random misclassification results when inaccuracies exist in the categorization of subjects by exposure or disease status but these inaccuracies occur in similar proportions in each of the study groups. Such misclassification is often present because there are so many difficulties inherent in the measurement of variables. For example, in the investigation of risks associated with different levels of smoking, categorization is usually based on the number of cigarettes smoked per day. This method does not account for differences related to brand of cigarettes, degree of inhalation, or the amount of each cigarette smoked. Consequently, some subjects classified as "light" smokers may, in fact, be "heavy" smokers in terms of amounts of tar or nicotine actually consumed, while other subjects classified as "heavy" smokers may be, in reality, "light" smokers. Similarly, occupational exposure is often classified using a proxy measure such as job title or duration of employment in an industry. While these may result in a certain degree of misclassification with respect to exposure to the actual agent under investigation, this misclassification is likely to be random or unrelated to the outcomes of interest.

The effect of random misclassification is to increase the similarity between the exposed and nonexposed groups, so that any true association between the exposure and outcome will be diluted or underestimated. As a result, the observed relative risk estimate will always be biased towards the null value of 1.0. Thus, random misclassification may obscure the true relationship between an exposure and disease but cannot be responsible for causing the observation of an association if one does not truly exist.

Differential or nonrandom misclassification, on the other hand, results when the errors in the classification of individuals by exposure or disease produce a differential accuracy or quality of information among the study groups. If, in a study of the role of smoking in the development of bronchitis, smokers sought medical attention more often than nonsmokers, bronchitis is likely to be more frequently or accurately diagnosed in those exposed than those nonexposed. This would result in an excess incidence of bronchitis observed among smokers due to the effect of the method of ascertainment of outcome rather than to the effect of the exposure itself. Depending on the situation, differential misclassification can result in a biased risk estimate that is either an underestimate, an overestimate, or, by chance, the same as the true measure of association.

The Effect of Losses to Follow-Up

The major source of bias in cohort studies relates to the necessity of following individuals for a period of time after exposure to determine the development of the outcome of interest. A number of members of the exposed and nonexposed groups will be lost to follow-up by the end of the study period. If this proportion is large, in the range of 30 to 40 percent, this would certainly raise serious doubts about the validity of the study results. However, the more difficult issue for interpretation is that even if the rate of loss is not that extreme, the probability of loss may be related to the exposure, to the outcome, or to both. For example, smokers may be more likely to move to another geographic location than nonsmokers, or those who develop lung cancer may be less likely to continue participating in a study than those who remain disease-free. To the extent that losses to follow-up are correlated with both exposure and disease—e.g., that smokers are more likely to leave the study area if they develop lung cancer than if a nonsmoker develops that disease—a biased estimate of the association may result.

Since it is extremely difficult to know the factors to which such losses are related, the best method of eliminating this source of bias in cohort studies is to keep losses to follow-up to an absolute minimum. For those who are lost, an assessment of as much outcome data as can be independently determined by the investigator should be made. This would include, at the very least, an assessment of mortality status using sources such as obituary listings, state vital statistics bureaus, contacts with relatives or neighbors, mail returns by the Post Office, and searches using the National Death Index. Previously collected data can also be examined to determine whether there are systematic differences in the exposure or other risk factors between those whose outcome is known and those who have been lost to follow-up. An indirect approach used to describe the extent of bias introduced by losses to follow-up is to calculate estimates of the exposure-disease association assuming the most extreme situations with respect to both exposure and outcome. One estimate would be based on the assumption that all those who were lost to follow-up developed the outcome of interest, while the other would assume that none developed it. The results of these calculations provide a range within which the true association will lie. If losses to follow-up are large, however, the observed range will be so wide as to provide little useful information. Again, the best method to eliminate this source of bias in cohort studies is prevention to minimize losses to follow-up.

The Effects of Nonparticipation

In virtually every cohort study, only a proportion of those who are eligible to participate actually agree to do so and are entered into the study. In the Nurses' Health Study [3], for example, of the approximately 172,000 female married nurses who received letters of invitation, approximately 122,000 or 71 percent were willing and eligible to participate. Similarly, in the Framingham Heart Study [9], 4469 (69 percent) of the 6507 persons in the initial sample actually underwent the first examination. Those who agree to participate are likely to differ from nonparticipants in a number of important ways, including basic levels of motivation and attitudes towards health [44] as well as risk factor status [4]. A number of studies have shown that nonparticipants are more likely than participants to be current smokers [11]. Moreover, in the Framingham study [17], a higher proportion of nonparticipants than participants died within the first 2 years after the initiation of the investigation. The effect of this difference between these groups concerns the generalizability of the study results. A positive finding in a particular study population would not preclude the possibility that such a relationship would not exist, or that it might exist to a different degree, among persons not included in the cohort. For example, in the Nurses' Health Study [43], risk of nonfatal myocardial infarction was found to be strongly related to current cigarette smoking. Whether this risk is believed to pertain to nurses who were unwilling to be in the study, to women who are not nurses, and to women not living in the United States, is solely a matter of judgment.

While the nature of subjects selected for investigation may limit the ability to generalize the study results, it will not usually affect their validity. The true relationship between exposure and disease will be biased only if nonresponse is related to both the exposure and other risk factors for the outcome under study. If the rate of nonresponse is related only to exposure—for example, if heavy smokers are less likely to cooperate than nonsmokers—the experience of the study cohort will accurately reflect the strength of the association between smoking and lung cancer but will also result in an underestimate of the proportion of heavy smokers in the population. Similarly, if the nonresponse is related only to outcome—if those who are in poor health are less likely to agree to be in the study—then again, the disease rates in the cohort will be an underestimate of those in the population, but the association between smoking and lung cancer observed in the study will be valid. However, if those who refuse to participate are both heavy smokers and, independent of their smoking, are at increased (or decreased) risk of developing lung cancer, then, and only then, would a biased estimate of the association between smoking and lung cancer result.

Usually, a direct assessment of whether the rate of nonresponse is related to the exposure, the outcome, or both, cannot be made. Sometimes, however, it is possible to argue indirectly concerning the likelihood that nonresponse may have accounted for an observed result. For example, approximately two-thirds of the British physicians who were initially sent questionnaires were willing and eligible to be included in the Doll and Hill cohort study of smoking and lung cancer [12]. Followup of these physicians revealed that heavy smokers were about 20 times more likely to die from lung cancer than nonsmokers. The tobacco companies have claimed that the risk observed for heavy smokers was not valid due to the high rate of nonresponse [39]. If, however, as the tobacco companies claim, smoking really has no effect on lung cancer, there would need to have been about a 30-fold protective effect of smoking among the one-third who were nonrespondents. Thus, among those who were included in the study, the results observed were valid, and the question then becomes whether the results are generalizable to those who did not participate in the study.

Another way of assessing the possible effects of nonresponse on either generalizability or validity involves a comparison of those who do and do not participate in a study. For many cohorts, the address lists, registries, or personnel records that were used to identify the study population may also include baseline information on age, sex, and other demographic characteristics. If those not included in the study are found to be similar to respondents with respect to known variables, it may then be possible to judge whether their other experience will also be similar. For example, in the Nurses' Health Study [3], the cohort was established with the collaboration of the American Nurses' Association (ANA). The ANA subsequently provided data from their national inventory [45] on age, education, status of residence, employment status and affiliation, and major practice area. These data permitted a comparison of respondents and nonrespondents to the initial enrollment questionnaire in 1976. These comparisons revealed high degrees of similarity between the more than 122,000 respondents and the 43,000 nonrespondents, allowing the investigators to conclude "that estimation of exposure-disease associations is unlikely to be affected by major bias due to non-response" in this cohort [2].

CONCLUSION

Like all epidemiologic design options, the cohort study has unique strengths and limitations that must be taken into account when choosing to use this approach for the evaluation of a particular research question or when interpreting published results. As summarized in Table 7-1, in many ways the advantages and disadvantages of cohort studies are the mirror image of those that were discussed for case-control studies. A principal advantage of cohort studies is that they are optimal for the investigation of the effects of rare exposures. With an uncommon exposure, it is unlikely that a sufficient number of exposed subjects could be identified in a case-control study even if the sample size were very large. Thus, the more efficient design is to select participants on the basis of their exposure status to ensure an adequate sample size to test the hypothesis. A second advantage of cohort studies is their ability to examine multiple effects of a single exposure, thus providing a picture of the range of health outcomes that could be related to a factor or factors of interest. Third, since the participants are disease-free at the time exposure status is identified, the temporal sequence between exposure and disease can be more clearly elucidated. Moreover, since in a prospective cohort study the outcomes of interest have not yet occurred at the time the study is begun, bias in the selection of subjects and ascertainment of exposure is minimized. For retrospective cohort studies, where all the relevant events have occurred when the study begins, the potential for these biases is similar to that of a case-control study. Finally, cohort studies allow the direct calculation of incidence rates of the outcomes under investigation in the exposed and nonexposed groups.

Table 7-1. Strengths and limitations of the cohort study design

Strengths
- Is of particular value when the exposure is rare
- Can examine multiple effects of a single exposure
- Can elucidate temporal relationship between exposure and disease
- If prospective, minimizes bias in the ascertainment of exposure
- Allows direct measurement of incidence of disease in the exposed and nonexposed groups

Limitations
- Is inefficient for the evaluation of rare diseases, unless the attributable-risk percent is high
- If prospective, can be extremely expensive and time consuming
- If retrospective, requires the availability of adequate records
- Validity of the results can be seriously affected by losses to follow-up

With respect to disadvantages, a cohort study is not an efficient design for the evaluation of a rare outcome unless the study population is extremely large or the outcome is common among those who are exposed. Moreover, if prospective, a cohort study is very expensive and time-consuming compared with either a case-control or retrospective study. Finally, the unique potential for bias in the cohort design is the problem of losses to follow-up. If the proportion of those lost to follow-up is high, or even if the proportion is low but is related to both the exposure and outcome under investigation, the study findings may not be valid.

Thus, as with the case-control design, the cohort study has unique advantages and disadvantages that must be considered in the design, conduct, analysis, and interpretation of each particular investigation. While, as we have emphasized, neither the case-control nor the cohort study is an inherently better design option, a well-designed and well-conducted cohort study is an extremely valuable strategy to obtain a valid estimate of the association between an exposure and disease.

STUDY QUESTIONS

1. Discuss the strengths and limitations of cohort studies.
2. Compare and contrast the design features of prospective and retrospective cohort studies.
3. What types of bias are particular concerns in cohort studies?

REFERENCES

1. Bain, C., Hennekens, C. H., Speizer, F. E., et al. Oral contraceptive use and malignant melanoma. *J.N.C.I.* 68:537, 1982.
2. Barton, J., Bain, C., Hennekens, C. H., et al. Characteristics of respondents and non-respondents to a mailed questionnaire. *Am. J. Public Health* 70:823, 1980.
3. Belanger, C. F., Hennekens, C. H., Rosner, R., et al. The Nurses' Health Study. *Am. J. Nurs.* 78:1039, 1978.
4. Bergstrand, R., Vedin, A., Wilhelmsson, C., et al. Bias due to non-participation and heterogenous sub-groups in population surveys. *J. Chronic Dis.* 36:725, 1983.
5. Boice, J. D., Jr., and Monson, R. R. Breast cancer in women after repeated fluoroscopic examination of the chest. *J.N.C.I.* 59:823, 1977.
6. Case, R. A. M. Tumours of the urinary tract as an occupational disease in several industries. *Ann. R. Coll. Surg. Engl.* 39:213, 1966.
7. Colditz, G. A., Martin, P., Stampfer, M. J., et al. Validation of questionnaire

information on risk factors and disease outcomes in a prospective cohort study of disease in women. *Am. J. Epidemiol.* 123:894, 1986.

8. Court Brown, W. M., and Doll, R. Mortality from cancer and other causes after radiotherapy for ankylosing spondylitis. *Br. Med. J.* 2:1327, 1965.

9. Dawber, T. R., Kannel, W. B., and Lyell, L. P. An approach to longitudinal studies in a community: The Framingham study. *Ann. N.Y. Acad. Sci.* 107:539, 1963.

10. Dawber, T. R. *The Framingham Study: The Epidemiology of Atherosclerotic Disease.* Cambridge, MA: Harvard University Press, 1980.

11. Doll, R., and Hill, A. B. Mortality in relation to smoking: Ten years' observation of British doctors. *Br. Med. J.* 1:1399, 1964.

12. Doll, R., and Hill, A. B. The mortality of doctors in relation to their smoking habits: A preliminary report. *Br. Med. J.* 1:1451, 1954.

13. Dyer, A. R., Stamler, J., Paul, O., et al. Alcohol consumption and 17-year mortality in the Chicago Western Electric Company Study. *Prev. Med.* 9:78, 1980.

14. Enterline, P. E. Mortality among asbestos products workers in the United States. *Ann. N.Y. Acad. Sci.* 132:156, 1965.

15. Ferris, B. G., Jr., Speizer, F. E., Spengler, J. D., et al. Effects of sulfur oxides and respirable particles on human health: Methodology and demography of populations in study. *Am. Rev. Respir. Dis.* 120:767, 1979.

16. Friedman, G. D., Kannel, W. B., and Dawber, T. R. The epidemiology of gallbladder disease: Observations in the Framingham study. *J. Chronic Dis.* 19:273, 1966.

17. Gordon, T., Moore, F. E., Shurtleff, D., et al. Some epidemiologic problems in the long-term study of cardiovascular disease. Observations on the Framingham study. *J. Chronic Dis.* 10:186, 1959.

18. Gunby, P. Military looks toward 1985 in ongoing defoliant study. *J.A.M.A.* 85:383, 1984.

19. Hall, A. P., Barry, P. E., Dawber, T. R., et al. Epidemiology of gout and hyperuricemia: A long term population study. *Am. J. Med.* 42:27, 1967.

20. Kannel, W. B., and Feinleib, M. Natural history of angina pectoris in the Framingham study. *Am. J. Cardiol.* 29:154, 1972.

21. Kannel, W. B., and Shurtleff, D. Cigarettes and the development of intermittent claudication: The Framingham study. *Geriatrics* 28:61, 1973.

22. Kannel, W. B., Dawber, T. R., Sorlie, P., et al. Components of blood pressure and risk of atherothrombotic brain infarction: The Framingham study. *Stroke* 7:327, 1976.

23. Kitigawa, E. M., and Hauser, P. M. *Differential Mortality in the United States.* Cambridge, MA: Harvard University Press, 1973.

24. Klatsky, A. L., Friedman, G. D., and Siegelaub, A. B. Alcohol consumption before myocardial infarction: Results from the Kaiser-Permanente epidemiologic study of myocardial infarction. *Ann. Intern. Med.* 81:294, 1974.

25. Lathrop, G. D., Wolfe, W. H., Albanese, R. A., et al. *Project Ranch Hand II. An Epidemiologic Investigation of Health Effects in Air Force Personnel Following Exposure to Herbicides: Baseline Morbidity Study Results.* San Antonio, TX: US Air Force School of Aerospace Medicine, Aerospace Medical Division, Brooks Air Force Base, 1984.

26. Leibowitz, H. M., Krueger, D. E., Maunder, L. R., et al. The Framingham Eye Study Monograph: An ophthalmological and epidemiologic study of cataract, glaucoma, diabetic retinopathy, macular degeneration and visual acuity in a general population of 2631 adults. *Surv. Ophthalmol.* 24(Suppl.):335, 1980.

27. Lipnick, R. J., Buring, J. E., Hennekens, C. H., et al. A prospective study of oral contraceptives and risk of breast cancer. *J.A.M.A.* 255:58, 1986.

28. Matanoski, G. M., Seltzer, R., Sartwell, P. E., et al. The current mortality rates of radiologists and other physician specialists: Specific causes of death. *Am. J. Epidemiol.* 101:199, 1975.

29. McKee, P. A., Castelli, W. P., McNamara, P., et al. The natural history of congestive heart failure. *N. Engl. J. Med.* 285:1141, 1971.

30. McMichael, A. J., Andjelkovich, D. A., and Tyroler, H. A. Cancer mortality among rubber workers: An epidemiologic study. *Ann. N.Y. Acad. Sci.* 271:125, 1976.

31. McMichael, A. J., Haynes, S. G., and Tyroler, H. A. Observations on the evaluation of occupational mortality data. *J. Occup. Med.* 17:128, 1975.

32. McMichael, A. J., Spirtas, R., and Kupper, L. L. An epidemiologic study of mortality within a cohort of rubber workers, 1964–72. *J. Occup. Med.* 16:458, 1974.

33. McMichael, A. J., Spirtas, R., Gamble, J. R., et al. Mortality among rubber workers: Relationship to specific jobs. *J. Occup. Med.* 18:178, 1976.

34. Monson, R., and Fine, L. J. Cancer mortality and morbidity among rubber workers. *J.N.C.I.* 61:1047, 1978.

35. Monson, R. R., and Nakano, K. K. Mortality among rubber workers: I. White male union employees in Akron, Ohio. *Am. J. Epidemiol.* 103:284, 1976.

36. Morris, J. N., Kagan, A., Pattison, D. C., et al. Incidence and prediction of ischaemic heart disease in London busmen. *Lancet* 2:553, 1966.

37. Paffenbarger, R. S., Wing, A. L., Hyde, R. T., et al. Physical activity and incidence of hypertension in college alumni. *Am. J. Epidemiol.* 117:245, 1983.

38. Paffenbarger, R. S., Jr., and Hale, W. E. Work activity and coronary heart disease mortality. *N. Engl. J. Med.* 292:545, 1975.

39. Peto, R. Personal communication, 1986.

40. Ram, W. N., and Lockey, J. E. Diffuse malignant mesothelioma: A review. *West. J. Med.* 137:548, 1982.

41. Reid, D. D., Hamilton, P. J. S., McCartney, P., et al. Smoking and other risk factors for coronary heart disease in British civil servants. *Lancet* 2:979, 1976.

42. Rogot, E. Smoking and mortality among U.S. veterans. *J. Chronic Dis.* 27:189, 1974.

43. Rosenberg, L., Hennekens, C. H., Rosner, B., et al. Oral contraceptive use in relation to non-fatal myocardial infarction. *Am. J. Epidemiol.* 111:59, 1980.

44. Rosenthal, R., and Rosnow, R. L. *The Volunteer Subject.* New York: Wylie-Interscience, 1975.

45. Roth, A., and Walder, A. *The Nation's Nurses: 1972 Inventory of Registered Nurses.* Kansas City: American Nurses' Association, 1974.

46. Selikoff, I. J., Hammond, E. C., and Seidman, H. Latency of asbestos disease among insulation workers in the United States and Canada. *Cancer* 46:2736, 1980.

47. Stokes, J., and Dawber, T. R. Rheumatic heart disease in the Framingham study. *N. Engl. J. Med.* 255:1228, 1956.
48. Willett, W., Bain, C., Hennekens, C. H., et al. Oral contraceptives and risk of ovarian cancer. *Cancer* 48:1684, 1981.

8

Intervention Studies

The intervention study, or clinical trial, is an epidemiologic design that can provide data of such high quality that it most closely resembles the controlled experiment done by basic science researchers. As in a cohort study, individuals are enrolled on the basis of their exposure status; however, the distinguishing characteristic of a clinical trial is that the investigators themselves allocate the exposure. The primary advantage of this feature is that if the treatments are allocated at random in a sample of sufficiently large size, intervention studies have the potential to provide a degree of assurance about the validity of a result that is simply not possible with any observational design option.

It is rare that the introduction of a new treatment or procedure is accompanied by benefits as striking and unequivocal as those that followed the introduction of the antibiotic penicillin, namely an immediate sixfold reduction in death rates from pneumococcal pneumonia, from about 95 to 15 percent. A randomized trial of the efficacy of penicillin seemed neither necessary nor, for ethical reasons, desirable, in part because the mortality reduction was so large and immediate that it seemed clearly due to the drug itself. Most often, however, the effects of therapeutic or preventive measures are small to moderate in size, on the order of 10- to 20-percent differences in disease outcomes. Such effects can be extremely important from a clinical or public health standpoint, especially when the outcome of interest is mortality from common diseases. While important, small to moderate differences are very difficult to establish reliably from observational studies, since the magnitude of the observed effect of the treatment or procedure may be about the same as the amount of uncontrolled confounding. In these circumstances, the conduct of a randomized trial will yield the strongest and most direct epidemiologic evidence on which to base a judgment of whether an observed association is one of cause and effect.

In this chapter, we focus on the general principles and methods of designing, conducting, and analyzing intervention studies.

TYPES OF INTERVENTION STUDIES

Intervention studies can generally be considered either therapeutic or preventive. Therapeutic (or secondary prevention) trials are conducted among patients with a particular disease to determine the ability of an agent or procedure to diminish symptoms, prevent recurrence, or decrease risk of death from that disease. For example, in the Coronary Artery Surgery Study (CASS) [6], 780 patients who had mild or moderate stable angina pectoris or who were free from angina but had a well-documented history of myocardial infarction more than 3 weeks previously were assigned at random to receive either coronary artery bypass surgery or medical therapy. After 5 years of follow-up, no significant differences were found in total or coronary heart disease (CHD) mortality rates between the two groups. One inference from these findings was that such patients could receive medical therapy and defer bypass surgery until symptoms worsened without decreasing their chances of survival. Similarly, two recent randomized trials [13, 14] among breast cancer patients have compared radical mastectomy with more limited resection. William Halsted, considered the father of American surgery, introduced the radical mastectomy for the treatment of breast cancer in the early twentieth century, based on his clinical impression that removal of the surrounding lymph nodes and muscles in addition to the tumor and breast would reduce risk of recurrence or spread of the cancer. For decades thereafter, this procedure was the standard treatment for this disease. Only in the 1970s did the scientific community begin to address whether less extensive surgery might be equally beneficial. Data from both trials showed that, in fact, rates of recurrence of cancer and 5-year mortality were very similar among those undergoing radical mastectomy and those receiving more limited resection.

A preventive (or primary prevention) trial involves the evaluation of whether an agent or procedure reduces the risk of developing disease among those free from that condition at enrollment. Thus, preventive trials can be conducted among healthy individuals at usual risk or those already recognized to be at high risk of developing a disease. For example, in the 1954 Francis field trial [15] of the poliomyelitis vaccine, healthy children from 11 states were assigned at random to one of two groups. While each child was given a series of three injections, one group received the active vaccine and the other was administered an inert placebo. The incidence of paralytic poliomyelitis in the vaccinated group was over 50-percent less than that among the children given placebo. This large and highly significant difference provided strong evidence on which to judge that the vaccine reduced the risk of poliomyelitis among healthy children. With respect to trials enrolling high-risk participants, the Coronary Primary Prevention Trial (CPPT) [26] tested the efficacy of the cholesterol-lowering drug cholestyramine in reducing the risk of CHD among 3806 men with elevated cholesterol levels. All participants followed a cholesterol-lowering diet and took either six packets of cholestyramine per day or an equal amount of a placebo. After 7 to 10 years of follow-up, the treated group experienced a statistically significant 19-percent reduction in risk of the combined end point of nonfatal myocardial infarction and fatal CHD. These data indicated that cholestyramine reduced the occurrence of CHD in men at high risk due to elevated blood cholesterol levels.

While therapeutic trials are virtually always conducted among individuals, primary prevention measures can be studied among either individuals, as in the Francis field trial of the polio vaccine and the CPPT of cholestyramine, or entire populations. One example of the latter, also termed a community trial, is the Newburgh-Kingston dental caries study [4], in which one entire community (Newburgh) was allocated at random to receiving sodium fluoride added to the water supply, while the other (Kingston) continued receiving water without supplementation. This trial indicated clinically important and statistically significant reductions in the development of decayed, missing, or filled teeth in the community receiving fluoridation.

UNIQUE PROBLEMS OF INTERVENTION STUDIES

While the investigator is merely a passive observer in observational analytic study designs, in the intervention study there is active assignment of participants to a particular treatment or procedure. Consequently, for reasons of both ethics and feasibility, there must be sufficient doubt about the particular agent to be tested to allow withholding it from half the subjects, and at the same time there must be sufficient belief in the agent's potential to justify exposing the remaining half of all willing and eligible participants. Ethical considerations preclude the evaluation of many treatments or procedures in an intervention study. Practices or substances already known to be harmful should not be allocated by an investigator, although such agents can be tested indirectly in trials of their removal, such as the effects of smoking cessation programs on subsequent morbidity and mortality. Similarly, therapies known to be beneficial, such as medical treatment of severe hypertension, should not be withheld from any affected individual. In many instances, however, there is insufficient evidence in either direction. In these circumstances, the question then becomes not whether it is ethical to conduct a trial, but whether it is ethical *not* to proceed with a randomized intervention.

The widespread adoption of measures by either the medical community or the general public can cause insurmountable problems of feasibility. It may become difficult to find a sufficiently large population of individuals willing to forego a treatment or practice believed to be beneficial for the duration of a trial, even if there is no sound evidence to support this view. For example, in recent years, there has been growing public awareness concerning the possibility that a number of micronutrients contained in multiple vitamin supplements may reduce risk of developing cancer [20]. To date, the scientific evidence is far from conclusive. Nonetheless, during the 1970s, even after adjustment for inflation, there was a several-fold increase in sales of vitamin pills in the United States [22]. Moreover, in 1981, 35 percent of middle-aged (35–60 years) female nurses in the U.S. used multivitamin supplements regularly [45], and by 1985, the corresponding figure among all women 19 to 50 years was 57 percent [39]. If randomized trials of the cancer chemoprevention potential of these micronutrients are not conducted in the next few years, vitamin consumption may become so generally widespread a practice that their conduct might no longer be feasible. Reliable evidence on this issue is essential, for if nutritional supplements do not reduce cancer risk, the proportion of the U.S. public using them may wish to alter their habit, while if there is a substantial benefit, the proportion not using them may wish to consider their use. Thus, for reasons of ethics and feasibility, it is optimal to conduct a randomized trial when any agent or procedure is first introduced rather than after it gains widespread acceptance and becomes considered a standard practice.

In addition to the unique ethical and feasibility problems of conducting intervention studies, there is also the question of cost. In the past, clinical trials have been generally much more expensive to conduct than observational studies; subjects usually have been evaluated and treated individually by study personnel and have returned to a hospital or clinic for periodic and extensive examinations. As a result, clinical trials of primary prevention have generally cost on the order of $3000 to $15,000 per randomized participant. In recent years, attention has begun to focus on conducting large trials with streamlined protocols carefully designed to minimize time and expense [29, 46]. In these circumstances, the cost of conducting an efficiently designed randomized clinical trial should be no greater than for observational studies of comparable sample sizes.

ISSUES IN THE DESIGN AND CONDUCT OF CLINICAL TRIALS

When issues of ethics, feasibility, and cost, all of which can add to the complexity of planning and conducting an intervention study, are addressed satisfactorily, the randomized clinical trial represents the "gold standard" for epidemiologic research. There are a number of issues to consider in the design and conduct of clinical trials to ensure that valid

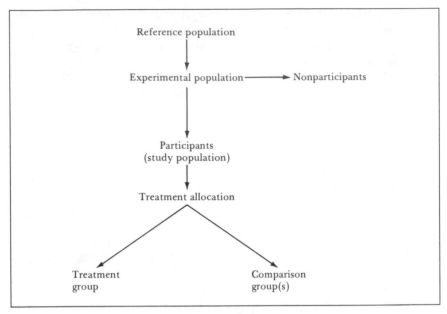

Fig. 8-1. Population hierarchy for an intervention study.

results are obtained. These include the selection of the study population, allocation of the treatment regimens, maintenance and assessment of compliance, and achieving high and uniform rates of ascertainment of outcomes.

Selection of a Study Population

The groups of individuals among whom an intervention study is conducted are derived from a number of interrelated populations, which can be considered as a population hierarchy (Fig. 8-1). The reference population is the general group to whom the investigators expect the results of the particular trial to be applicable. The reference population may include all human beings, if it seems likely that the study findings are universally applicable. Conversely, the reference population may be restricted by geography, age, sex, or any other characteristic that is thought to modify the existence or magnitude of the effects seen in the trial. Thus, the reference population represents the scope of the public health impact of the intervention. For example, the Physicians' Health Study [19] is a randomized trial of aspirin in the reduction of total cardiovascular mortality and beta-carotene in decreasing cancer incidence that is being conducted among over 22,000 male physicians aged 40 to 84 years in the U.S. There seems to be no reason to believe that the effects of either aspirin or beta-carotene would be inherently different among male physicians in the U.S. than in a comparable group of males who are not physicians or even among those who do not live in the U.S. Therefore, the reference population of this trial may reasonably include all men 40 years of age and older. While some may consider the reference population to be as broad as all people over 40 years of age, others might be unwilling to generalize the findings of this trial to women. Thus, the reference population is related to the issue of generalizability, which involves a judgment about an intervention based on considerations beyond the data from an individual trial.

The experimental population is the actual group in which the trial is conducted. While, in general, it is preferable that this group not differ from the reference population in such a way that generalizability to the latter is not possible, the primary consideration in the design of the trial should always be to obtain a valid result. The selection of the experimental population is crucial to achieving that aim and involves consideration of each of several important issues. First, it is essential to determine whether the proposed experimental population is sufficiently large to achieve the necessary sample size for the trial. For example, in considering design features for a trial of intravenous streptokinase therapy in acute myocardial infarction to decrease subsequent cardiovascular mortality, a single hospital would certainly not admit enough patients to permit enrollment of the requisite number of participants to test the hypothesis of a small to moderate benefit, even within a study period of several years. It would therefore be necessary to design a multicenter trial, including a number of hospitals in the community, across the country, or throughout the world. Such a study is currently underway in 15 countries and expects to enroll perhaps 20,000 patients over 2 years [24].

Analogously, it is essential to choose an experimental population that will experience a sufficient number of the end points or outcomes of interest to permit meaningful comparisons between various treatments or procedures within a reasonable period of time. For example, if a primary prevention trial of regular aspirin consumption in reducing the risk of total cardiovascular mortality were conducted among a group of 20,000 women under age 40, it would take several decades to accumulate sufficient end points to test the hypothesis because of the relatively low frequency of this disease in this population. In contrast, a similar trial conducted among men aged 40 and over could provide sound evidence on this question after several years, since total cardiovascular disease death rates are several-fold higher in men than women and increase markedly in middle age. A third major concern is the likelihood of obtaining complete and accurate follow-up information for the duration of the trial. A long-term trial conducted among a highly mobile group such as college students or a study requiring frequent clinic visits among a group of infirm elderly subjects might result in low follow-up rates, which would render the findings uninterpretable.

In designing the Physicians' Health Study [19], for example, the considerations described above contributed to the choice of doctors as the experimental population. The number of willing and eligible physicians in the age groups at risk of death from cardiovascular disease as well as the development of cancer seemed sufficient for an adequate test of each hypothesis. Moreover, because of their training, doctors would be able to recognize any side effects of the agents promptly. They are also well aware of their medical history and health status and would report this information with a high degree of accuracy and detail. Finally, since physicians are less mobile and easier to trace than members of the general population, a high rate of follow-up could be attained, even for an extended duration of the trial. Pilot studies conducted among random samples of this group also indicated a high degree of compliance with the study regimen as well as adherence to the trial protocol, which included the completion of follow-up questionnaires. Thus, the trial could be conducted entirely by mail at a small fraction of the usual cost for previous intervention studies of primary prevention [18]. These general considerations must all be addressed in the design phase of any trial, to avoid the possibility of wasting valuable time and resources on studies that cannot provide either a definitive positive finding or a null result that is truly informative.

Once the experimental population has been defined, subjects must then be invited to participate after being fully informed as to the purposes of the trial, the study procedures, and the possible risks and benefits. If appropriate, this information will include knowledge that they may be allocated to a group receiving no active treatment and that they may not know the treatment they received until the end of the trial. Those willing to participate must then be screened for eligibility according to predetermined criteria. Reasons for exclusion from the trial may include factors such as a previous history of any end points under study, a definite need for the study treatments, as well as contraindications to their use. Those who are eventually determined to be both willing and eligible to enroll in the trial compose the actual study population and are often a relatively small subgroup of the experimental population. For example, as shown in Figure 8-2, in the Hypertension Detection and Follow-Up Program (HDFP) [23], a randomized trial testing a stepped-care approach compared with usual medical care to treat hypertension, an initial enumeration of the populations of the 14 participating communities identified a total of 178,009 men and women in the eligible age range, 30 to 69 years. Of these potentially eligible subjects, 158,906 completed a first screen, and 22,978 were found to have diastolic blood pressures of at least 95 mm Hg. Subsequently, 17,476 of these individuals completed a second screen to establish the final study population of

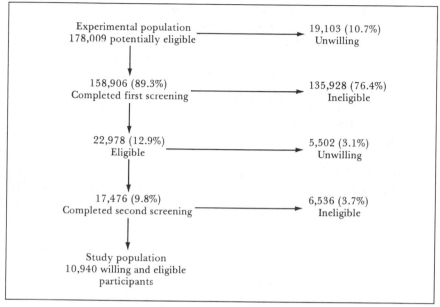

Fig. 8-2. Population hierarchy for hypertension detection and follow-up program. (From Hypertension Detection and Follow-up Program Cooperative Group, Five-year findings of the Hypertension Detection and Follow-up Program: I. Reduction in mortality of persons with high blood pressure, including mild hypertension. *J.A.M.A.* 242:2562, 1979.)

10,940 persons with diastolic blood pressures greater than or equal to 90 mm Hg who were both willing and eligible to participate in the trial. Thus, only 6.1 percent of the total experimental population formed the study population for the HDFP.

The actual study population of a trial is often not only a relatively small but also a select subgroup of the experimental population. It is well recognized that those who participate in an intervention study are very likely to differ from nonparticipants in many ways that may affect the rate of development of the end points under investigation [16]. Among all who are eligible, those willing to participate in clinical trials tend to experience lower morbidity and mortality rates than those who do not, regardless not only of the hypothesis under study, but of the actual treatment to which they are assigned [44]. Volunteerism is likely to be associated with age, sex, socioeconomic status, education and other, less well-defined correlates of health consciousness that might significantly influence subsequent morbidity and mortality. Whether the subgroup of participants is representative of the entire experimental population will not affect the validity of the results of a trial conducted among that group. It may, however, affect the ability to generalize those results to either the experimental or the reference population.

If it is possible to obtain baseline data and/or to ascertain outcomes for subjects who are eligible but unwilling to participate, such information is extremely valuable to assess the presence and extent of differences between participants and nonparticipants in a particular trial. This will aid in the judgment of whether the results among trial participants are generalizable to the reference population. For example, in the previously discussed CASS trial [6], 780 patients at 11 participating institutions entered the trial and were randomized to either coronary artery bypass surgery or medical management. An additional 1315 patients at the same institutions met the randomization criteria but were unwilling to participate. Of these 1315 eligible but unwilling patients, 435 started with surgical therapy, and 880 received medical treatment. These 1315 eligible/unwilling patients were compared with the 780 eligible/willing patients regarding a number of baseline characteristics such as demographic factors, medical history, extent of disease, and life-style variables, and all were followed for an average of 5 years. The investigators found that the entry characteristics of randomized patients were generally similar to those of eligible but unwilling patients. Moreover, mortality rates in both the randomized and nonrandomized groups of medically treated patients were similar, as were those for the two groups of surgically treated subjects [7]. These data indicate that those who were willing to enter the CASS trial do not appear to have been a special subset of those eligible for randomization but seemed representative of all eligible patients. The availability of these data strengthen the belief that the study results are generalizable beyond the trial population.

Allocation of Study Regimens

Since participants and nonparticipants may differ in important ways related to the outcome under study, allocation into the various treatment groups should take place only after subjects have been determined to be eligible and have expressed a willingness to participate (see Fig. 8-1). The effects of a treatment, procedure, or program can be compared with those of one or more of a variety of groups, such as another dosage of the same drug, another therapy or program, continuation of standard medical practice, or a placebo. To maximize the probability that the groups receiving these differing interventions will be comparable, assignment to a study group should be at random. Random assignment implies that each individual has the same chance of receiving each of the possible treatments and that the probability that a given subject will receive a particular allocation is independent of the probability that any other subject will receive the same treatment assignment. The two methods most commonly used to achieve this objective are the use of a table of random numbers or the use of a computer-generated randomization list. In addition, when the outcome under study is anticipated to vary appreciably in frequency among subgroups of the study population, for instance, between men and women, or when response is likely to differ markedly between subjects, such as those with different stages of disease, the efficiency of the study might be increased by ensuring that treatment groups are approximately equal or balanced with respect to such characteristics. This can be accomplished by a somewhat more complex form of randomization, called blocking, in which every participant is classified with respect to each such variable before allocation and then randomized within the subgroup. Since randomization of large samples virtually guarantees comparability of treatment groups, blocking has particular relevance when the study size is limited [31, 32].

Randomization has many unique advantages when compared with other methods of allocation. First, if randomization is properly done, nobody either involved in deciding whether a patient is eligible to enter into a trial or responsible for the allocation procedure will know the assigned treatment group. Thus, the potential for bias in allocation to study groups is removed, and investigators can be confident that observed differences are not due to the selection of particular patients to receive a given therapy. Whenever a system can be predicted, as with the use of any other procedure to allocate treatment, there is the potential for manipulation. For example, alternate assignment to study and comparison groups is often used but is always liable to potential bias. Specifically, if two willing and eligible subjects presented at the same time with different prognoses, a physician might, consciously or not, enter them into the study in the order that would allow the more seriously ill patient to receive the treatment the physician already believed to be more (or perhaps even less) promising. If a large proportion of subjects were entered in this way, a serious imbalance in the treatment groups with respect to factors affecting the outcome under study would result. A truly more promising treatment could in fact appear less effective than the alternative simply because it was administered to a group less likely to benefit from any form of therapy than the individuals who were systematically assigned to the alternative being studied. Allocation on the basis of day of the week is also subject to a systematic bias, especially for patients presenting at or near midnight.

Another unique advantage of randomization is that on average, the study groups will tend to be comparable with respect to all variables except for the interventions being studied. "On average" implies that the larger the sample size, the more successful the randomization process will be in distributing these factors equally among the groups. For example, the total population of 10,940 participants in the HDFP [23] consisted of 34.3 percent white males, 25.9 percent regular smokers, 26.0 percent current takers of antihypertensive medications, and 5.2 percent

Table 8-1. Selected baseline characteristics of the total study population and the two treatment groups of the Hypertension Detection and Follow-up Program (HDFP)

Baseline characteristics	Total HDFP ($n = 10,940$)	Stepped care ($n = 5485$)	Referred care ($n = 5455$)
White male	34.3%	34.5%	34.1%
Regular smoker	25.9%	25.6%	26.2%
Currently taking antihypertensive medication	26.0%	26.3%	25.7%
History of myocardial infarction	5.2%	5.1%	5.2%

Source: Hypertension Detection and Follow-up Program Cooperative Group, Five-year findings of the Hypertension Detection and Follow-up Program: I. Reduction in mortality of persons with high blood pressure, including mild hypertension. *J.A.M.A.* 242:2562, 1979.

with a history of myocardial infarction. Randomization resulted in two study groups of 5485 (stepped care) and 5455 (referred care) with virtually identical proportions of each of these factors (Table 8-1).

This feature of randomization is important because all baseline characteristics that affect risk and differ between the treatment groups could potentially confound the relationship between exposure and disease. An even more crucial implication, however, is that on average not only will all known confounding variables be equally distributed, but so will all potential confounders that are unsuspected by the investigator because of limitations of biologic knowledge at the time the trial is initiated. Variables that are not identifiable cannot be dealt with by any direct procedures. Consequently, the only possible way to achieve control for any influence of unknown variables is through randomization. When the sample size is sufficiently large, both known and unknown confounding factors are distributed equally among treatment groups. Thus, randomization can provide a degree of assurance about the comparability of the study groups that is simply not possible in any observational study design.

Finally, a significant advantage of randomization is the deservedly favorable impression that this design strategy may have on those reading the published results of a trial. When exposure is assigned by a method other than randomization, the burden of proof is on the investigator to show that all possible biases in the allocation of patients to a study group or confounding effects of known or unknown factors that may differ between the study groups did not account for the observed result. Thus, there is an inherent confidence in the results of a well-designed and conducted randomized trial that cannot be achieved with any alternative allocation scheme [16].

A type of nonrandomized intervention study that is sometimes seen in the literature is one in which the comparison group is historical. In this instance, the experience of a group of hospitalized patients allocated to a new agent or procedure is compared with that of other patients in the same hospital who had been exposed to the preexisting standard form of treatment. In general, such observational comparisons can provide reliable evidence when there is a relatively large effect of the new treatment compared with previous standard therapy. For example, the efficacy of treatment of malignant hypertension was demonstrated by observing a far lower mortality experience of newly treated patients with those previously untreated [12]. However, in the more common circumstance, where the effects are small to moderate, it is difficult to distinguish reliably such differences between the study groups. Since data on the new treatment and the standard therapy are collected during two different time periods, there may have been changes in the patient population admitted to the hospital, other advances in diagnostic or treatment methods, or even general modifications of health behavior. Any or all such factors may result in changes in the frequency of the disease that are totally unrelated to the intervention being tested.

Maintenance and Assessment of Compliance

By definition, an intervention study requires the active participation and cooperation of the study subjects. After agreeing to participate, subjects in a trial of medical therapy may deviate from the protocol for a variety of reasons, including developing side effects, forgetting to take their medication, or simply withdrawing their consent after randomization. Analogously, in a trial of surgical therapy, those who were randomized to one group may choose to obtain the alternative treatment on their own initiative. In addition, there will be instances where participants cannot comply, such as when the condition of a randomized patient rapidly worsens to the point where therapy becomes contraindicated. Consequently, the problem of achieving and maintaining high compliance is an issue in the design and conduct of all clinical trials.

The extent of noncompliance in any trial is related to the length of time that participants are expected to adhere to the intervention, as well as to the complexity of the study protocol. There are a number of possible strategies that can be adopted to try to enhance compliance among the participants in a trial. As discussed earlier, selection of a population of individuals who are both interested and reliable can enhance compliance rates. For example, the CPPT [26] was conducted among men with elevated blood cholesterol levels, who were consequently at increased risk of developing CHD. Such individuals in general have a much stronger motivation to comply with a study regimen than those at usual risk. Other ways of attempting to increase compliance include frequent contact with participants by home or clinic visit, telephone, or mail; the use of calendar packs of study medication, in which each pill is labelled with the day it is to be taken; and the use of incentives such as detailed medical information not ordinarily available from their usual source of health care.

Monitoring compliance is important because noncompliance will decrease the statistical power of a trial to detect any true effect of the study treatment. Thus, the interpretation of any trial result must take into account the extent to which there was adherence to the intervention regimen. To the extent that participants in the alternative treatment group receive the intervention under study or those in the intervention group do not actually adhere to their assigned regimen, the two groups will become very similar in terms of exposure. Consequently, any true magnitude of effect of the intervention may be obscured. For example, in the Multiple Risk Factor Intervention Trial (MRFIT) [27], 12,866 healthy men, aged 35 to 57 years, who were at high risk of developing CHD on the basis of current cigarette smoking, elevated blood pressure, and high blood cholesterol were randomized either to a special intervention program designed to promote the reduction of these three risk factors or to their usual sources of health care in the community. After 7 years of follow-up, there was a nonsignificant 7-percent decrease in deaths from CHD in the special intervention group compared with those allocated to usual medical care. One factor that contributed to the inability of the study to detect a significant difference despite sizeable reductions in the levels of all three risk factors in the special intervention group was that a large proportion of individuals in the usual care group also stopped smoking, received antihypertensive medication, and lowered their serum cholesterol through weight loss or dietary changes. Although it is not possible to know for certain why these men assigned to receiving usual care became "noncompliant" with their treatment regimen, it seems likely that it was due to the increasing awareness of the general public of the adverse effects of smoking, hypertension, and high cholesterol and attempts to alter these risk factors.

The higher the degree of compliance with the offered program, the greater the extent to which observed differences between those allocated to alternative therapies reflect real differences in the effects of the treatments themselves. Thus, compliance levels must be measured, which is generally not easy. All of the measures available to estimate compliance have inherent limitations. The simplest measure is a self-report. In fact, for some interventions, such as exercise programs or behavior modifications, this may be the only practical way to assess compliance. In trials of pharmacologic agents, pill counts have been used, where participants bring unused medication to each clinic visit or return it to the investigators at specified intervals. For example, participants in the CPPT brought unused packets of cholestyramine or placebo to each follow-up visit [26]. Although this method may eliminate inaccuracies due to poor memory, it assumes that the subject has ingested all medication that has not been returned to the clinic. A more objective means of assessing compliance, which is also expensive and logistically difficult, is the use of biochemical parameters to validate self-reports. Laboratory determinations on either blood or urine can frequently detect the presence of active drugs or metabolites. In cases where drugs or metabolites are difficult to measure, or for subjects taking an inert placebo, a safe biochemical marker such as trace amounts of riboflavin can be added to the treatment. Laboratory determinations are limited, however, in that they usually only reflect whether medication was taken in the preceding day or two and thus cannot be used as a reliable measure for long-term compliance.

Inevitably, some proportion of participants in a trial will become noncompliant despite all reasonable efforts. In such instances, maintaining any level of compliance is preferable to complete noncompliance. Moreover, as will be discussed, every randomized subject should be included in the primary analysis of any intervention study, so that it is essential to obtain as complete follow-up information as possible on those who have discontinued the treatment program. Investigators should pursue follow-up data on outcome for such individuals for the duration of the trial in a manner identical to that for subjects who continue to comply.

Uniform and High Rates of Ascertainment of Outcome

Another crucial issue to be considered in the design and conduct of an intervention study is the ascertainment of the outcome(s) of interest. The primary objective is to ensure that results are not biased by the collection of more complete or accurate information from one or another of the study groups. In addition to the need for uniform ascertainment of outcome is the requirement for complete follow-up of study participants over the duration of the trial. For some research questions, ascertainment of the outcome may require only a short follow-up period, as in a study of in-hospital mortality after treatment for acute myocardial infarction or in a trial assessing the acute toxicity following administration of a new chemotherapeutic agent. In these circumstances, it is often relatively easy to maintain contact with all participants during the entire study period. Often, however, many years of follow-up will be needed, especially for trials of treatments or other interventions that affect the risk of developing or dying from chronic diseases. As the period of time over which subjects must be followed increases, maintaining complete ascertainment of outcomes becomes more difficult. When outcomes for a proportion of study subjects are not identified but that proportion is similar for all treatment groups, the smaller the losses, the greater the likelihood that the magnitude of a bias will be small. On the other hand, if the proportion of outcomes that are not ascertained is large or differs among the study groups, the result could be an under- or overestimate or even, by chance, reflect the true effect. To avoid this situation, where it is not possible to know the magnitude or direction of the bias, it is crucial to keep the number of individuals lost to follow-up to an absolute minimum. For studies with mortality as an end point, the availability of the U.S. National Death Index has enabled researchers, at the very least, to assess the vital status on every individual entered into a trial [37]. Methods to maintain high follow-up rates in intervention studies are identical to those used in prospective cohort studies, which have been described in Chapter 7.

The potential for observation bias in ascertainment of outcome can exist in an intervention study in that knowledge of a participant's treatment status might, consciously or not, influence the identification or reporting of relevant events. The likelihood of such bias is directly related to the subjectivity of the outcomes under study. If the end point being considered is total mortality, observation bias is unlikely, since the fact of death is objective and indisputable and cannot be affected by knowledge of a patient's treatment regimen. In contrast, ascertainment of a specific cause of death may be less clear-cut and thus may be influenced by a clinician's knowledge of treatment assignment. Moreover, there are trials in which the end points of interest may include subjective outcomes such as severity of illness, frequency of side effects, increased mobility, or decreased pain. In all these circumstances, it is especially important to utilize methods to minimize the likelihood of any systematic difference in the ascertainment of outcomes between study groups.

One such approach is to keep the study participants and/or the investigators blinded so far as possible to the identity of the interventions until data collection has been completed. In a double-blind design, neither the participants nor the investigators responsible for assessment of outcomes know to which treatment group an individual has been assigned. The ability to conduct a double-blind trial is dependent on having treatment and comparison programs that are as nearly identical as possible. Consequently, in many trials, especially of drug therapies, the comparison group is assigned to receiving a placebo, which is an inert agent indistinguishable from the active treatment. By making it extremely difficult, if not impossible, to differentiate between the treatment and comparison groups, the use of a placebo will minimize bias in the ascertainment of both subjective disease outcomes and side effects.

One problem in the evaluation of such end points is the well-documented tendency for individuals to report a favorable response to any therapy regardless of the physiologic efficacy of what they receive. This phenomenon is referred to as the placebo effect. If a study does not use placebo control, it is impossible to tell whether subjective outcomes are due to the actual trial treatments, to the extra attention participants receive, or merely to their belief that the treatment will help. For example, in 1962, Wangensteen and colleagues [43] introduced a new technique for the treatment of duodenal ulcer, gastric "freezing," in which a coolant was administered by nasogastric tube to suppress secretions. In their case series of 31 patients, all reported marked or complete relief of pain following this procedure. Despite the fact that the data were descriptive and therefore could not test the hypothesis, gastric freezing began to be used in many clinical centers. Subsequently, concern about its efficacy and safety led to the initiation of a randomized trial [36]. Specifically, of 137 patients with duodenal ulcer, 69 were assigned at random to gastric freezing and 68 received a placebo, in that the nasogastric tube was inserted but coolant applied only as far as the upper esophagus. Using these procedures, all patients were aware of the presence of the coolant, but in the placebo group, no direct effect on gastric secretions was possible. The trial showed similar proportions of marked or complete relief of pain, suppression of secretions, as well as frequency and severity of recurrence between those who received the actual freezing procedure and those who did not. These statistically nonsignificant results suggested that the relief of symptoms reported by all subjects in the case series may have been due to the psychological effect of the procedure rather than any true physiologic benefits.

On the other hand, persons taking a drug or undergoing a medical procedure may be sensitized to their physical condition and tend to ascribe every symptom or unusual occurrence to their treatment. For example, in the Veterans Administration Cooperative Study of Antihypertensive Agents [42], 186 men were randomized to a combination of hydrochlorothiazide, reserpine, and hydralazine, and 194 were assigned to placebo. One of the anticipated side effects of these agents is impotence. Nevertheless, the proportions of subjects reporting this outcome at any time during the study period were virtually identical in the treatment and placebo groups (29% and 28%, respectively). Similarly, in the Aspirin Myocardial Infarction Study [3], 23.7 percent of subjects randomized to receiving 1 gm of aspirin per day reported symptoms suggestive of peptic ulcer, gastritis, or erosion of gastric mucosa, whereas 14.9 percent of those receiving placebo reported similar symptoms. If the trial had not used placebo control, an erroneously high rate of gastrointestinal side effects would have been attributed to aspirin, whereas in actuality the rate was 23.7 percent minus 14.9 percent, or 8.8 percent. The use of a placebo will ensure that all aspects of the program offered to participants are identical except for the actual experimental treatment. Consequently, by comparing the proportions of individuals in the active treatment and placebo groups who report a particular symptom or outcome, the true incidence of subjective treatment-related effects can be determined.

Thus, the primary strength of a double-blind design is to eliminate the potential for observation bias. Of course, a concomitant limitation is that such trials are usually more complex and difficult to conduct. Procedures must be established for immediate "unblinding" of a participant's physician in the event of serious side effects or other clinical emergencies in which this information seems essential. Moreover, in some circumstances, it is not possible to "blind" both the participants and the investigators to the allocated treatment regimen. It is very difficult to design a double-blind trial for the evaluation of programs involving substantial changes in life-style, such as exercise, cigarette smoking or diet, surgical procedures, or drugs with characteristic side effects. In these circumstances, a single-blind or unblinded trial may be necessary. In a single-blind design, the investigator alone is aware of which intervention a subject is receiving, while in an unblinded or open trial, both the subject and the investigator know to which study group the individual has been assigned.

Single-blind or unblinded trials are simpler to execute than double-blind studies and may be more acceptable both to physicians randomizing their patients and to participants. Of course, these designs also have special problems. For example, subjects aware that they are not on the new or experimental program may become dissatisfied and drop out of the trial, thus resulting in differential compliance or loss to follow-up. Moreover, as discussed earlier, knowledge of the intervention to which the participant has been assigned again raises the potential for observation bias in the reporting of side effects or assessment of outcomes. Thus, when a double-blind design is not possible, it is imperative that special precautions be taken to reduce the potential for observation bias. For measurement of both side effects and end points, objective criteria should be used, and the study groups should be followed with equal intensity by independent examiners who are unaware of the subjects' treatment status.

Use of a Factorial Design

In this chapter, we have thus far considered issues in the design of intervention trials of a single factor, where one treatment or regimen is compared with one or more alternatives or placebo. Given the cost and feasibility issues in designing clinical trials, one technique to improve efficiency is to test two or more hypotheses simultaneously in a factorial design. A clinical trial of two hypotheses can utilize a two-by-two factorial design, in which subjects are first randomized to treatments α or β to address one hypothesis, and then within each treatment group there is further randomization to treatments A or B to evaluate a second ques-

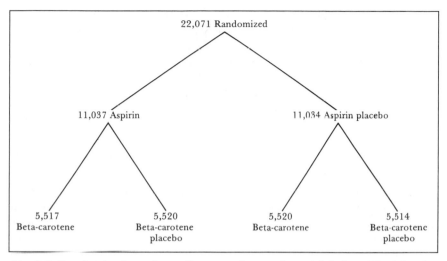

Fig. 8-3. Randomization scheme for a two-by-two factorial design: Physicians' Health Study.

tion. Similarly, in a two-by-two-by-two factorial design, each of these subgroups would be further randomized into two additional intervention groups to address a third hypothesis, and so on.

The Physicians' Health Study [19, 38] utilizes a two-by-two factorial design to evaluate the two hypotheses that consumption of low-dose aspirin reduces cardiovascular mortality and that beta-carotene consumption decreases cancer incidence. As shown in Figure 8-3, the more than 22,000 willing and eligible physicians were first randomized into two groups, one receiving aspirin and the other aspirin placebo. Each of these treatment groups was further randomized to receiving either beta-carotene or its placebo. Thus, physicians in the trial were allocated to one of four possible regimens: aspirin alone, beta-carotene alone, both active agents, or both placebos.

The principal advantage of the factorial design is its ability to answer two or more questions in a single trial for only a marginal increase in cost. Moreover, as in the Physicians' Health Study, the use of a factorial design can allow testing a less mature hypothesis together with a more mature question having reliable evidence available to justify its evaluation. The Physicians' Health Study sought primarily to test the hypothesis that a single 325-mg aspirin tablet taken every other day could reduce total cardiovascular mortality among men with no history of a prior myocardial infarction. Since there was a large body of laboratory and observational epidemiologic data, as well as information from trials of aspirin among those with a history of myocardial infarction or unstable angina [2, 25], a primary prevention trial of aspirin seemed warranted. Whether beta-carotene could decrease cancer incidence, however, was a promising but as yet immature hypothesis [20, 21, 33]. Nevertheless, as discussed earlier, because of the continuing widespread use of multivitamin supplements in the U.S., for reasons of feasibility it seemed important that a trial of beta-carotene be conducted as soon as possible. By using a two-by-two factorial design, the carotene hypothesis could also be tested in the Physicians' Health Study without materially affecting the sensitivity or the cost of the aspirin component.

Ideally, of course, the additional treatments in a factorial design should not complicate trial operations, materially affect eligibility requirements, or cause side effects that could lead to poor compliance or losses to follow-up. In addition, the possibility of an interaction between treatment regimens must be considered. Fortunately, such interactions tend to affect the magnitude of observed treatment effects rather than changing their direction from benefit to harm or vice versa. Moreover, while the effects of interactions could be viewed as a potential limitation of a factorial trial, this design in fact facilitates the identification of their existence [38]. For example, in the Second International Study of Infarct Survival [24], the two major questions of interest are the efficacy of intravenous streptokinase and of low-dose oral aspirin in the reduction of cardiovascular mortality after an acute myocardial infarction. It may well be that any benefit of the thrombolytic agent intravenous streptokinase would be greater in the presence of the antiplatelet drug aspirin than in its absence. The use of a two-by-two factorial design allows for the assessment of such an interaction, which could not be done in a single-factor study.

STOPPING RULES: DECISION FOR EARLY TERMINATION OF A TRIAL

In the design phase of a trial, there is a need to develop guidelines for deciding whether a trial should be modified or terminated before originally scheduled. In addition, in some trials of preventive and therapeutic regimens, individuals enter the study over an extended period of time, and the experience of the early participants becomes available while later individuals are still being enrolled. To assure that the welfare of the participants is protected, interim results should be monitored by a group that is independent of the investigators conducting the trial. If the data indicate a clear and extreme benefit on the primary end point due to the intervention, or if one treatment is clearly harmful, then early termination of the trial must be considered. For example, the Beta-Blocker Heart Attack Trial [10] was a randomized, double-blind study comparing propranolol with placebo in 3837 patients with a recent myocardial infarction. The trial was terminated 9 months before the scheduled closing date on the recommendation of an external data monitoring board. At that time, the propranolol group had a highly statistically significant ($P = 0.005$) 26-percent reduction in the primary end point, total mortality, when compared with the placebo group. The emergence of such an extreme result raised the question of whether it would be ethical to continue withholding propranolol from the placebo group.

Of at least equal importance, it would also seem unethical to stop a trial prematurely based solely on emerging trends from a small number of patients. Such findings might well be only transient and disappear or even reverse after data have accumulated from a larger sample. For example, on three occasions during the first 30 months of the Coronary Drug Project (CDP) trial [9], the mortality of the group receiving clofibrate was significantly lower, at the conventional $P = 0.05$ level, than that of the placebo group. However, the finding did not achieve the extreme level of significance recommended for consideration of early termination [31, 32]. The study group therefore decided not to stop the trial but to continue to monitor the results closely. On this basis, the scheduled follow-up period was completed, and when the final results were analyzed, the mortality of the clofibrate group was, in fact, identical to that of the placebo group (25.5% versus 25.4%).

Thus, a decision to terminate a study early is based on a number of complex issues and must be made with a great deal of caution. There are a variety of sophisticated statistical methods that are currently available for monitoring the accumulating data from a clinical trial. As a general rule, the first requirement for even considering modification or early termination of an ongoing trial is the observation of a sustained statistical association that is so extreme, and, therefore, so highly significant, that it is virtually impossible to arise by chance alone [1, 16, 31, 34]. While a statistical test should not normally be used as the sole basis for the decision to stop or continue a trial, it serves an important function to alert those responsible for monitoring interim data to the possibility that there may be cause for concern. The observed association must then be considered in the context of the totality of evidence, including known or postulated biologic mechanisms that might explain such an effect, if it was unanticipated; results from other randomized trials and, to a lesser extent, those from observational studies; and an assessment of how the observed association would affect the overall risk-to-benefit ratio of the intervention. Similarly, the specific statistical criterion used to alert investigators to the need to consider these issues cannot be specified exactly for all trials. In fact, there are many different views of what constitutes sufficient proof that an observed association in interim data does not represent a temporary, random fluctuation. Moreover, some investigators feel that this criterion should not be equally stringent for beneficial and harmful effects, or with respect to anticipated and unanticipated findings. Whatever the specific guideline, however, the aim is to achieve an equitable balance between, on the one hand, protection of randomized participants against real harm and, on the other, minimizing the risk of mistakenly modifying or stopping the trial prematurely. Detailed discussions of the issues involved in such decisions can be found elsewhere [1, 9, 10, 16, 31, 34].

SAMPLE SIZE CONSIDERATIONS: STATISTICAL POWER

Although sample size must be addressed early in the planning stage of any analytic epidemiologic investigation, it has particular importance in an intervention study. Observational analytic study designs can most reliably study large effects, so that the sample may be moderate in size. In contrast, a trial must have a sufficient sample size to have adequate statistical power or ability to detect reliably the small to moderate but clinically important differences between treatment groups that are most likely to occur [47]. Peto [29] has stated that most of the roughly 2000 randomized clinical trials currently underway worldwide are of "little or no scientific value," based primarily on the fact that these studies are of inadequate sample size to detect such effects reliably. We believe that such trials actually have the potential for great scientific harm, especially if their results are misinterpreted as demonstrating that an intervention has no effect when in fact the sample size was not sufficient to provide an informative null result. Even if an investigator feels confident that a new intervention will have a large benefit (i.e., a 50% or greater reduction in the primary end point), it is far preferable to design a trial to test the more likely small to moderate benefit (i.e., 10–20%) and stop the trial early than to anticipate a larger effect and have no ability to detect smaller but nonetheless clinically important differences.

In designing a clinical trial, investigators often devote much time and effort to increasing the total number of participants enrolled. However, the statistical power of a trial to detect a postulated difference between treatment groups, if one truly exists, is dependent not simply on the sample size, but more specifically on two factors: (1) the total number of end points experienced by the study population and (2) the difference in compliance between the treatment groups [29].

Accumulation Of Adequate End Points

To accumulate sufficient numbers of end points, two major strategies may be considered: first, selecting a high-risk population for study and, second, ensuring an adequate duration of follow-up.

Selection of a High-Risk Population

A primary strategy to ensure the accumulation of an adequate number of end points is to select individuals at increased risk of developing the outcomes of interest. With respect to the general population, a simple but important criterion for this selection is age. Since the frequency of most outcomes rises with increasing age, the impact of this factor can be dramatic. For example, in a study of mortality from CHD, 10,000 men aged 45 and 54 would be expected to experience only about 27 coronary deaths during a 1-year follow-up period, while a comparable group of men aged 65 to 74 followed for 1 year would yield about 167 such fatalities [40]. Other risk factors on which selection of a study population might be based include sex, occupation, geographic area, or one or more medical or life-style variables. As mentioned earlier, the CPPT [26] was conducted among middle-aged men at increased risk of CHD due to elevated blood cholesterol levels (above 265 mg/dl). Similarly, MRFIT [27] selected men aged 35 to 57 years who were in the upper 15 percent of a risk score distribution based on combined levels of cigarette smoking, blood cholesterol, and/or blood pressure.

The collection of baseline data can be planned to allow the identification of particular subgroups who might experience different effects of an intervention. For example, in the Physicians' Health Study, if the true reduction in cancer incidence due to beta-carotene is 30 percent or greater, there is excellent power to detect that difference among the total of more than 22,000 randomized physicians. On the other hand, if the overall reduction in risk is only 10 percent, it would not be possible to detect such an effect with great assurance. However, a 10-percent overall reduction could result from a much larger effect confined exclusively to a particular subgroup, in this case, those with the lowest levels of beta-carotene or vitamin A at baseline [30]. This finding could easily be detected if participants were stratified by baseline levels of these parameters. For this reason, prerandomization blood specimens were collected by mail from 14,916 of the participating physicians, to be analyzed for baseline levels of retinol, carotene, retinol-binding protein, as well as other relevant parameters. The availability of these prerandomization blood specimens will increase the sensitivity of the trial to identify which particular subgroup of doctors, if any, stands to benefit most from beta-carotene. If there is a benefit confined to those having low baseline levels, then future public health interventions could be aimed at that target population. Conversely, if there is no true effect of beta-carotene supplementation on cancer incidence, this strategy would in fact produce a more convincing and truly informative null result, for then it could be stated that not only was there no significant overall effect observed, but in addition, no effect of supplementation with this agent was apparent regardless of initial blood levels. Despite the fact that such hypotheses are formulated before data collection, it remains important to keep in mind that such comparisons are not strictly randomized.

Length of the Follow-Up Period

The length of any planned follow-up period should always consider that the actual rate of accrual of end points will be less than projected. This situation is not unusual in clinical trials and may occur for reasons beyond the control of the investigators. First, as discussed previously, those who volunteer to participate in intervention studies are a self-selected group who also tend to experience generally lower morbidity and mortality rates than those who do not take part, regardless of the hypothesis under study or the treatment allocated at random. For example, in planning the Physicians' Health Study, we considered the likelihood that the relatively small proportion of all potential participants who were actually both willing and eligible to enroll would have substantially lower rates of cardiovascular mortality and cancer than the general population, due to the generally better health and habits of U.S. doctors as a whole, to the impact of our exclusion criteria, and to the "healthy volunteer effect." We therefore postulated that the rates of these end points in the trial would be about half those that might be expected. In fact, mortality rates during the first year were less than 20 percent of what would have been expected among a general population with the same age distribution, or about 40 percent of our projection for the initially planned duration of the study (3.5 years). The only way to compensate for this deficit in expected end points would be to extend the length of the follow-up period. In fact, with the continued cooperation and permission of participating doctors, we have doubled the length of follow-up and expect to accrue about four times the number of end points.

Moreover, there may be secular changes in disease rates during the course of the trial, sometimes as great as that due to the intervention studied. For example, as discussed previously, MRFIT [27] was designed to evaluate whether the combined effects of cessation of smoking, control of hypertension, and reduction of cholesterol would decrease the mortality rate from CHD. During the decade in which this trial was conducted, the entire U.S. population, including all MRFIT participants, experienced a marked 25- to 30-percent decline in CHD mortality [17]. In part due to this secular trend, the observed numbers of deaths in the trial were less than two-thirds the numbers expected for the 6-year follow-up period. Extending the length of follow-up would have increased the number of end points, thereby increasing the power of the trial.

The choice of duration of the follow-up period must also take into consideration the postulated mechanism by which the study agent exerts its effects. In the Physicians' Health Study, for example, any benefit from aspirin in reducing cardiovascular mortality is likely to be acute, since the postulated mechanism relates to immediate effects on platelet aggregability. On the other hand, if the beneficial effect of beta-carotene supplementation is analogous to the effect of cessation of cigarette smoking on reduction of lung cancer risk, where it may take 2 years before any decrease begins to become apparent and 6 to 9 before the effect becomes maximal [11], then a much longer period of follow-up is required.

While every effort should be made to incorporate an adequate length of follow-up during the planning phase of a trial, the emergence of new evidence on mechanisms, changes in rates of disease within the general population, and even, on occasion, the failure to achieve a sufficient sample size or enough end points within the trial itself may all, for the reasons discussed above, raise the question of increasing the duration beyond the planned period of follow-up. Any such decision should be made as early in the trial as possible to maintain the scientific credibility of the study and avoid the implication that the change in study design was based on last-minute efforts to achieve statistical significance [16]. For this reason, with the consent of the participating doctors, the Physicians' Health Study research group was able, at an early stage of the study, to secure funding to extend the duration of the trial, based primarily on far lower than expected mortality rates among trial participants. Additional issues that should be considered in making a decision regarding extensions of a trial can be found elsewhere [16].

The Effect of Compliance

In addition to the number of end points accrued, the second major factor influencing the power of the study to detect a true difference between treatment groups is compliance. It is important to remember that the assessment of whether compliance is adequate must include all the study participants, regardless of their particular treatment assignment. The effect of noncompliance in any participant is to make the intervention and comparison groups more alike, which has the result of decreasing the ability of the trial to detect any true differences between the groups. For example, in MRFIT, while the compliance among participants in the special intervention program was generally higher than expected, individuals in the usual care group also stopped smoking, reduced their blood pressure, and lowered their cholesterol to an extent unanticipated by the investigators. As a result, the small differences in risk factors between the groups could only result in a 22-percent reduction in CHD mortality. When coupled with secular decreases in mortality from CHD in the general population, this study did not have adequate power to detect this small effect [27].

The impact of noncompliance is illustrated in Figure 8-4, which shows power curves calculated for various postulated reductions in risk of mortality from CHD due to aspirin in the Physicians' Health Study. The top

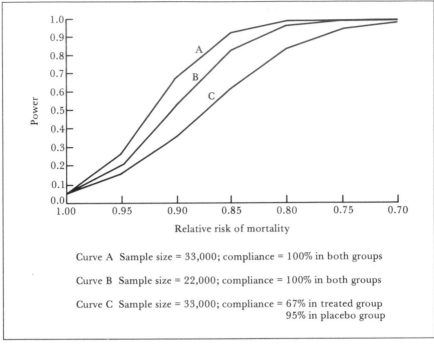

Fig. 8-4. Power curves for various postulated reductions in risk of mortality, total sample sizes, and levels of compliance in those receiving active treatment and placebo.

curve *(A)* represents the power for a total sample size of 33,000 and 100-percent compliance in the active aspirin and placebo groups. The bottom curve *(C)* shows the decrease in power that results when the same number of subjects are randomized, but the compliance rates are only 67 percent among those in the active aspirin group and 95 percent for those taking placebo. The shapes of both curves are approximately the same, but with noncompliance there is less power for the detection of an effect of any size. Moreover, the greatest reduction in power is for the most plausible relative risks, which are on the order of 0.8 to 0.9.

One strategy to maximize compliance that has been used infrequently to date in intervention studies but could have wide applicability in clinical trials is the implementation of a run-in or "wash-out" period prior to actual randomization. All participants receive either the active treatment or placebo for a number of weeks or months before formal randomization to a treatment group. This permits potentially eligible participants who have difficulty adhering to the intervention program or those perceiving adverse effects to withdraw before randomization without affecting the validity of the study [5, 18]. Such a strategy seems particularly attractive in trials where it is not necessary for an intervention to begin during or immediately following an acute event. The effects on power of reducing the sample size in this way is illustrated in Figure 8-4. The middle curve *(B)* represents the power associated with a sample size that is one-third smaller than the 33,000 enrollees in the Physicians' Health Study, or 22,000 subjects, but again with compliance rates of 100 percent in both groups. This results in an intermediate power curve, with less power than if a larger number of good compliers had been randomized, but considerably more than if a larger, mixed group of compliers and noncompliers were randomized. Consequently, the use of techniques to maintain high compliance, such as the use of a run-in period, will maximize the power of a clinical trial to detect small to moderate effects between treatment groups [5].

The actual format of the run-in period will depend on the particular hypotheses being tested. For example, in the Veterans Administration Cooperative Group Study on Antihypertensive Agents [41], male patients whose diastolic blood pressures averaged 90 to 129 mm Hg were considered for admission to a randomized trial of active drug (hydrochlorothiazide plus reserpine plus hydralazine hydrochloride) versus placebo treatment. Following discharge from the hospital, the patients entered a prerandomization phase, where for 2 to 4 months they took daily tablets of a placebo containing a fluorescent biochemical marker (riboflavin) and were seen in the clinic at monthly intervals. Failure to appear for a clinic appointment, failure of the urine to exhibit fluorescence, or a count of returned tablets outside a specific range excluded a potential participant from randomization into the actual trial. Using this procedure, nearly 50 percent of the patients initially eligible for this trial were excluded before randomization for one of these reasons. While decreasing the actual sample size, this technique resulted in a study of greater power due to the exclusion of noncompliers before randomization.

Both the postulated mechanisms of action and frequency of side effects should be considered in determining the specific agents for a run-in period. In the Physicians' Health Study, the postulated beneficial effects of aspirin are acute and side effects common [35], so that it was desirable to expose all willing and eligible subjects to active aspirin during a run-in prior to randomization. On the other hand, as the possible beneficial effects of beta-carotene are cumulative and side effects minimal [21, 33], a placebo rather than active agent was given. Thus, during the 18-week run-in period, all 33,211 physicians who were initially willing and eligible to enroll in the trial took a daily pill from calendar packs containing active aspirin alternating with beta-carotene placebo. At the end of that time, each physician was sent a questionnaire to identify doctors reporting side effects or a desire to discontinue participation, those who wished to continue but whose self-reported compliance was considered inadequate by the investigators, and those who developed a cardiovascular or cancer end point during this period. Using these criteria, about 35 percent of enrolled physicians were deemed ineligible to be randomized and were excluded from the trial. The remaining 22,071 willing and eligible physicians who were proven good compliers were then randomized into one of the four treatment groups.

One possible limitation of a run-in is that by restricting a trial to a group of proven good compliers, the study subjects may differ from the general population with respect to factors that might affect the development of the outcomes of interest. Of course, to the extent that the noncompliers who were eliminated can be followed, this question can be evaluated directly. From a more theoretic perspective, however, this issue relates solely to the generalizability of study findings to the total experimental or reference populations. In that regard, as has been discussed previously, the primary goal in the design of a trial is to ensure that the results obtained are valid. Consequently, any procedure that maximizes compliance, thus increasing the chances of obtaining a valid result, will positively affect the ability to generalize that finding to other populations. The proven good compliers resulting from a run-in period who contribute to a valid result are a far greater asset to the generalizability of the trial results than would be a more representative study population who were unable to maintain adequate compliance for the duration of the study. Such an investigation would lead to an invalid result and, therefore, one that has no potential for generalizability despite having been conducted among a representative population.

ISSUES IN ANALYSIS AND INTERPRETATION

The basic approach to the analysis of intervention studies is similar to that discussed for cohort studies (see Chap. 7), where the fundamental comparison is between the rates of the outcome of interest in the treated group(s) and the corresponding rates in the comparison group(s). As for any analytic epidemiologic study, the roles of chance, bias, and confounding must be evaluated as possible alternative explanations for the findings. Clinical trials, however, have unique design features with special implications for their analysis and interpretation.

As regards chance, a sufficient sample size addresses this issue in a manner analogous to other analytic designs. Moreover, randomization minimizes the potential for bias in the allocation of participants to treatment group, and bias in the observation of outcomes of interest can be minimized by using blind or double-blind procedures. With respect to confounding, randomization tends to distribute both known and unknown confounders evenly among the treatment groups. If the sample size is large, this comparability is virtually guaranteed. However, as discussed previously, with a small sample size or even, in the rare instance, as a result of the play of chance in a large sample, randomization may not always result in groups that are alike with respect to every factor except the treatment under study. Consequently, one important early step in the analysis of any clinical trial is to compare the relevant characteristics of the randomized treatment and comparison groups to assure that balance was achieved. This comparison should always be presented as one of the first tables in the report of the study findings.

For example, Table 8-2 shows the baseline distribution of subjects in the CASS trial [6] for a number of potentially important risk factors for subsequent mortality and the development of CHD. Additional comparisons were made of electrocardiographic, arteriographic, and ventriculographic characteristics. There were no imbalances between patients assigned to receive surgical and those allocated to medical therapy with respect to any of these baseline characteristics. Thus, randomization was effective in establishing two study groups that were similar with respect to other factors that could independently affect the outcome under study. If such a comparison had indicated that randomization was not effective and that there were imbalances between the study groups with respect to known confounding factors, such discrepancies could be controlled in the analysis using statistical techniques analogous to those employed in observational cohort studies (see Chap. 12).

A second important issue that often arises in clinical trials is the question of which subjects to include in the analysis. Some investigators remove from the analysis subjects who were determined to be ineligible after randomization or who did not comply with the study protocol. We believe, however, that the exclusion of any randomized patients from the analysis can lead to biased results. It may be particularly appealing, intuitively, to eliminate those who become noncompliant. However, it is unwarranted and incorrect to perform a fundamental analysis that compares the outcome rates of only those individuals who actually received that treatment with only those who did not.

First, in most trials, perfect compliers represent only a fraction of the total study population. As with losses to follow-up, noncompliance may be related to factors that also affect the risk of the outcome under study, and failure to analyze data on all randomized participants could introduce bias. For example, as mentioned earlier, when all randomized subjects in the Coronary Drug Project trial of clofibrate in the reduction of mortality following myocardial infarction were included in the major analysis, the 5-year total mortality rates in the two groups were very similar (18.0% versus 19.5%) [9]. To explore the effect of compliance on

Table 8-2. Baseline characteristics of participants in the
Coronary Artery Surgery Study, by treatment group

Variable	Medical group ($n = 390$)	Surgical group ($n = 390$)
Sex		
Male	90.0%	90.5%
Female	7.5	7.3
Race: White	98.7	98.0
Work status		
Full-time	64.1	71.0
Part-time	4.6	4.6
Retired or quit	22.8	19.5
Other	8.5	4.9
Angina		
None	21.5	22.1
Class I	12.1	16.9
Class III–IV	0.0	0.0
Nonexertional	4.1	5.4
Cigarette use		
Present smoker	40.8	38.7
Former smoker	43.6	44.4
Never smoked	15.6	16.9
Medical history		
Prior MI	62.6	57.2
Hypertension	29.4	32.7
Congestive failure	2.3	3.9
Diabetes mellitus	8.1	9.3
Stroke	2.1	2.1
Peripheral artery disease	9.3	7.3
Use of medications		
Nitroglycerin	54.9	56.2
Long-acting nitrates	44.6	47.3
Beta-blockers	42.6	44.1
Antiarrhythmics	9.0	9.7

Source: Coronary Artery Surgery Study (CASS), A randomized trial of
coronary artery bypass surgery: Comparability of entry characteristics and
survival in randomized patients and nonrandomized patients meeting
randomization criteria. *J.A.C.C.* 3:114, 1984.

this outcome, the investigators then analyzed the mortality experience within the clofibrate group and found that those whose compliance was at least 80 percent had a mortality rate of 15.0 percent, compared with 24.6 percent among those who were poor compliers. Such a finding might be erroneously interpreted to indicate that clofibrate reduces mortality. Indeed, a similar analysis within the placebo group found a comparable disparity in mortality among compliers and noncompliers, with rates of 15.1 and 28.2 percent, respectively [8]. These data do indicate that in both the active and placebo groups, compliers are different from noncompliers in ways that affect their prognosis. Even after controlling for 40 known possible confounders, there was still a difference in the mortality rates in the placebo group between good (16.4%) and poor (25.8%) compliers. Thus, there must be additional but unknown variables associated with both compliance and mortality in this trial. These data clearly show that subgroup comparisons of compliers did not provide valid results.

A second limitation in evaluating data on only those subjects who comply with the study regimen is that such an analysis does not address the actual research question being posed in an intervention study—whether the *offering* of a treatment program is of benefit. While we wish to study the actual effect of the treatment, we are in fact randomizing only on the basis of the offering of treatment, so that we must analyze the data on this basis to preserve the power of randomization. It is only the entire groups allocated by randomization that are truly comparable. Once participants are randomized to a treatment group, their subsequent health experience must be assessed and analyzed along with all others in that group, regardless of whether they comply with their assigned regimen. This methodologic issue emphasizes the need to maintain high compliance with their assigned regimen among all study participants. It is also important to keep in mind that if a particular regimen is so difficult and uncomfortable that it is likely to be accepted and used by only a small proportion of the reference population, it may not be practical to recommend its use, no matter how effective the actual treatment may be.

Thus, in all circumstances, the comparison that is optimal to estimate the true benefit to be obtained from the intervention program is to analyze by intention to treat—in other words, "once randomized, always analyzed." For this reason, it is imperative to maintain high levels of compliance, keep losses to follow-up at a minimum, and to collect complete information on all randomized subjects. Those who are no longer complying with the study regimen should continue to provide all follow-up information whenever possible, or at the very least, their vital status should be ascertained. Subsequent analyses can certainly be performed based on that subgroup of participants who actually received their assigned treatment. However, if this is done, while it is possible to perform analyses that achieve balance in the distribution of known confounders, it is impossible to regain the control of unknown confounders that had been achieved originally through randomization.

The need to perform randomized comparisons in the analyses of data from a trial is equally important when subgroups are identified on the basis of other characteristics besides compliance. Investigators are often tempted to examine differences in treatment effects among those with various baseline characteristics, such as age, prognostic factors, or previous medical history. For example, in MRFIT [28], a subgroup analysis by presence or absence of resting electrocardiogram abnormalities suggested that among men with such abnormalities at baseline, those receiving the special intervention program actually had an increased risk of death from CHD relative to those in the group allocated to usual medical care. This finding led to a further exploration of the effects of the intervention among those with various levels of hypertension. The investigators wisely concluded that "subgroup analyses must be interpreted with caution, particularly those that go beyond the randomized clinical trial design by the MRFIT" and added that "these findings pose hypotheses for investigation by other researchers in systemic hypertension" [28].

In general, the caveats needed to compare subgroups defined a priori by baseline characteristics are far less than those required when comparisons are made on the basis of variables chosen after randomization such as compliance. As regards the former, a minor concern involves a loss of statistical power because only subgroups of the total number of randomized subjects are being compared. A greater concern, however, is to ensure adequate control of variables that may no longer be distributed at random among the subgroups. With respect to analyses of subgroups defined a posteriori on the basis of information accumulated after randomization, they can only raise data-derived hypotheses, not test particular research questions.

CONCLUSION

The ultimate goal of any intervention study is to provide either a definitive positive result on which public policy can be based or a reliable and informative null finding that can then safely permit the redistribution of resources to other important areas of research. Intervention studies certainly can be more difficult to design and conduct than observational epidemiologic studies, due to their unique problems of ethics, feasibility, and costs. However, trials that are sufficiently large, randomized, and carefully designed, conducted, and analyzed can provide the strongest and most direct epidemiologic evidence on which to make a judgment about the existence of a cause-effect relationship.

STUDY QUESTIONS

1. In the Physicians' Health Study [19], 22,071 male physicians were randomized and mortality was postulated to be 70 percent that of white males in the general population. During the first 2 years, mortality was less than 25 percent rather than the anticipated 70 percent.
   a. How do you explain these findings?
   b. What could be done at that stage of the trial to increase the power of the study to maximize the chances of observing the small to moderate effects anticipated, which include a 20-percent reduction in total cardiovascular mortality, a 10-percent reduction in mortality from all causes, and a 30-percent reduction in cancer rates?
2. During the planning phase of the Physicians' Health Study, which restricted admission to male physicians between the ages of 40 and 84, it was suggested that female physicians be included to study the effect of aspirin in women and to see if there was a different effect in women as compared with men. Discuss the advantages and disadvantages of including female physicians in the trial.
3. As discussed earlier, in the MRFIT trial [27], 480 end points were anticipated, and only 260 were observed. Consequently, at the end of the trial, the reduction in cardiovascular deaths was statistically non-significant.
   a. What factors contributed to these findings?
   b. What changes in the study design might have enabled MRFIT to report a more definitive result?

REFERENCES

1. Armitage, P. *Sequential Medical Trials* (2nd ed.). New York: Wiley, 1975.
2. Aspirin for heart patients. *FDA Drug Bulletin* 15:34, 1985.
3. Aspirin Myocardial Infarction Study Research Group. A randomized, controlled trial of aspirin in persons recovered from myocardial infarction. *J.A.M.A.* 243:661, 1980.
4. Ast, D. B., Finn, S. B., and McCaffrey, I. The Newburgh-Kingston Caries Fluorine Study: I. Dental findings after three years of water fluoridation. *Am. J. Public Health* 40:716, 1950.
5. Buring, J. E., and Hennekens, C. H. Sample Size and Compliance in Randomized Trials. In M. A. Sestili and J. G. Dell (eds.), *Chemoprevention Clinical Trials: Problems and Solutions, 1984*. N.I.H. Publication No. 85-2715. Hyattsville, MD: U.S. D.H.H.S., 1985. Pp. 7–11.
6. Coronary Artery Surgery Study (CASS). A randomized trial of coronary artery bypass surgery. *Circulation* 68:939, 1983.
7. Coronary Artery Surgery Study (CASS). A randomized trial of coronary artery bypass surgery: Comparability of entry characteristics and survival in

randomized patients and nonrandomized patients meeting randomization criteria. *J.A.C.C.* 3:114, 1984.

8. Coronary Drug Project Research Group. Influence of adherence to treatment and response of cholesterol on mortality in the Coronary Drug Project. *N. Engl. J. Med.* 303:1038, 1980.

9. Coronary Drug Project Research Group. Practical aspects of decision making in clinical trials: The Coronary Drug Project as a case study. *Controlled Clin. Trials* 1:363, 1981.

10. DeMets, D. L., Hardy, R., Friedman, L. M., et al. Statistical aspects of early termination in the Beta-Blocker Heart Attack Trial. *Controlled Clin. Trials* 5:362, 1984.

11. Doll, R., and Peto, R. Cigarette smoking and bronchial carcinoma: Dose and time relationships among regular smokers and lifelong non-smokers. *J. Epidemiol. Community Health* 32:303, 1978.

12. Dustan, H. P., Schneckloth, R. E., Corcoran, A. S., et al. The effectiveness of long-term treatment of malignant hypertension. *Circulation* 18:644, 1958.

13. Fisher, B., Bauer, M., Margolese, R., et al. Five-year results of a randomized clinical trial comparing total mastectomy and segmental mastectomy with or without radiation in the treatment of breast cancer. *N. Engl. J. Med.* 312:665, 1985.

14. Fisher, B., Redmond, C., Fisher, E. R., et al. Ten-year results of a randomized clinical trial comparing radical mastectomy and total mastectomy with or without radiation. *N. Engl. J. Med.* 312:674, 1985.

15. Francis, T., Jr., Korns, F. T., Voight, R. B., et al. An evaluation of the 1954 poliomyelitis vaccine trials: Summary report. *Am. J. Public Health* 45:1, 1955.

16. Friedman, L. M., Furberg, C. D., and DeMets, D. L. *Fundamentals of Clinical Trials* (2nd ed.). Littleton, MA: PSG, 1985.

17. Havlik, R. J., and Feinleib, M. (eds.). *Proceedings of the Conference on the Decline in Coronary Heart Disease Mortality.* U.S. D.H.E.W., N.I.H. Publication No. 79-1610, 1979.

18. Hennekens, C. H. Issues in the design and conduct of clinical trials. *J.N.C.I.* 73:1473, 1984.

19. Hennekens, C. H., and Eberlein, K., for the Physicians' Health Study Research Group. A randomized trial of aspirin and beta-carotene among U.S. physicians. *Prev. Med.* 14:165-8, 1985.

20. Hennekens, C. H., Stampfer, M., and Willett, W. Micronutrients and cancer chemoprevention. *Cancer Detect. Prev.* 7:147, 1984.

21. Hennekens, C. H. Vitamin A Analogues in Cancer Chemoprevention. In V. T. Devita, Jr., S. Hellman, and S. A. Rosenberg (eds.), *Important Advances in Oncology.* Philadelphia: Lippincott, 1986. Pp. 867–71.

22. Herbert, V. The vitamin craze. *Arch. Intern. Med.* 140:173, 1980.

23. Hypertension Detection and Follow-Up Program Cooperative Group. Five-year findings of the Hypertension Detection and Follow-up Program: I. Reduction in mortality of persons with high blood pressure, including mild hypertension. *J.A.M.A.* 242:2562, 1979.

24. ISIS-2 Steering Committee (P. Sleight, Chairman; R. Collins, Coordinator; R. Peto, Statistician). Personal communication, 1986.

25. Lewis, H. D., Jr., Davis, J. W., Archibald, D. G., et al. Protective effects of

aspirin against acute myocardial infarction and death in men with unstable angina: Results of a Veterans Administration Cooperative Study. *N. Engl. J. Med.* 309:396, 1983.

26. Lipid Research Clinics Program. The Lipid Research Clinics Coronary Primary Prevention Trial results: I. Reduction of incidence of CHD. *J.A.M.A.* 251:351, 1984.

27. Multiple Risk Factor Intervention Trial Research Group. Multiple Risk Factor Intervention Trial: Risk factor changes and morbidity results. *J.A.M.A.* 248:1465, 1982.

28. Multiple Risk Factor Intervention Trial Research Group. Baseline rest electrocardiographic abnormalities, antihypertensive treatment, and mortality in the Multiple Risk Factor Intervention Trial. *Am. J. Cardiol.* 55:1, 1985.

29. Peto, R. Statistics of Cancer Trials. In K. E. Halnan (ed.), *Treatment of Cancer.* London: Chapman and Hall, 1982. Pp. 867–71.

30. Peto, R. The marked differences between carotenoids and retinoids: Methodological implications for biochemical epidemiology. *Cancer Surv.* 2:327, 1983.

31. Peto, R., Pike, M. C., Armitage, P., et al. Design and analysis of randomized clinical trials requiring prolonged observation of each patient: I. Introduction and design. *Br. J. Cancer* 34:585, 1976.

32. Peto, R., Pike, M. C., Armitage, P., et al. Design and analysis of randomized clinical trials requiring prolonged observation of each patient: II. Analyses and examples. *Br. J. Cancer* 35:1, 1977.

33. Peto, R., Doll, R., Buckley, J. D., et al. Can dietary beta-carotene materially reduce human cancer rates? *Nature* 290:201, 1981.

34. Pocock, S. J. Group sequential methods in the design and analysis of clinical trials. *Biometrika* 64:191, 1977.

35. Rees, W. D., and Turnberg, L. A. Reappraisal of the effects of aspirin on the stomach. *Lancet* 2:410, 1980.

36. Ruffin, J. M., Grizzle, J. E., Hightower, N. C., et al. A cooperative double-blind evaluation of gastric "freezing" in the treatment of duodenal ulcer. *N. Engl. J. Med.* 281:16, 1969.

37. Stampfer, M. J., Willett, W. C., Speizer, F. E., et al. Test of the National Death Index. *Am. J. Epidemiol.* 119:837, 1984.

38. Stampfer, M., Buring, J. E., Willett, W., et al. The 2×2 factorial design: Its application to a randomized trial of aspirin and beta-carotene in US physicians. *Stat. Med.* 4:111, 1985.

39. U.S.D.A. *Nationwide Food Consumption Survey: Continuing Survey of Food Intakes by Individuals. Women 19–50 Years and Their Children 1–5 Years.* Nutrition Monitoring Report No. 85-1. Hyattsville, MD: Human Nutrition Information Service, 1985.

40. U.S. D.H.H.S. *Health United States 1984.* D.H.H.S. Publication No. (P.H.S.) 85-1232. Hyattsville, MD: National Center for Health Statistics, 1984.

41. Veterans Administration Cooperative Study Group on Antihypertensive Agents. Effects of treatment on morbidity in hypertension: Results in patients with diastolic blood pressures averaging 115 through 129 mm Hg. *J.A.M.A.* 202:1028, 1967.

42. Veterans Administration Cooperative Study Group on Antihypertensive

Agents. Effect of treatment on morbidity in hypertension: III. Influence of age, diastolic pressure, and prior cardiovascular disease; further analysis of side effects. *Circulation* 45:991, 1972.

43. Wangensteen, O. H., Peter, E. T., Bernstein, E. F., et al. Can physiological gastrectomy be achieved by gastric freezing? *Ann. Surg.* 156:579, 1962.

44. Wilhelmsen, L., Ljungberg, S., Wedel, H., et al. A comparison between participants and non-participants in a primary preventive trial. *J. Chronic Dis.* 29:331, 1976.

45. Willett, W., Sampson, L., Bain, C., et al. Vitamin supplementation use among registered nurses. *Am. J. Clin. Nutr.* 34:1121, 1981.

46. Yusuf, S., Collins, R., and Peto, R. Why do we need large, simple randomized trials? *Stat. Med.* 3:409, 1984.

III. DESCRIPTION AND ANALYSIS OF EPIDEMIOLOGIC DATA

9

Presentation and Summarization of Data

In the first section of this book, we emphasized how all epidemiologic investigations, whether descriptive or analytic, rely on the quantification of the health status and disease patterns of human populations. For any single study, this may involve collection of information on many variables for a large number of individuals, so that presentation of all the original, or raw, data can be cumbersome and even unintelligible. Descriptive statistics are used to summarize data in a form that permits the clearest presentation of the most information and facilitates useful comparisons between study groups or populations. Since this summarization involves a reduction in the amount of data presented, there is inevitably some loss of information. It is therefore particularly important to be aware of the various descriptive statistics that are available in order to choose the one most appropriate for a particular situation. In this chapter, we will review the basic methods most frequently used for presenting and summarizing data in epidemiologic research.

TYPES OF VARIABLES

The presentation and summarization of data first requires an understanding of the types of variables that are encountered in epidemiologic research and how they are measured. Any variable can generally be considered as one of two basic types: discrete or continuous. Discrete variables are those having values that can fall into only a limited number of separate categories with no possible intermediate levels. There are several different subtypes of discrete variables. In the simplest form, values of a discrete variable can be categorized as one of only two alternatives. Such dichotomous or "either/or" variables include gender (male or female), survival status (alive or dead), and exposure status (exposed or nonexposed). When more than two alternative categories are possible, the variables are termed multichotomous. Such variables include blood type (A, B, AB, O), race (white, black, oriental, hispanic, other), and marital status (single, married, divorced, widowed). There is no inherent order associated with the individual categories in these examples of dichotomous and multichotomous variables; consequently, such variables represent what is called a nominal scale. When the possible responses have a natural order or progression, the variables are termed ordinal. These would include stage of disease at diagnosis (Stage I through IV for breast cancer), improvement in mobility (none, slight, moderate, considerable), and level of current cigarette smoking (none, light, moderate, heavy). Finally, the most complex form of discrete data is called numerical discrete, in which the categories into which the values of the variables fall are not qualitative, as in the above examples, but quantitative. Such variables would include the number of bacteria in a culture, the number of episodes of angina during a 6-month period, or a woman's total number of live births (parity). These are classified as discrete because the values, although numerical, cannot take on any intermediate levels (i.e., it is not possible to experience half an attack of angina or have a fraction of a live birth).

In contrast, continuous variables are those that theoretically can assume all possible values along a continuum within a specified range. Many clinical parameters are continuous, including height, weight, blood cholesterol levels, and blood pressure. Such variables are not restricted to particular values and, in fact, are limited only by the accuracy and precision of the measuring instrument. Because of this, continuous variables allow the greatest degree of quantification of data.

The classification of variables into discrete or continuous provides a convenient basis for the presentation and analysis of data. In addition to distinguishing between the two on the basis of the types of values each can assume, it is useful to consider the basic questions each can address. With discrete variables, whether categorical or numerical, the basic analysis will involve comparison of the proportions of subjects falling into the various categories. Thus, questions of interest might be whether the proportion of leukemia patients who survive for 5 years following treatment A differs from the corresponding proportion among those who receive treatment B, whether those with blood group O are more likely to develop duodenal ulcer than those with blood group A, or whether, within a given industry, the proportion of men reporting respiratory symptoms is greater among heavy smokers than among nonsmokers. With continuous variables, groups are often compared in terms of average values of the variables. For example, the average birthweight of children born to women who smoke can be compared with that of infants born to nonsmokers. Similarly, in a trial designed to test the efficacy of a drug in reducing blood cholesterol, the average cholesterol level in the treated group could be compared with that of a group receiving either nonpharmacologic therapy or a placebo.

Data Reduction

Although certain variables can, by their very nature, be classified in only one way, many other measures can be considered in a number of forms. For example, the sex of a study participant can be classified only as male or female. As regards age, however, an individual who is 58½ years old could be categorized in a number of ways, such as "55 to 59," "greater than 50" or "middle-aged." The level of detail or precision needed for analysis will depend on the research questions under study. For example, in evaluating risk factors for osteoporotic hip fractures, it would be necessary to distinguish between women in various decades of life because such fractures are rare before age 40 and rise steadily during middle age and exponentially after age 70 [1]. In contrast, to compare rates of coronary heart disease among pre- and postmenopausal women, dichotomizing age as less than or greater than 54 years, the average age of menopause in the U.S., would be an adequate first step [3]. Even in the same study, the categorization of age to evaluate one hypothesis may not be the same as that required to evaluate another. For example, in a study of maternal age and risk of various reproductive outcomes, to evaluate Down's syndrome, which is rare among children of younger women and increases in frequency after age 30, maternal age could be classified as "less than 30 years," "30 to 34," "35 to 39," and "40+ years." This categorization would not, however, be adequate to evaluate complications of pregnancy, since teenage mothers are at particular risk [16] and could not be identified in an age category as broad as "less than 30 years."

As these examples illustrate, reducing or collapsing the multiple values of a variable into fewer discrete categories in the analysis of a study may well be sufficient to evaluate a particular hypothesis. Nevertheless, as was shown in the example of age and complications of pregnancy, it is important to keep in mind that while data reduction often increases the ease of presentation and may simplify the subsequent statistical analyses, there is always an accompanying loss of detail from the original observations that may mask important information or trends. Moreover, while data can always be reduced to a simpler form, it is never possible to reconstruct more detailed information from data that were originally recorded only in categories. For example, in a study of coronary heart disease, it would not be possible to evaluate the risks associated with varying levels of total blood cholesterol if these values had been recorded initially only as the dichotomy of normal or elevated. If, however, the actual cholesterol levels had been recorded, a subsequent analysis comparing individuals with normal or elevated levels could easily be performed. It is therefore important to consider carefully all research questions that might possibly be of interest before beginning data collection, so that the necessary level of detail can be obtained. The reduction of data, if necessary or desirable, can then be done in the analysis of the study.

DATA PRESENTATION

In most epidemiologic studies, the number of subjects is too large to permit reporting the actual data for each individual. What is needed is a way to present data in a manner that will communicate the maximum amount of information in the most efficient format. The most common forms for presenting data include tables, such as frequency and cumulative frequency distributions, and graphs, such as histograms and frequency polygons. These formats provide complementary information, with tables giving more specific detail about the individual values and graphs a general depiction of the overall pattern.

Frequency Distributions

A frequency distribution lists, for each value (or small range of values) of a variable, the number or proportion of times that observation occurs in the study population. This is illustrated in Table 9-1, which shows the frequency distribution of oral contraceptive (OC) use among cases and controls from a study of OC use and risk of breast cancer [6]. Of the 989

Table 9-1. Frequency distribution of oral contraceptive (OC) use among cases of breast cancer and controls

	Cases	Controls
OC use	Number (%)	Number (%)
Ever use	273 (27.6)	2641 (26.7)
Duration (months)		
1–11	81 (8.2)	735 (7.4)
12–35	77 (7.8)	664 (6.7)
36–59	30 (3.0)	403 (4.1)
60–119	73 (7.4)	672 (6.8)
120+	12 (1.2)	167 (1.7)
Never use	716 (72.4)	7260 (73.3)
Total	989 (100.0)	9901 (100.0)

Data from: Hennekens, C. H., Speizer, F. E., Lipnick, R. J., et al., A case-control study of oral contraceptive use and breast cancer. *J.N.C.I.* 72:39, 1984.

Table 9-2. Two-by-two table summarizing data from a case-control study of oral contraceptive (OC) use and breast cancer

| | Breast cancer | | |
	Cases	Controls	Total
OC use			
Ever	273	2641	2914
Never	716	7260	7976
Total	989	9901	10,890

Data from: Hennekens, C. H., Speizer, F. E., Lipnick, R. J., et al., A case-control study of oral contraceptive use and breast cancer. *J.N.C.I.* 72:39, 1984.

women with breast cancer, 273, or 27.6 percent, had ever used OCs, while 716, or 72.4 percent, had never used these agents. For the controls, the corresponding percentages were 26.7 percent and 73.3 percent. With respect to duration of use, 1.2 percent of the cases and 1.7 percent of the controls reported long-term use, defined as 120 months or more.

When presenting discrete data, as in Table 9-1, an alternative and more commonly used format is the contingency table introduced in Chapter 4. In its general form, the *r*-by-*c* contingency table contains counts of observations arranged in *r* rows and *c* columns, representing the various levels of exposure and disease. For dichotomous variables such as "diseased/nondiseased" and "exposed/nonexposed," there are two rows and two columns and the table is referred to as a two-by-two or fourfold table. As shown in Table 9-2, the case-control data on ever use of OCs and risk of breast cancer can be summarized using this format, with the rows representing exposure status (ever versus never use of OCs) and the columns represent disease status (cases or controls).

Analogously, the data on duration of use can be presented in a six-by-two table (Table 9-3), with the six rows representing the one category of never users and the five duration of use categories, while the two columns represent those with and without the disease.

While frequency distributions can be used to present discrete data, as shown in Table 9-3, they provide the most complete and convenient way to summarize quantitative continuous variables. In fact, as the data increase in terms of both number of subjects and amount of information recorded, the relative efficiency of this method of presentation also increases. Because of the number of values a continuous variable can theoretically assume, it is often necessary to define classes of values and record the number of observations that fall within each category. For example, Table 9-4 shows the frequency distribution of total blood cholesterol values for a group of 209 healthy men under the age of 75 from

Table 9-3. Six-by-two table summarizing data on duration of oral contraceptive (OC) use in a case-control study of breast cancer

	Breast cancer		Total
Duration	Cases	Controls	
Never use	716	7260	7976
Ever use (months)			
1–11	81	735	816
12–35	77	664	741
36–59	30	403	433
60–119	73	672	745
120+	12	167	179
Total	989	9901	10,890

Data from: Hennekens, C. H., Speizer, F. E., Lipnick, R. J., et al., A case-control study of oral contraceptive use and breast cancer. *J.N.C.I.* 72:39, 1984.

the Boston Area Health Study [2], a case-control study of the interrelationships of alcohol, diet, and other risk factors for myocardial infarction. Levels of blood cholesterol, a continuous variable, have been divided into 14 mutually exclusive classes. As can readily be seen from the table, while the observed values range from 100 to 379 mg/dl, the majority of the men have total blood cholesterol levels between 160 and 259 mg/dl.

The choice of the number of categories in which to group such continuous data for presentation in a frequency distribution is not clear-cut. The use of too many classes is tantamount to tabulating the raw data. On the other hand, too few classes can easily obscure important information. For example, Table 9-5 presents the same data as were shown in Table 9-4, but with the cholesterol levels grouped into only 3 categories rather than 14. Using this categorization, 37.8 percent of the values fall between 100 and 199 mg/dl. This might be erroneously interpreted to imply a fairly uniform spread of the observed levels throughout this range, while in fact, as shown in Table 9-4, 69 of 79 or 88 percent are actually between 160 and 199 mg/dl. Similarly, reporting that 5.7 percent of the men have cholesterol levels between 300 and 399 mg/dl obscures the important information that 92 percent of these values are between 300 and 319 mg/dl and that only one individual in this population had a cholesterol level over 320 mg/dl. Thus, as stated earlier, to examine adequately any research question for a particular variable, it is advisable to consider collecting a greater amount of detail, that is, a larger number of small categories that can then be combined into broader classes of data, rather than beginning with broad classes and subsequently being unable to reconstruct and investigate the appropriate level of detail. It is also useful to examine the full frequency distri-

Table 9-4. Frequency distribution of total blood
cholesterol levels in healthy men (Boston Area Health Study)

Total blood cholesterol level (mg/dl)	Number	Percent
100–119	2	0.95
120–139	2	0.95
140–159	6	2.9
160–179	33	15.8
180–199	36	17.2
200–219	40	19.1
220–239	29	13.9
240–259	27	12.9
260–279	13	6.2
280–299	9	4.3
300–319	11	5.3
320–339	0	0
340–359	0	0
360–379	1	0.5
Total	209	100.0

Table 9-5. Frequency distribution of total blood cholesterol levels in healthy
men (Boston Area Health Study), with data divided into three classes

Total blood cholesterol level (mg/dl)	Number	Percent
100–199	79	37.8
200–299	118	56.5
300–399	12	5.7
Total	209	100.0

bution in the context of the particular question before selecting the most
appropriate level of data classification.

In addition to presenting the numbers and percentages of observations that fall within classes of values of a variable, frequency distributions can also include the numbers or percentages of observations that
fall above or below a particular value or category. Table 9-6 presents the
cumulative frequency distribution of total blood cholesterol levels from
the Boston Area Health Study, indicating the number and percentage
of subjects having values less than or equal to the upper bound of each

Table 9-6. Cumulative frequency distribution of total blood
cholesterol levels in healthy men (Boston Area Health Study)

Total blood cholesterol level (mg/dl)	Frequency distribution		Cumulative frequency distribution	
	Number	Percent	Number	Percent
100–119	2	0.95	2	0.95
120–139	2	0.95	4	1.9
140–159	6	2.9	10	4.8
160–179	33	15.8	43	20.6
180–199	36	17.2	79	37.8
200–219	40	19.1	119	56.9
220–239	29	13.9	148	70.8
240–259	27	12.9	175ʳ	83.7
260–279	13	6.2	188	89.9
280–299	9	4.3	197	94.2
300–319	11	5.3	208	99.5
320–339	0	0	208	99.5
340–359	0	0	208	99.5
360–379	1	0.5	209	100.0
Total	209	100.0		

category. In these data, approximately 5 percent of the subjects had total cholesterol levels of 159 mg/dl or lower, while almost 90 percent had values less than or equal to 279 mg/dl. A cumulative frequency distribution can also be used to calculate the numbers and percentages of values greater than or equal to the lower bound of a category. The percentage of men with cholesterol levels greater than or equal to 300 mg/dl can be calculated from the table as 100 percent minus 94.2 percent, or 5.8 percent. Such cumulative frequency distributions can be used to provide answers to a number of types of research questions, including what proportion of the U.S. population is over the age of 65, how many residents of a city have an annual income under $5000, or what proportion of families in a community have more than three children. They can also be used to relate individual test scores or measures of growth, such as height or weight in children, to the distribution of those variables in a broader population.

Histograms

A frequency distribution can be displayed graphically as a histogram, or bar graph, with the values of the variable on the horizontal axis and the frequencies of observation for each value on the vertical axis. The height

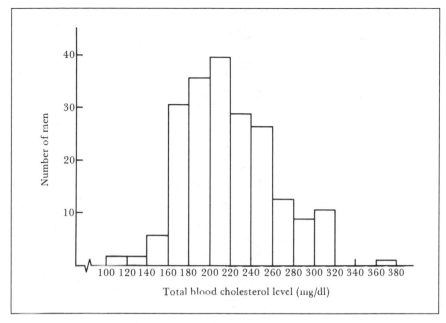

Fig. 9-1. Histogram of the frequency distribution of total blood cholesterol levels among 209 healthy men (Boston Area Health Study).

of each bar represents the number or proportion of subjects for each value of the variable or class interval. When intervals of values are used on the horizontal axis, each bar is centered over the midpoint of the class. For example, a histogram depicting the distribution of total cholesterol levels in Table 9-4 is shown in Figure 9-1.

A key point to remember with histograms is that it is the area of each bar that depicts the frequency of subjects observed. If all bars represent intervals of the same width, as in Figure 9-1, then the area is proportional to the height, and the frequencies in different categories can be directly compared by examining the relative height of the respective bars. If, however, the class intervals are not all of equal width, it is necessary to make adjustments so that the total area remains in proper proportion and direct comparisons can be made.

To illustrate how misleading such a graph can be if appropriate adjustments are not made, Figure 9-2 depicts the same data as the histogram in Figure 9-1, except that instead of grouping the cholesterol values into classes of equal width, each including 20 units of measurement, the classes are not all of equal size. Specifically, the categories 180 to 199 mg/dl and 200 to 219 mg/dl have been combined into a single interval, 40 units wide. If the height of that bar is made to represent the total of 76 values falling into the category 180 to 219 mg/dl, that category will appear greatly out of proportion compared with the pattern illustrated

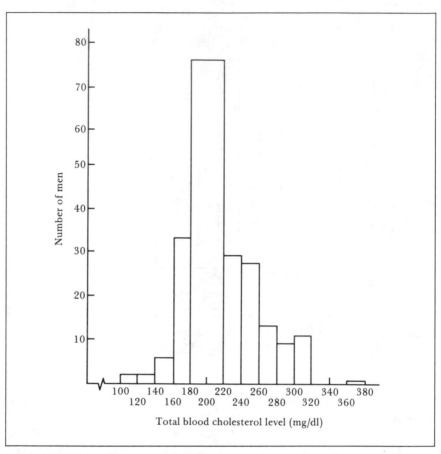

Fig. 9-2. Incorrect histogram of the frequency distribution of total blood cholesterol levels of 209 healthy men (Boston Area Health Study) with classes of unequal width.

in the original histogram. To correct this distortion, it is necessary to determine the relative widths of the classes and adjust each in proportion to the narrowest, in this case, 20 units. Since the class 180 to 219 mg/dl is twice as wide as the other intervals, the frequency of that class of values (i.e., 76) must be divided by two, giving an average frequency of 38 for each of the two equal segments, and the adjusted height graphed as illustrated in Figure 9-3. When this rectangle is compared with the histogram in Figure 9-1, it is clear that the adjusted area represents the true pattern of frequencies more accurately than the unadjusted bar. As a general rule, it is always best to use intervals of equal width whenever possible to minimize the potential for misinterpretation.

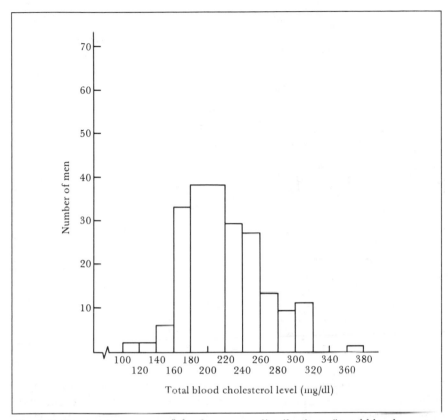

Fig. 9-3. Correct histogram of the frequency distribution of total blood cholesterol levels of 209 healthy men (Boston Area Health Study) with classes of unequal width.

Frequency Polygons

Frequency polygons or curves are another type of graphic representation of frequency distributions that are used primarily for continuous variables. As with a histogram, the values of the variable are represented along the horizontal axis and their frequencies along the vertical axis. However, instead of using rectangles to represent the data, the midpoints of the top of each bar of the histogram are simply plotted and connected with straight lines. Figure 9-4 illustrates a frequency polygon for the data on total cholesterol levels shown in Table 9-4. As with the histogram, when plotting class intervals of unequal width on a frequency polygon, the height of the point representing the frequency must be adjusted so that the area under the curve at that interval remains in proper proportion.

One major advantage of using frequency polygons is that curves for

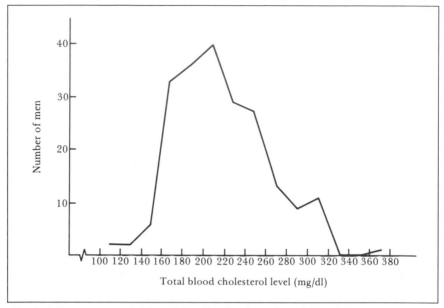

Fig. 9-4. Frequency polygon of the distribution of total blood cholesterol levels among 209 healthy men (Boston Area Health Study).

two or more sets of data can easily be constructed on the same graph to facilitate direct comparisons. For example, Figure 9-5 shows the age-adjusted death rates among men for nine cancer sites in the U.S. between 1930 and 1981 [14]. The most striking observation is that while the death rates for most cancers have remained relatively stable over this 50-year period, two cancers show a dramatically different pattern. Specifically, death rates from stomach cancer decreased from about 38 per 100,000 men in 1930 to about 9 per 100,000 in 1981, while in contrast, lung cancer mortality rates increased from about 5 per 100,000 men to about 71 per 100,000 during the same time period, an approximately 14-fold increase.

Frequency polygons can also present a simple picture of the shape of the distribution of observations and thus provide information about the underlying characteristics of the data. For example, Figure 9-6 presents a frequency polygon for the distribution of diastolic blood pressure values observed among a group of 500 men [15]. The distribution of diastolic blood pressures approximates the so-called normal or bell-shaped curve, with the majority of observations clustered around a central value and smaller but similar numbers at each interval above and below the central value. Such a curve, with equal proportions on either side of the central point or peak, is termed symmetric.

The values of many biologic variables in the underlying population can best be described by the normal distribution, including height,

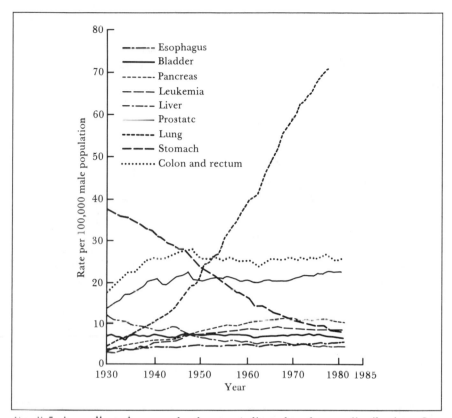

Fig. 9-5. Age-adjusted cancer death rates (adjusted to the age distribution of the 1970 U.S. census population) for selected sites among males, United States, 1930–1981. (From E. Silverberg, Cancer statistics, 1985. *CA.* 35:19, 1985.)

weight, and white blood count. For other variables the distributions of observations are not symmetric, because extreme high and low values are not equally common. Moreover, even variables that are normally distributed in the general population may not be so in the particular sample selected for study. When a greater proportion of observations fall at one end or tail of the distribution than at the other, the distribution is considered to be skewed. For example, Figure 9-7 depicts the frequency distribution of white blood cell (WBC) counts in a sample of blood specimens from a hospital laboratory. As might be expected, this distribution is markedly skewed toward higher values (i.e., positively skewed), due, at least in part, to the greater than average proportion of individuals with infection in a hospital population. In such circumstances, it is possible to transform each of the original observations into a form that is

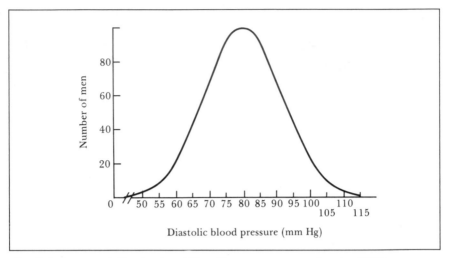

Fig. 9-6. A normal distribution: Diastolic blood pressure levels of 500 men. (From T. D. V. Swinscow, *Statistics at Square One*. London: British Medical Association, 1976.)

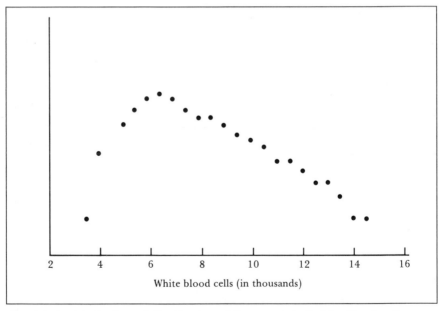

Fig. 9-7. Positively skewed distribution of frequencies of white blood cell (WBC) counts in a sample of blood specimens.

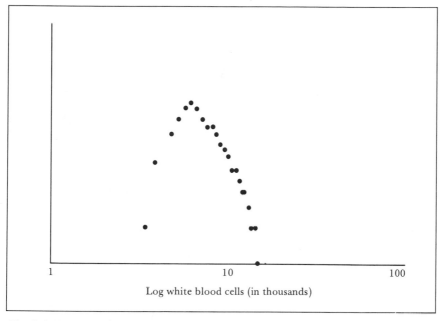

Fig. 9-8. Log transformation of the distribution of frequencies of white blood cell (WBC) counts in a sample of blood specimens.

more normally distributed and thus amenable to standard statistical testing. One common adjustment procedure is the logarithmic or log transformation, which uses the logarithm of each observation rather than the actual value. This process tends to stretch out smaller values of observations and compress very large values. For example, Figure 9-8 depicts the log transformation of the WBC count distribution in Figure 9-7. In the second graph, while there are still more values in the right half of the curve, the shape is more nearly symmetric, and the distribution of the logs of WBCs can be considered approximately normal.

SUMMARY STATISTICS

While tables are a convenient way to present specific information about individual values of a variable and graphs can provide a general picture of the pattern of the observations, it is often useful to provide, in addition, a numerical summary of the important characteristics of the distribution of a variable. Such summary statistics are also necessary for precise and efficient comparisons of different sets of data. For discrete variables, the most informative summary measure is simply the propor-

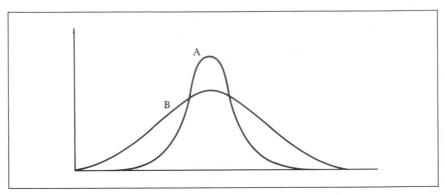

Fig. 9-9. Two distributions with the same central location but different spread.

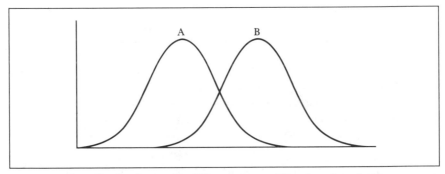

Fig. 9-10. Two distributions with different central locations but the same spread.

tion of individuals falling within each category. Continuous variables, however, generally require the use of at least two parameters. The first is a measure of central tendency or location of the observations, and the second is a measure of their variability or spread. Information on both these parameters is necessary to describe completely the shape of the distribution of the observations, as demonstrated by the graphs presented in Figures 9-9 and 9-10. Specifically, Figure 9-9 shows two distributions that are centrally located at the same value on the horizontal axis, but have substantially different amounts of variability. Distribution *A* is narrower, indicating that a larger proportion of observed values cluster around the point of central tendency than in curve *B*. In contrast, Figure 9-10 shows two distributions that have the same shape, indicating the same amount of variability, but very different locations. The measure of central tendency does not provide any information about the shape of the distribution, and the amount of variability alone does not indicate the central location. Thus, both measures are needed to describe the distribution of a continuous variable.

Measures of Central Tendency

There are three measures of central tendency that are frequently used in the literature: the mean, the median, and the mode. Each has advantages and disadvantages in describing a "typical" value for a given continuous variable in a specific population.

Mean

The most commonly used measure of central tendency is the mean, or arithmetic average. It is calculated simply by adding all the observed values and dividing by the total sample size of the group. Denoting each individual observation by x, the total number of observations by n, and the process of summation by the Greek capital letter sigma (Σ), the calculation of the mean of a sample ($\bar{x}$) is expressed as:

$$\bar{x} = \Sigma x / n$$

As an example, Table 9-7 presents total cholesterol levels for a sample of 20 men, selected at random from the group of 209 healthy males presented in Table 9-4. The mean cholesterol level for this sample can be calculated as follows:

$$\bar{x} = \frac{179 + 184 + 186 + \ldots + 296}{20}$$

$$= \frac{4406}{20}$$

$$= 220.3 \text{ mg/dl}$$

The mean has a number of desirable theoretic properties that allow it to be used as the basis for a large proportion of statistical tests, as will be illustrated in Chapter 10. As a solely descriptive measure, however, the mean has the potentially serious disadvantage of being very sensitive to extreme values, or outliers, which may distort its representation of the typical value of a variable. For example, if five women in a group weighed 105, 110, 112, 115, and 227 pounds, the mean weight of the women would be 669/5, or 133.8 pounds. Given that four of the five observed weights are actually 115 pounds or less, however, the mean of this sample is not a good indication of a "typical" observation. Thus, the more asymmetric the distribution, the less desirable it is to summarize the observations by using the mean.

Table 9-7. Calculation of the mean, median, and mode of total blood cholesterol levels for a sample of 20 healthy men (Boston Area Health Study)

Rank	Total blood cholesterol (mg/dl) x
1	179
2	184
3	186
4	189
5	192
6	196
7	203
8	204
9	206
10	211
11	219
12	222
13	227
14	237
15	238
16	241
17	246
18	248
19	282
20	296
Total	4406

Mean: $\Sigma x/n = 4406/20 = 220.3$ mg/dl
Median: $(211 + 219)/2 = 215$ mg/dl
Mode: None

Median

The median, or 50th percentile, describes the literal "middle" of the data. It is defined as the value above or below which half the observations fall. To identify the median, the individual observations are first listed in ascending or descending order. If the number of observations is odd, the position or rank of the median is determined by the formula $(n + 1)/2$, where n equals the total sample size. Thus, for a series of 51 observations, the median would be the value of the observation corresponding to the 52/2 or 26th rank. For an even number of observations, the median is the arithmetic average of the values located at the two positions ($n/2$) and [($n/2$) + 1]. For example, the median total cholesterol level for the 20 subjects listed in Table 9-6 would be calculated as the mean of the observations ranked 10th (20/2) and 11th (20/2 + 1). Thus, the median total cholesterol level in this sample is (211 + 219)/2, or 215 mg/dl.

The advantage of the median as a measure of central tendency is that it is unaffected by extreme values. For example, for the five subjects whose weights were listed above (105, 110, 112, 115, and 227 pounds), the median weight would be 112 pounds, a value much more representative of the fact that four of the five values are 115 pounds or less than the mean value of 133.8 pounds. Similarly, in a case-control study investigating risk factors among homosexual men for the development of Kaposi's sarcoma and *Pneumocystis carinii* pneumonia, the median number of different sexual partners was reported among the cases as 61 per year, compared with 27 per year among controls identified from a sexually transmitted diseases clinic [7]. The median rather than the mean number of partners was reported because some cases had reported more than 90 different sexual partners per month during the year prior to diagnosis [9]. The mean would be highly distorted by such outliers, resulting in an average value that was not at all reflective of the typical observations. The disadvantage of the median, however, is that since its value is determined solely by its rank, it provides no information about any of the other values within the distribution. Moreover, from a mathematical perspective, it is far less amenable than the mean to tests of statistical significance.

Mode

The mode of a distribution is the value that is observed most frequently in a given data set. The mode is rarely used as the sole descriptive measure of central tendency, since with a small number of observations, it is likely that each value will occur only once, and there may be no mode. This is true of the distribution of total cholesterol values on the sample of 20 men presented in Table 9-7. Moreover, the mode is even less amenable to statistical manipulation than the median.

As discussed in Chapter 5, however, examination of the mode can sometimes be used to provide insights into the possible etiology of a disease. For example, the observation that the distribution of the incidence rates of Hodgkin's disease by age was bimodal—that is, had two distinct modes, one around age 29 and the other around age 73—raised the possibility that "Hodgkin's disease" might actually consist of two separate disease entities [8]. In fact, subsequent analytic studies have shown that Hodgkin's disease among young adults seems to be an inflammatory process, while among the elderly its course more closely resembles a neoplastic process [4].

One problem, however, is that positively skewed distributions can

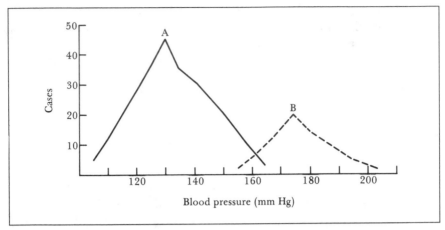

Fig. 9-11. Systolic blood pressure levels in a population, represented as a bimodal distribution. (From R. Platt, The nature of essential hypertension [letter]. *Lancet* 1:1189, 1960.)

sometimes be misinterpreted as being bimodal. Perhaps the classic example of this formed the basis for an extended controversy on the nature of essential hypertension. Sir Robert Platt [12, 13] advocated the view that primary hypertension was a genetic disorder based on his interpretation of the frequency distribution of blood pressures in a population (Figure 9-11). He interpreted this distribution as bimodal with curve *A* representing the population of normotensive individuals and curve *B* representing those genetically disposed to hypertension. In contrast to this commonly held view, Sir George Pickering [11] reasoned that blood pressure was in fact a continuous variable with a single, unimodal distribution positively skewed toward higher values, as illustrated in Figure 9-12. This interpretation supported the now commonly accepted view of hypertension as largely environmentally rather than genetically determined.

Choice of Measures of Central Tendency

The choice of a measure of central tendency will depend in large part on the nature of the distribution of the observations. For continuous variables with a unimodal (single-peaked) and symmetric distribution, the mean, median, and mode will be identical. With a distribution that is skewed, however, the median may be a more informative descriptive measure than the mean. For statistical analyses and tests of significance, however, the mean is preferable whenever possible, since it includes information from all observations and its theoretic properties provide for more powerful statistical tests. If the data are considerably skewed and there is no function that will transform the observations into a form that

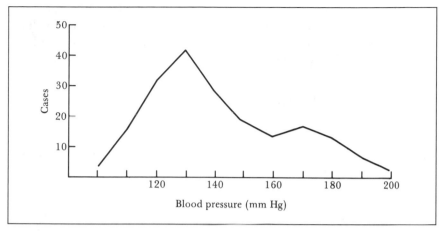

Fig. 9-12. Systolic blood pressure levels in a population, represented as a positively skewed, unimodal distribution. (From G. Pickering, *The Nature of Essential Hypertension*. New York: Grune & Stratton, 1961.)

is more symmetric, specialized methods of statistical analysis based on the median may need to be considered [10].

Measures of Spread or Variability

In addition to a measure of central tendency, in describing a distribution it is important to provide information concerning the relative position of other data points in the sample, that is, a measure of spread or variability.

One simple descriptive measure of variability is the range, calculated by subtracting the lowest observed value from the highest. For example, the range of total cholesterol levels for the sample of 20 men presented in Table 9-7 is 296 minus 179, or 117 mg/dl. While the range is both simple to calculate and easy to understand, it is far from optimal as a measure of variabilty. First, the range is not a stable estimate, because as sample size increases, the range also tends to increase. Second, it is not amenable to statistical procedures and testing. Finally, since the range is derived from only the most extreme values, a sample may have a large range even when the majority of the observations are fairly close in value. Thus, a preferable measure of variability would include the distribution of all observed values, not just those at the extremes.

The most informative and frequently employed measures of variability are the variance and its related function, the standard deviation. Each of these parameters provides a summary of the dispersion of individual observations around the mean. The variance of a sample is computed by first calculating the difference between each observation *(x)* and the mean ($\bar{x}$). Next, these differences are squared ($[x - \bar{x}]^2$), so that negative and positive deviations will not cancel each other out, and the resultant quantities are added together ($\Sigma[x - \bar{x}]^2$). The sum of the squared deviations is then divided by the total number of observations minus one ($n - 1$). The formula for the variance (V) can thus be written as follows:

$$V = \Sigma \frac{(x - \bar{x})^2}{n - 1}$$

The standard deviation (SD) is simply the square root of the variance:

$$SD = \sqrt{V}$$

$$= \sqrt{\frac{\Sigma (x - \bar{x})^2}{n - 1}}$$

The term $n - 1$ rather than n is used in the denominator to adjust for the fact that the mean of the sample is used as an estimate of the mean of the underlying population. If data are available from the entire population rather than only a sample, $n - 1$ can be replaced by n in these calculations.

Table 9-8 illustrates the calculations of the variance and standard deviation for the sample of blood cholesterol levels. For this sample of 20 healthy men, the mean cholesterol level was 220.3 mg/dl, the variance 1024.3 (mg/dl)^2, and the standard deviation 32.0 mg/dl. Although both these parameters are used in statistical testing, the standard deviation, which is expressed in the same units as the original data (in this case, mg/dl), is more commonly reported. Thus, the distribution of the total blood cholesterol levels from this sample could be described by presenting the mean ± 1 SD, or 220.3 ± 32.0 mg/dl.

There are two additional points to note concerning the formulas for the calculation of the variance and standard deviation presented in this section. First, as illustrated in Table 9-8, there is an algebraically equivalent formula for determining the variance, which can be computed using the functions available on most pocket calculators:

$$V = \frac{\Sigma (x - \bar{x})^2}{n - 1}$$

$$= \frac{\Sigma x^2 - (\Sigma x)^2/n}{n - 1}$$

In applying this formula, it is important to note the distinction between Σx^2 and $(\Sigma x)^2$. The former, Σx^2, means to take each observation, square it, then sum the squares. The latter, $(\Sigma x)^2$, means to take all the observations, add them together, and then square the sum. Second, the for-

Table 9-8. Calculation of the variance and standard deviation of total blood cholesterol levels for a sample of 20 healthy men (Boston Area Health Study)

Total blood cholesterol (mg/dl) x	$x - \bar{x}$	$(x - \bar{x})^2$	x^2
179	−41.3	1705.69	32,041
184	−36.3	1317.69	33,856
186	−34.3	1176.49	34,596
189	−31.3	979.69	35,721
192	−28.3	800.89	36,864
196	−24.3	590.49	38,416
203	−17.3	299.29	41,209
204	−16.3	265.69	41,616
206	−14.3	204.49	42,436
211	−9.3	86.49	44,521
219	−1.3	1.69	47,961
222	1.7	2.89	49,284
227	6.7	44.89	51,529
237	16.7	278.89	56,169
238	17.7	313.29	56,644
241	20.7	428.49	58,081
246	25.7	660.49	60,516
248	27.7	767.29	61,504
282	61.7	3806.89	79,524
296	75.7	5730.49	87,616
4406	0	19,462.20	990,104

Mean: $\bar{x} = \Sigma x/n = 4406/20 = 220.3$ mg/dl

Variance: $V = \dfrac{\Sigma(x - \bar{x})^2}{(n - 1)}$ or $V = \dfrac{\Sigma x^2 - (\Sigma x)^2/n}{n - 1}$

$= 19462.2/19$

$= 1024.3$ (mg/dl)^2

$= \dfrac{990104 - (4406)^2/20}{19}$

$= \dfrac{19462.2}{19}$

$= 1024.3$ (mg/dl)^2

Standard deviation: $SD = \sqrt{V} = \sqrt{1024.3}$

$= 32.0$ mg/dl

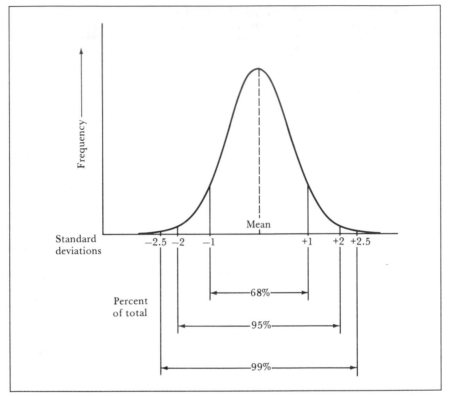

Fig. 9-13. Percentages of observations falling within 1, 2, and 2.5 standard deviations of the mean for a unimodal and symmetric (normal) distribution.

mulas presented in this section for calculating the variance and standard deviation can be applied directly when actual data values are available. When the values of the observations have been combined into class intervals, as in the frequency distribution shown in Table 9-4, analogous formulas for grouped data are available [5].

For distributions that are approximately normal—that is, unimodal and roughly symmetric (following a bell-shaped curve)—the standard deviation and the mean together provide sufficient information to describe the distribution totally. A very useful property of the normal distribution is that, as illustrated in Figure 9-13, 68 percent of the individual observations in such distributions will lie within 1 standard deviation of the mean (± 1 SD), approximately 95 percent within 2 standard deviations (± 2 SD), and roughly 99 percent within 2½ standard deviations (± 2½ SD). Thus, knowledge of the mean and standard deviation of a distribution will permit the estimation of ranges of values that would be expected to include a certain proportion of the observed values, such as the "normal" range of a biochemical measurement, which usually includes the values within which 95 percent of the observations from a given population will lie.

It is also sometimes of interest to compare the degree of variability in the distribution of a factor from two different populations or of two different variables from the same population. For example, an investigator might wish to know whether there is more variability in systolic blood pressure among children than adults, or whether among adults, the distribution of systolic blood pressure has more spread than that of diastolic. Since the standard deviation is the variability around the mean of the distribution, a direct comparison of standard deviations for samples with different means, as in both these examples, would not be informative. Even if the absolute magnitudes of the deviations are equal, the degree of variability relative to each mean could be very different. For example, the relative degree of variability in a distribution with a mean of 10 and a standard deviation of 5 would be much larger than that of the distribution of another variable with the same standard deviation but a mean of 100. One measure that takes this into account is the coefficient of variation (CV), which expresses the standard deviation as a proportion of the mean and is calculated as:

$$CV = (SD/\bar{x}) \times 100$$

The coefficients of variation can then be compared directly. When two distributions have means of different magnitudes, a comparison of their coefficients of variation is therefore much more meaningful than a comparison of their respective standard deviations.

The Standard Error of the Mean

An additional measure of variability, the standard error of the mean, is commonly encountered—and often used incorrectly—in the medical literature. While the standard error is related to the standard deviation, they actually measure two very different things. The standard deviation quantifies the spread of the individual observations of a value of a variable around the mean value of the sample, while the standard error measures the variability of the mean of the sample as an estimate of the true value of the mean for the population from which the sample was drawn.

To understand this distinction, it is important to recognize that the value of the mean computed from a single sample (such as the 20 healthy men selected from the Boston Area Health Study) can be used to provide an estimate of the mean of the entire population from which the sample was selected. If another sample of 20 individuals from the population were drawn, it is unlikely that the mean of this sample would be equal to that of the first group of 20. Both, however, would be estimates of the same population mean, and the average of these sample means would be a more accurate estimate of the population value than either one considered individually. If we continue to draw samples and calculate the mean of the observations for each group of subjects, we will have a series of means. If the number of samples is large, the distribution of the sample means will be approximately normal, regardless of the distribution of values in the original population from which the samples were drawn, and the mean value of the group of all possible sample means will approximate the true population mean. This is referred to as the central limit theorem, which is described more fully elsewhere [5]. Just as we measured the variability of the individual observations around the mean of the sample by calculating the standard deviation, we can estimate an analogous measure of the variability of the sample means around the true population mean. This parameter is called the standard error (SE) and indicates the degree to which the sample mean reflects the true population parameter.

The precision with which we can estimate the true population mean is dependent on both the variability in the original population and the size of the sample on which the estimate is based. Although the true amount of variation in the underlying population cannot usually be determined, the variability of the sample, as represented by the standard deviation, provides a reasonable estimate. The formula for calculating the standard error of the mean is as follows:

$$SE(\bar{x}) = SD/\sqrt{n}$$

where SD is the standard deviation of the sample and n equals the size of the sample.

For example, we have already calculated the mean and standard deviation of the cholesterol values of the random sample of 20 healthy men from the Boston Area Health Study (see Table 9-8). The sample mean was 220.3 mg/dl, with a standard deviation of 32.0 mg/dl. The standard error of the mean can be calculated:

$$SE(\bar{x}) = 32.0/\sqrt{20}$$
$$= 7.16 \text{ mg/dl}$$

The standard error is used to describe an interval within which we can say with a given level of certainty that the true population mean lies, or to compare means in different populations. Note, however, that both these issues relate to the distribution of the mean of the sample. When describing the distribution of individual observations in the population, the appropriate measure of variability under the usual assumption of normality is the standard deviation.

CONCLUSION

In this chapter, we have considered a variety of ways to describe epidemiologic data. In this context, data description includes both presentation of actual values in tables or graphs and summarization of the characteristics of the distribution of observed values, including measures of central tendency and variability. A major issue in deciding which measures to use in a given situation is balancing the need to present the data efficiently with that of maintaining the level of detail necessary to answer adequately a particular research question. Summary statistics are very useful tools, but if applied incorrectly, they may be uninformative or even misleading.

In addition to simply describing a single set of data, the descriptive measures presented in this chapter can also facilitate the comparison of different groups of observations. In this capacity, knowledge of the properties of distributions and their measures is essential to an understanding of tests of statistical significance. These tests are used to evaluate the role of chance as an alternative explanation for observed differences between study groups, as will be discussed in Chapter 10.

STUDY QUESTIONS

1. Define discrete and continuous variables and discuss ways of presenting data of each type.
2. Discuss the rationale for presenting raw data versus descriptive statistics.
3. Compare and contrast the utility of frequency distributions and frequency polygons.
4. Discuss the rationale for the choice of various measures of
   a. Central tendency
   b. Variability

REFERENCES

1. Brody, J. A., Farmer, M. E., and White, L. R. Absence of menopausal effect on hip fracture occurrence in white females. *Am. J. Public Health* 74:1397, 1984.
2. Buring, J. E., Willett, W., Goldhaber, S. Z., et al. Alcohol and HDL in nonfatal myocardial infarction: Preliminary results from a case-control study. *Circulation* 68:227, 1983.
3. Colditz, G. A., Willett, W. C., Stampfer, M. J., et al. Menopause and risk of coronary heart disease in women. *N. Engl. J. Med.* 316:1105, 1987.
4. Cole, P., MacMahon, B., and Aisenberg, A. Mortality from Hodgkin's disease

in the United States: Evidence for the multiple-aetiology hypothesis. *Lancet* 2:1371, 1968.

5. Colton, T. *Statistics in Medicine*. Boston: Little, Brown, 1974.

6. Hennekens, C. H., Speizer, F. E., Lipnick, R. J., et al. A case-control study of oral contraceptive use and breast cancer. *J.N.C.I.* 72:39, 1984.

7. Jaffe, H. W., Cho, K., Thomas, P. A., et al. National case-control study of Kaposi's sarcoma and *Pneumocystis carinii* pneumonia in homosexual men: Part 1. Epidemiologic results. *Ann. Intern. Med.* 99:145, 1983.

8. MacMahon, B. Epidemiologic evidence on the nature of Hodgkin's disease. *Cancer* 10:1045, 1957.

9. Marmor, M., Friedman-Kien, A. E., Laubenstein, L., et al. Risk factors for Kaposi's sarcoma in homosexual men. *Lancet* 1:1083, 1982.

10. Mosteller, F., and Tukey, J. W. *Data Analysis and Regression: A Second Course in Statistics*. Reading, MA: Addison-Wesley, 1971.

11. Pickering, G. *The Nature of Essential Hypertension*. New York: Grune & Stratton, 1961.

12. Platt, R. The nature of essential hypertension. *Lancet* 2:55, 1959.

13. Platt, R. The nature of essential hypertension (letter). *Lancet* 1:1189, 1960.

14. Silverberg, E. Cancer statistics, 1985. *CA* 35:19, 1985.

15. Swinscow, T. D. V. *Statistics at Square One*. London: British Medical Association, 1976.

16. U.S. D.H.H.S. *Health United States 1984*. D.H.H.S. Publication No. (P.H.S.) 85-1232. Hyattsville, MD: National Center for Health Statistics, 1984.

10

Analysis of Epidemiologic Studies: Evaluating the Role of Chance

In previous chapters, we have considered various design strategies for epidemiologic studies as well as methods for the presentation and summarization of results. The next step in the evaluation of an epidemiologic hypothesis is an assessment of the validity of the findings. As discussed in Chapter 3, this process involves consideration of whether an observed association between an exposure and a disease is due to alternative explanations, in particular, to chance, bias, or confounding. The first of these, evaluating the role of chance, consists of two separate but related components: hypothesis testing, or performing a test of statistical significance to determine the likelihood that sampling variability can be considered an explanation of the observed results, and estimation of the confidence interval to indicate the range within which the true estimate of effect is likely to lie with a given degree of assurance.

In this chapter, we will discuss the principles underlying tests of statistical significance and confidence intervals and illustrate their use as well as the interpretation of the results. In addition, we will discuss consideration of the role of chance in the design of a study with regard to sample size and power, as well as the use of statistical overviews or meta-analyses to minimize the role of chance in interpreting the results from several individual investigations.

INFERENCE

To understand the need for assessing the role of chance as an alternative explanation of an observed association, it is first necessary to consider the concept of inference. Inference involves making a generalization about a larger group of individuals on the basis of a subset or sample. Whenever an inference about the characteristics of a population is made using information obtained from a sample, there is always the possibility that the inference will be either inaccurate or imprecise, simply because of the play of chance or sampling variability. On the other hand, this possibility will decrease as the size of the sample on which the inference is based increases. For example, suppose we have a bag of 100 marbles, of which half are red and half blue and we wish to infer the true proportions of the different colored marbles in the entire bag by drawing a sample. If we were to draw only two marbles, there would be about one chance in four $[(\frac{1}{2})^2]$ that both marbles would be blue. This means that 25 percent of the time we would incorrectly conclude that all the marbles in the bag were blue given that only half were, based on a sample size of two. By drawing even five marbles instead of two, the probability of observing all five to be blue drops to about 3 in 100 $[(\frac{1}{2})^5]$. Thus, as the sample size increases, the likelihood that we will incorrectly infer from the sample the true characteristics of the entire population decreases.

Similarly, in epidemiology, investigators rarely evaluate every member of an entire population. Most often, an inference concerning the true relationship between an exposure and disease is made from observations on a sample. Thus, for example, the magnitude of an association between obesity and myocardial infarction (MI) would not be assessed in a case-control design by obtaining height and weight on every individual in a community who has had an MI and every individual who has not. More commonly, a sample of those with an MI would be taken as well as a sample of those who had not experienced this end point, and the heights and weights for those individuals would be compared. As a result, as in the previous example with the marbles, there is always a possibility that the resultant estimate will differ from the true magnitude of the association between obesity and MI simply because of chance or sampling variability. Again, however, as in the marbles example, the smaller the sample on which the inference is made, the more variability there will be in the estimate and the less likely the findings will be to reflect the experience of the total population. Conversely, the larger the sample on which the estimate is based, the less variability and the more reliable the inference. In all instances, the play of chance must be considered as an alternative explanation when assessing the validity of the study findings.

HYPOTHESIS TESTING

Hypothesis testing involves conducting a test of statistical significance and quantifying the degree to which sampling variability may account for the results observed in a particular study. This requires making an explicit statement of the hypothesis to be tested, or the null hypothesis. Denoted as H_0, the null hypothesis represents the assertion that there is no relationship between exposure and disease. The alternative hypothesis, denoted as H_1 or H_A, is the assertion that there is some relation between the exposure and disease. For example, if, in a cohort study, we denote the proportion who develop a particular outcome in the nonexposed group as p_0 and the corresponding proportion in the exposed as p_1, the null hypothesis of no association between the exposure and disease would imply that these two proportions are equal or that the relative risk is 1.0. This could be expressed as:

$$H_0: \quad p_0 = p_1$$

or $\quad H_0: \quad \text{RR} = 1$

The alternative hypothesis, that there is an association, could then be expressed as follows:

$$H_1: \quad p_0 \neq p_1$$

or $\quad H_1: \quad \text{RR} \neq 1$

Once H_0 and H_1 have been specified, a test of statistical significance can be performed. There are a number of specific formulas available that are applicable to particular situations. However, all have the same basic structure in that each test statistic is a function of the difference between the values that were observed in the study and those that would have been expected if the null hypothesis were true as well as the amount of variability in the sample. It is therefore possible to consider any significance test as a fraction with two components: a numerator, which increases as the difference between the observed values and those expected under the null hypothesis increases, and a denominator, the variability of the estimate, which decreases as the size of the sample increases.

In addition to sharing a conceptual structure, all tests of statistical significance lead to a probability statement or P value. This statement is based on the principle that if the mean and standard deviation of any normally distributed variable are specified, it is possible to calculate the exact probabilities of specified events, such as the probability of observing a specific value or one more extreme. Specifically, the P value indicates the probability or likelihood of obtaining a result at least as extreme as that observed in a study by chance alone, assuming that there is truly no association between the exposure and outcome under consideration (i.e., H_0 is true). The larger the value for the test of statistical significance, the lower the level of the P value. The particular level of the P value that indicates an association is statistically significant is arbitrarily determined; for medical research, it is usually set, by convention, at 0.05. Thus, any value of P less than or equal to 0.05 ($P \leq 0.05$) indicates that there is, at most, a 5-percent or 1 in 20 probability of observing an association as large or larger than that found in the study by chance alone, given that there is really no association between the exposure and disease. This is taken to mean that chance is an unlikely explanation of the findings, and thus we reject the null hypothesis and conclude that there is a statistically significant association between the exposure and disease under study. Similarly, if the P value is greater than 0.05 ($P > 0.05$), we consider that chance cannot be excluded as a likely explanation for the findings, the null hypothesis is not rejected, and we state that the findings are not statistically significant at that level.

Most commonly, the P value reported from a specific statistical test will represent the probability of observing a difference between the two study groups without specification of direction. Such two-sided or two-tailed P values are the most commonly used in epidemiologic analyses because they allow for the uncertainty about the direction of an effect that is often present. It is, however, also possible to determine a one-sided or one-tailed P value, which represents the probability of observing a difference between study groups of a given magnitude as well as direction. One-sided P values are used only when there is a strong prior hypothesis and the goal of the study is to increase the precision of an estimate where the direction is known, or when a study is conducted specifically to refute the findings of a previous investigation. As long as the results are clearly specified as being one-sided or two-sided, the conversion can be made from one to the other based on the particular needs of the reader.

Despite the conceptual similarity of all hypothesis tests, not all are equally appropriate for any given situation. The selection of a particular statistical test depends on the specific hypothesis being evaluated as well as the type and characteristics of the data collected. We will summarize the methods for calculating only the t test for continuous data and the chi-square test for discrete data, since these are the two most frequently encountered tests of statistical significance in the medical literature [7]. The other tests available are described in detail in textbooks of biostatistics [5, 23].

t *Test*

For continuous data, hypothesis testing involves determining the statistical significance of an observed difference between the mean values of the study groups. This can be accomplished by the use of the normal distribution (if the variance of the measurements in the underlying population is known or the sample size is large) or, most commonly, by use of a t distribution. Denoting the means of two independent study groups as $\bar{x}_1$ and $\bar{x}_0$, the null hypothesis for such a comparison can be expressed as

$$H_0: \quad \bar{x}_1 = \bar{x}_0$$

The corresponding two-sided alternative hypothesis is

H_1: $\bar{x}_1 \neq \bar{x}_0$

To perform a test of statistical significance, the t statistic or critical ratio would be calculated as follows:

$$t_{(df)} = \frac{(\bar{x}_1 - \bar{x}_0) - 0}{\sqrt{s_p^2 \left(\dfrac{1}{n_1} + \dfrac{1}{n_0}\right)}}$$

The numerator of the t test compares the difference between the means of the two study groups ($\bar{x}_1 - \bar{x}_0$) with the difference that would be expected under the null hypothesis (i.e., $\bar{x}_1 - \bar{x}_0 = 0$). The denominator includes the sample size of each study group (n_1 and n_0), as well as the pooled estimate of the common variance (s_p^2), which estimates the overall variance of the entire study population. This is calculated by weighting the two sample or study group variances (s_1^2 and s_0^2) according to the number of observations in each. If the two study groups are the same size ($n_1 = n_0$), the weights are equal and the pooled variance is simply the arithmetic average of the two individual variances ($s_p^2 = [s_1^2 + s_0^2]/2$). If the two groups are of unequal size ($n_1 \neq n_0$), the pooled variance is calculated using the following formula:

$$s_p^2 = \frac{(n_1 - 1)s_1^2 + (n_0 - 1)s_0^2}{n_1 + n_0 - 2}$$

This critical ratio follows a t distribution with ($n_1 + n_0 - 2$) degrees of freedom (df), since there are ($n_1 + n_0 - 2$) total independent pieces of information on which we are basing our estimate.

The calculation of the t test can be illustrated using data from a study of oral contraceptive (OC) use in which fasting triglyceride levels were measured among 190 white women, aged 21 to 39 years, who were classified as current OC users or nonusers [12]. As shown in Table 10-1, the mean fasting triglyceride level among the 86 current OC users was 95 ± 42.4 mg/dl, while that among the 104 nonusers was 73 ± 53.9 mg/dl. The pooled variance can be calculated as follows:

$$s_p^2 = \frac{(n_1 - 1)s_1^2 + (n_0 - 1)s_0^2}{n_1 + n_0 - 2}$$

$$= \frac{(86 - 1)(42.4^2) + (104 - 1)(53.9^2)}{86 + 104 - 2}$$

$$= 2404.5$$

Table 10-1. Mean fasting triglyceride levels among 190 white
women, aged 21–39, by current use of oral contraceptives (OCs)

	Mean fasting triglyceride (mg/dl)	Standard deviation (mg/dl)
Current OC users (n = 86)	95	42.4
OC nonusers (n = 104)	73	53.9

Data from: C. H. Hennekens, D. A. Evans, W. P. Castelli, J. O. Taylor, B. Rosner, and E. H. Kass. Oral contraceptive use and fasting triglyceride, plasma cholesterol and HDL cholesterol. *Circulation* 60:486–489. 1979.

The t test, based on $(86 + 104 - 2)$ or 188 degrees of freedom, can then be performed to determine whether the observed 22 mg/dl difference between mean triglyceride levels is statistically significant:

$$t_{(df)} = \frac{\bar{x}_1 - \bar{x}_0}{\sqrt{s_p^2 \left(\frac{1}{n_1} + \frac{1}{n_0} \right)}}$$

$$= \frac{95 - 73}{\sqrt{2404.5 \left(\frac{1}{86} + \frac{1}{104} \right)}}$$

$$= 3.08$$

To convert this t statistic into a probability statement or P value, we would look up the value of t, in this case 3.08, in a t table (see Appendix A, Table A-3) by locating the row with the appropriate degrees of freedom and finding the value closest to 3.08. In this instance $df = 188$ and thus the last row (marked ∞) would be used. A value of t of 3.08 would correspond to a two-sided P value of less than 0.01 but greater than 0.001. Stated algebraically, the result is $0.001 < P < 0.01$. Thus, there is less than a 1 in 100 probability of observing a difference in triglyceride levels at least as large as 22 mg/dl by chance alone if there is truly no association between current OC use and fasting triglyceride level. We would therefore conclude that the observed mean difference was unlikely to be due to chance and consider the finding statistically significant.

Table 10-2. Presentation of data in a two-by-two table: observed values

| | Disease | | |
	Yes	No	Total
Exposure			
Yes	a	b	$a + b$
No	c	d	$c + d$
Total	$a + c$	$b + d$	$T*$

$*T = a + b + c + d.$

Chi-Square Test

For discrete data, the simplest and most common method to determine whether observed differences in proportions between study groups are statistically significant is the use of the chi-square test. The general form of the chi-square can be expressed as follows:

$$\chi^2_{(df)} = \sum \frac{(O - E)^2}{E}$$

in which O = the observed count in a category, E = the expected count in that category under the null hypothesis, Σ = the sum of all categories, and df = the degrees of freedom associated with the test statistic. As with all tests of statistical significance, this formula includes components of the magnitude of the difference between the study groups as well as a measure of the variability of the estimates.

The expected values for each category are determined based on the assumption that the null hypothesis of no difference between the study groups in the proportions of the factor of interest is true. In a case-control study, this would mean that the proportion with the outcome is the same for those exposed and nonexposed. This assumption can be applied to data that are presented in the form of a two-by-two table (Table 10-2). Cell a represents the observed number of exposed cases. If there were no association between the exposure and disease, the proportion of cases that were exposed would be the same as the proportion of the entire study population that was exposed. Specifically, the expected number of exposed cases would be calculated as the product of the exposure rate in the study—$(a + b)/T$—times the total number of cases in the study—$(a + c)$. The expected values for the other cells in the table would be calculated analogously, as summarized in Table 10-3.

To convert the chi-square statistic into a *P* value involves determining the relevant degrees of freedom and looking up the value in a table of

Table 10-3. Calculation of expected values in a two-by-two table

	Disease	
	Yes	No
Exposure		
Yes	$\dfrac{(a+b)(a+c)}{T}$	$\dfrac{(a+b)(b+d)}{T}$
No	$\dfrac{(c+d)(a+c)}{T}$	$\dfrac{(c+d)(b+d)}{T}$

the chi-square distribution. In general, the degrees of freedom for an r-by-c contingency table is equal to the product of the number of rows in the table minus one times the number of columns minus one, which is expressed as $(r-1)\,(c-1)$. Thus, for any two-by-two table, the degrees of freedom equals $(2-1)(2-1)$ or 1. This value represents the fact that in a two-by-two table, given that the margins are known, knowledge of the number in only one of the cells is necessary to permit the calculation of the numbers in the other three cells by subtraction. The P value associated with a chi-square statistic with 1 degree of freedom can alternatively be determined by using the fact that the square root of the statistic is distributed as a standard normal distribution, using the two-tailed percentage cutoffs. Consequently, either the chi-square or standard normal table can be used to determine the corresponding P value.

The use of the chi-square test can be illustrated using data from a study of the association between current postmenopausal hormone use and risk of nonfatal myocardial infarction (MI), in which 88 women reporting a diagnosis of MI and 1873 healthy control subjects were identified from a large population of married, female registered nurses, aged 30 to 55 years [2]. This study found a relative risk of 0.73 for MI associated with current use of female hormones. These data are presented in Table 10-4, along with calculations of the expected numbers under the null hypothesis. To test the hypothesis that there is no association between use of postmenopausal hormones and risk of MI, the corresponding chi-square statistic can be calculated as follows:

$$\chi^2_{(1)} = \sum \frac{(O - E)^2}{E}$$

$$= \frac{(32 - 38.5)^2}{38.5} + \frac{(825 - 818.5)^2}{818.5} + \frac{(56 - 49.5)^2}{49.5} + \frac{(1048 - 1054.5)^2}{1054.5}$$

$$= 1.10 + 0.05 + 0.85 + 0.04$$

$$= 2.04$$

Table 10-4. Observed and expected values for a case-control study of current use of postmenopausal hormones in relation to risk of nonfatal myocardial infarction (MI)

	Observed		
	Cases	Controls	Total
OC use			
Current use	32	825	857
Never use	56	1048	1104
Total	88	1873	1961

	Expected	
	Cases	Controls
OC use		
Current use	(857)(88)/1961 = 38.5	(857)(1873)/1961 = 818.5
Never use	(1104)(88)/1961 = 49.5	(1104)(1873)/1961 = 1054.5

Data from: Bain, C., Willett, W., Hennekens, C. H., Rosner, B., Belanger, C., and Speizer, F. E. S. Use of postmenopausal hormones and risk of myocardial infarction. *Circulation* 64:42–46, 1981.

Using the table of the chi-square distribution (Appendix A, Table A-4), the observed value of 2.04 with 1 *df* is smaller than the smallest listed value, 2.71. The *P* value would therefore be greater than 0.10 (*P* > 0.10). A more precise *P* value can be obtained from the table of the standard normal distribution (Appendix A, Table A-2) by using the square root of the chi-square value, or $\sqrt{2.04} = 1.43$. A critical ratio or *z* value of 1.43 corresponds to a two-sided *P* value of 0.15. This *P* value indicates that we would expect to observe an association between post-menopausal hormones and risk of MI as strong or stronger than that observed in this study at least 15 percent of the time due to chance alone if there really were no relationship between the exposure and disease. Thus, there is not a significant association between current use of post-menopausal hormones and MI at the *P* = 0.05 level in these data.

The chi-square statistic for a two-by-two table can also be calculated using one of two mathematically equivalent but computationally simpler formulas:

$$\chi^2_{(1)} = \frac{[a - (a + b)(a + c)/T]^2}{\dfrac{(a + b)(c + d)(a + c)(b + d)}{T^2(T - 1)}}$$

or $\quad \chi^2_{(1)} = \dfrac{(ad - bc)^2(T)}{(a + b)(c + d)(a + c)(b + d)}$

Using the data on postmenopausal hormone use and MI from Table 10-4, this would be

$$\chi^2_{(1)} = \frac{[32 - (857)(88)/1961]^2}{\dfrac{(857)(1104)(88)(1873)}{1961^2(1960)}}$$

$$= 2.02$$

or $$\chi^2_{(1)} = \frac{[(32)(1048) - (825)(56)]^2(1961)}{(857)(1104)(88)(1873)} = 2.02$$

There are other versions of each of these two formulas that contain a "continuity correction," first derived by Yates [29] in an attempt to obtain a more precise result in small sample sizes. Formulas with and without the Yates correction will be encountered in the literature. Some authors have argued against the use of such a correction, while others continue to advocate its use, particularly in tests of data from small samples, where it provides a more conservative P value [6, 18, 20].

ESTIMATION: CONFIDENCE INTERVALS

As the basic structure of every test of statistical significance indicates, the size of the P value is a function of two factors: the magnitude of the difference between the groups or the strength of the association, and the size of the sample. Consequently, even a very small difference may be statistically significant, or deemed unlikely to be due to chance, if the sample size is sufficiently large and, conversely, a large effect may not achieve statistical significance if there is substantial variability due to a small sample size.

For this reason, the P value should be considered as a guide to action rather than a hard and fast rule on which to base a conclusion about the role of a factor. It is always advisable to report the actual P value rather than merely that the results did or did not achieve statistical significance. P values of 0.60 and 0.06 would both be reported as nonsignificant at the conventional level of $P = 0.05$. However, the P value of 0.06 is very close to achieving significance and likely would have done so if the sample size had been larger. Thus, the judgment could be made to continue to evaluate that factor in another investigation of adequate sample size.

To overcome the difficulty arising because the P value reflects both the size of the sample and the magnitude of the effect, a related but far more informative measure to evaluate the role of chance, the confidence interval (CI), can be reported. The confidence interval represents the range within which the true magnitude of effect lies with a certain degree of assurance. For example, in evaluating the relationship of smoking with bladder cancer in men, instead of simply reporting that those who smoked had a statistically significant increased risk (RR = 1.9) of bladder cancer compared with those who did not, the 95 percent confidence interval of (1.3–2.8) would also be presented. This indicates that the best estimate of the increased risk of bladder cancer associated with smoking is 1.9; however, we are 95 percent confident that the true relative risk is no less than 1.3 and no greater than 2.8.

The confidence interval can provide all the information of the *P* value in terms of whether the association is statistically significant at a specified level. If the null value (e.g., 1.0 for the relative risk estimate) is included in a 95 percent confidence interval, then the corresponding *P* value is, by definition, greater than 0.05. If the null value is not included in the interval, then the corresponding *P* value is less than 0.05 and the association is statistically significant. In the above example, the 95-percent confidence interval was (1.3–2.8). Since this does not include the null value of 1.0, we can conclude that the *P* value from the test of significance would be less than 0.05 and there is a statistically significant association between smoking and bladder cancer.

In addition, the width of the confidence interval indicates the amount of variability inherent in the estimate and thus the effect of sample size. The larger the study sample, the more stable the estimate, and the narrower the confidence interval. The wider the confidence interval, the greater was the variability in the estimate of the effect and the smaller the sample size. For example, a confidence interval of (1.3–1.8) indicates a much smaller degree of variability than one of (1.2–7.6) and is much more informative about the true magnitude of the relative risk associated with a particular exposure. The information provided by the confidence interval is particularly important when interpreting the results of studies that are not statistically significant (i.e., null findings). A narrow confidence interval will add support to the belief that there is actually no true increased risk, whereas a wide interval suggests that the data are compatible with a true increased (or decreased) risk but that the sample size was simply not sufficient to have adequate statistical power to exclude chance as a likely explanation of the findings.

Thus, the *P* value and confidence interval together provide the most information about the role of chance. As with tests of statistical significance, there is a wide variety of formulas available for the calculation of confidence intervals [5, 15, 23, 25, 27]. In the next two sections, we present formulas for the confidence interval around a difference in means and a relative risk.

Construction of the Confidence Interval: Difference in Means

The confidence interval around a difference in means of two independent populations may be calculated using the following formula:

$$\text{CI} = (\bar{x}_1 - \bar{x}_0) \pm t_{(df)} \sqrt{s_p^2 \left(\frac{1}{n_1} + \frac{1}{n_0} \right)}$$

where, as previously, s_p^2 represents the pooled variance, $\bar{x}_1$, $\bar{x}_0$, n_1, and n_0 the means and sample sizes, respectively, of the two groups, and t the value of the t distribution, given the appropriate degrees of freedom, that corresponds to the significance level of interest (such as 0.05 for a 95% confidence interval).

For example, a 95-percent confidence interval can be constructed around the observed difference in the mean fasting triglyceride levels for users and nonusers of OCs (see Table 10-1) as follows:

$$95\% \text{ CI} = (\bar{x}_1 - \bar{x}_0) \pm t_{(n_1 + n_0 - 2)} \sqrt{s_p^2 \left(\frac{1}{n_1} + \frac{1}{n_0} \right)}$$

$$= (95 - 73) \pm 1.96 \sqrt{2404.5 \left(\frac{1}{86} + \frac{1}{104} \right)}$$

$$= 22 \pm 14.01$$

$$= 7.99, 36.01$$

This range indicates that we can rule out a true difference in mean triglyceride levels between users and nonusers of OCs that is smaller than 8 or larger than 36 mg/dl with 95% confidence. Since this confidence interval does not include zero, the value for the difference in means that would be expected under the null hypothesis, the observed difference is statistically significant at the $P = 0.05$ level.

Construction of the Confidence Interval: Relative Risk

There are a number of methods commonly used to construct a confidence interval around an estimate of the relative risk. Formulas for the confidence interval around this estimate of effect must take into account the fact that the distribution of possible values for the relative risk is highly skewed to the right: relative risk estimates can never be less than zero, but they can theoretically assume any positive value up to infinity. However, applying a transformation to the individual relative risks—specifically, taking the natural logarithm (denoted ln) of each—will result in a distribution that is approximately normal in shape. Then, using formulas analogous to those presented in the previous section for means, the upper and lower bounds of the confidence interval can be constructed around the value of the ln RR rather than the relative risk itself. To get back to the actual relative risk involves simply taking the antilogarithm of the ln RR (written as exp[ln RR] or $e^{\ln RR}$). Thus, the upper and lower bounds of the confidence interval for the relative risk can be calculated by taking antilogarithms of the corresponding values for the interval for ln RR. This can all be done in one step by using the general formula

$$CI = (RR)\exp[\pm z \sqrt{Variance(\ln RR)}]$$

where z is the value of the standard normal distribution associated with the desired level of confidence.

For the relative risk calculated as the odds ratio from a case-control study [27, 28], the variance can be approximated using a Taylor series expansion, and the formula for the confidence interval can be expressed as follows:

$$CI = (ad/bc)\exp[\pm z \sqrt{(1/a + 1/b + 1/c + 1/d)}]$$

Referring to the previously cited study of postmenopausal hormones and risk of MI (see Table 10-4), the 95-percent confidence interval would be calculated as follows:

$$95\% \ CI = (ad/bc)\exp(\pm 1.96 \sqrt{1/a + 1/b + 1/c + 1/d})$$

$$= \frac{32 \ (1048)}{825 \ (56)}\exp(\pm 1.96 \sqrt{1/32 + 1/825 + 1/56 + 1/1048})$$

$$= (0.73) \exp(\pm 0.44) \ or \ (0.73)e^{\pm 0.44}$$

Lower bound $= (0.73)e^{-0.44} = (0.73) \ (0.64)$

$$= 0.47$$

Upper bound $= (0.73)e^{+0.44} = (0.73) \ (1.55)$

$$= 1.13$$

Thus, in these data, the best estimate of the risk of MI associated with current use of postmenopausal hormones is 0.73. That is, women who are current users of postmenopausal hormones have 73% the risk of MI of women who do not use these agents. However, with 95% confidence the true relative risk lies between 0.47 and 1.13. Since this interval includes the null value (RR = 1), the observed association is not statistically significant at the 0.05 level. In fact, the totality of the evidence favors a 50-percent or greater statistically significant reduction in cardiovascular mortality among women who use postmenopausal hormones, a value that is compatible with results of the example above since it lies within the 95-percent confidence interval.

One alternative approach to the method used previously for the calculation of the confidence interval is a test-based method [21] that uses the square root of the chi-square value calculated in the test of significance, denoted as chi or χ, to approximate the variance. The upper and lower bounds of the confidence interval estimated in this way are

$$CI = RR^{(1 \pm z/\chi)}$$

where z is the value of the standard normal distribution associated with the desired level of confidence and $\chi = \sqrt{\chi^2_{(1)}}$ from the test of statistical significance. This is a very easy formula to compute with a simple pocket calculator, and in addition, software is available for programmable calculators [24].

For the example of current use of postmenopausal hormones and MI, the test-based 95-percent confidence interval would be calculated as follows:

$$CI = RR^{(1 \pm z/\chi)}$$
$$= 0.73^{(1 \pm 1.96/\sqrt{2.04})}$$
$$= 0.73^{(1 \pm 1.37)}$$
$$\text{Lower bound} = 0.73^{(2.37)}$$
$$= 0.47$$
$$\text{Upper bound} = 0.73^{(-0.37)}$$
$$= 1.12$$

These limits are virtually identical to those calculated by the previous method, although this is not always so. The intervals obtained by a Taylor series expansion in general tend to be a little wider, or more conservative, than the corresponding test-based intervals. This discrepancy is usually negligible when the sample size is large or when the relative risk estimate is near to the null value. For small samples, neither method is optimal, and the calculation of exact confidence intervals is preferable [15, 25, 27].

The 95-percent confidence interval is the most common, but other limits can easily be constructed simply by changing the z value. As the level of desired confidence increases, the width of the confidence interval will also increase so that more values are included. Thus, a 95-percent confidence interval will be wider than the corresponding 90-percent confidence interval.

Analogous formulas are available for the construction of the confidence interval around the relative risk calculated from a cohort study as well as around other measures of effect [25].

Issues in Interpreting Results of Tests of Statistical Significance

There are a number of issues that are important to keep in mind when interpreting the results of a test of statistical significance. First, the P value should be considered not as a hard and fast rule for establishing the role of chance, but as a guide to the likelihood that chance is an explanation of the findings. No P value, however small, excludes chance completely. Even if the P value were 0.0001, meaning that the probability of observing that particular result or one more extreme by chance alone given that there is truly no association between the exposure and disease is only 1 in 10,000, there would still be 1 time out of 10,000 when it would occur by chance. However, in this circumstance, chance can be considered an unlikely explanation for the findings. Moreover, no P value, however large, can be taken to mean that the observed finding was due to chance, only that chance cannot be excluded as a likely explanation. The absolute magnitude of the P value, as well as the contribution of sample size as seen from the confidence interval, must be considered in interpreting the results.

Second, the statistical significance of an association between an exposure and disease must be distinguished from the question of its biologic or clinical significance. Even a very small difference that is not clinically meaningful may achieve statistical significance—that is, appear unlikely to be due to chance—if the sample size is sufficiently large. Conversely, a large and clinically meaningful difference may not achieve statistical significance if the sample size is small.

Third, investigators often collect data pertaining to a large number of potentially important risk factors. In such instances, multiple tests of statistical significance are commonly performed to determine whether any of these variables is significantly associated with the disease or outcome of interest. However, as the number of variables tested is increased, so is the likelihood of finding a statistically significant difference solely due to the play of chance. For this reason, any unanticipated association that achieves statistical significance when the data are analyzed must be interpreted with caution. For example, in a case-control study of pancreatic cancer [17], cigarette smoking and alcohol consumption were specified a priori to be tested as risk factors for the disease. In addition, information was collected on coffee and tea consumption. In these data, coffee consumption was observed to be statistically significantly associated with an increased risk of pancreatic cancer. Since this finding was unexpected, the most appropriate interpretation is that these data provide evidence that can be used for formulate the hypothesis that coffee consumption is associated with pancreatic cancer and thus furnish a promising lead to be explored in further studies. Similarly, a case-control study designed specifically to test the hypothesis that coffee consumption increases mortality from coronary heart disease [11] showed no association but a subsequent analysis found a possible relation of retirement and coronary death [4]. Since this study had not been designed a priori to evaluate this latter issue, the authors concluded that their data raised a question to be addressed by other independent investigations using different methodology.

Finally, it must be clearly kept in mind that tests of statistical significance and confidence intervals evaluate only the role of chance as an alternative explanation of an observed association between an exposure and disease. While an examination of the P value and/or confidence interval may lead to the conclusion that chance is an unlikely explanation for the findings, this provides absolutely no information concerning the possibility that the observed association is due to the effects of uncontrolled bias or confounding. All three possible alternative explanations must always be considered in the interpretation of the results of every study.

STUDY DESIGN ISSUES: SAMPLE SIZE AND POWER

In this chapter, we have emphasized that the size of a study influences the magnitude of the P value and thus the likelihood that any observed difference will attain statistical significance. Consequently, a crucial question researchers must address during the planning phase of a study is how many subjects are needed to assure a given probability of detecting a statistically significant effect of a given magnitude if one truly exists. If, as is usually the case, only a limited pool of subjects is available for study, the more relevant question becomes how likely is it that a statistically significant effect of a given magnitude can be identified among this group of subjects if it is really there. The first question is addressed by sample size calculations and the second by power calculations.

In contrast to hypothesis testing, where all of the work proceeds from the assumption that the null hypothesis is true, for sample size and power calculations, we begin with the assumption that the null hypothesis is not true or, more specifically, that a particular alternative hypothesis is true. In other words, we need to have some general idea about how big the effect we are studying is likely to be, or at least the size of the smallest effect we think is worth detecting. For example, in a case-control study of hypertension as a risk factor for MI, we might be interested in detecting a relative risk of 1.5 or more—that is, that individuals with hypertension have at least a 50-percent increase in risk of developing coronary heart disease compared with those with normal

Table 10-5. Four possible outcomes of hypothesis testing

Conclusion of test of significance	Truth	
	H_0 True	H_1 True
Do not reject H_0 (not statistically significant)	Correct: H_0 is true, and we do not reject H_0	Type II or beta error: H_1 is true, but we do not reject H_0
Reject H_0 (statistically significant)	Type I or alpha error: H_0 is true, but we reject H_0	Correct: H_1 is true, and we reject H_0

blood pressure levels. We could then write the null and alternative hypotheses as follows:

H_0: RR = 1.0

H_1: RR ≥ 1.5

As we have seen, on the basis of the data collected in the study, we will then decide whether or not to reject the null hypothesis in favor of the alternative hypothesis. There are two possible decisions we can make, and two possible outcomes of each decision. These possibilities can be presented in a two-by two table (Table 10-5).

As illustrated in the table, if we reject the null hypothesis when the alternative hypothesis is true, or we fail to reject the null hypothesis when H_0 is true, there is no error made. However, in two situations there will be an error in rejecting or not rejecting the null hypothesis. Type I error refers to the situation in which the null hypothesis is rejected when it is in fact true. The probability of making a type I error is equal to the P value and is represented by the Greek letter alpha (α); for example, an alpha level of 0.05 would indicate that the likelihood of erroneously rejecting the null hypothesis is 5 percent (or 1 in 20) and $P = 0.05$. Type II error, in contrast, refers to a mistaken failure to reject the null hypothesis when the alternative hypothesis is true and there is a real difference between the study groups. The probability of making a type II error is represented by the Greek letter beta (β). The power of a study is defined as the probability of rejecting the null hypothesis and concluding that there is a statistically significance difference between the study groups if one truly exists and is calculated as $1 - \beta$. Thus, if beta is set at 0.20—that is, there is a 20 percent chance of making a type II error and failing to reject H_0 given that H_1 is true—the power of the study would equal $1 - 0.20$, or 0.80. This means there is an 80 percent chance of detecting a difference of the magnitude specified if one truly exists.

In designing a study, both types of error should, ideally, be minimized. However, due to their interrelationship, a decrease in the probability of one type of error is often achieved at the expense of an increase in the probability of the other. Because of sampling variability, it is unlikely that we would observe a relative risk of exactly 1.0 even if the null hypothesis were true, or of exactly 1.5 even if the alternative hypothesis were true. However, we would consider larger values of the relative risk as more compatible with H_1 and smaller values as more compatible with H_0. Suppose the observed result were RR = 1.3. If we judge that this result is more compatible with H_1, our chance of being wrong—that is, that the result really came from the H_0 distribution—is the type I error. If, instead, we judged the result to be more compatible with H_0, the chance of being wrong is the type II error. For a given magnitude of effect, the type II error can be decreased only by increasing the degree of precision of the measurements. This is most often accomplished by increasing the sample size.

Sample Size Determination

In calculating the required sample size for a given study, it is necessary to specify the desired values for the probabilities of type I (alpha) and type II (beta) errors, the proportion of the baseline population that is exposed to the factor of interest (for case-control studies) or has the disease under study (for cohort or intervention studies), and the magnitude of the expected effect. The estimates of the baseline proportions are usually based on previously published reports. The expected magnitude of effect may also be estimated from these sources or, if unavailable, may be taken to represent the minimum effect that the investigators would consider meaningful. Once these values have been specified, the necessary sample size can be determined using one of a number of standard formulas [5, 14, 15, 23, 27]. The specific formula chosen, like the particular test of significance, is dictated by features of the study design, the particular research question being addressed, as well as the type of data that will be collected. In the following example, we illustrate the calculation of the sample size for a case-control study with discrete data in which the measure of effect represents the difference in exposure proportions between the study groups.

Suppose that we wish to undertake a case-control study of current OC use in relation to risk of MI among women of childbearing age. From previous studies [22], we know that about 10 percent of such women in the United States are currently using OCs, and that the relative risk associated with the incidence of MI among current OC users is approximately 1.8. We would be interested in the conventional alpha level of

Table 10-6. Formula for the calculation of sample size in a case-control study evaluating the difference between exposure proportions

$$n(\text{each group}) = \frac{(p_0 q_0 + p_1 q_1)(z_{1-\alpha/2} + z_{1-\beta})^2}{(p_1 - p_0)^2}$$

in which: p_1 = the proportion of exposure among cases

p_0 = the proportion of exposure among controls

$q_1 = 1 - p_1$

$q_0 = 1 - p_0$

$z_{1-\alpha/2}$ = value of the standard normal distribution corresponding to a significance level of alpha (e.g., 1.96 for a two-sided test at the 0.05 level)

$z_{1-\beta}$ = value of the standard normal distribution corresponding to the desired level of power (e.g., 0.84 for a power of 80%)

0.05 and beta level of 0.20, representing a power of 80 percent to detect an effect of this magnitude if one truly exists. The sample size for such a study would be calculated using the formula shown in Table 10-6.

Assuming an expected relative risk of 1.8, the following values would be used to compute the required sample size:

p_0 = proportion of controls who are current OC users = 0.10

p_1 = proportion of cases who are current OC users =

$(P_0)(\text{RR}) = (0.10)(1.8) = 0.18$

$q_0 = 1.0 - 0.10 = 0.90$

$q_1 = 1.0 - 0.18 = 0.82$

$z_{1-\alpha/2} = 1.96$

$z_{1-\beta} = 0.84$

These values can then be entered into the sample size formula as follows:

$$n \ (\text{each group}) = \frac{[(0.1) \ (0.9) + (0.18) \ (0.82)] \ [1.96 + 0.84]^2}{(0.18 - 0.10)^2}$$

$$= \frac{(0.2376) \ (7.84)}{0.0064}$$

$$= 291.06$$

Table 10-7. Sample size estimates for a
case-control study of OC use and MI among women

Postulated relative risks	Required sample size in each group*
1.2	3834
1.3	1769
1.5	682
1.8	291
2.0	196
2.5	97
3.0	59

*Assuming proportion of current OC use in general population of women of childbearing age = 10%, power = 80%, type I error (two-sided) = 5%.

Thus, we would need at least 291 cases and 291 controls to detect a relative risk of MI associated with current OC use of 1.8 with a type II error of 0.20 (80% power) and a type I error of 5 percent.

In many instances, it is also of interest to know what sample sizes will be required if the true relative risk is higher or lower than anticipated. For example, we might be interested in being able to detect a smaller relative risk in our study of OC use and MI, given the high frequency of both the risk factor and the outcome in the United States. Similarly, the true relative risk might be much higher. It is therefore useful to construct a table of sample sizes that would be required for different postulated relative risks if the power is held at the conventional level of 80 percent and the proportion of exposure among the controls remains constant. As shown in Table 10-7, as the relative risk approaches 1.0— that is, as the magnitude of the difference between the groups that is of interest becomes smaller—the sample size that would be required to achieve the same power increases dramatically, so that to have adequate power to observe a 20-percent increase in risk associated with OC use, we would need at least 3834 subjects in each study group. Similarly, as the magnitude of effect becomes more extreme, the necessary sample size decreases, so that to detect a relative risk of 3.0, we would need only 59 subjects in each group.

These sample sizes should be interpreted as providing merely a minimum estimate of the desired sample sizes for the study because this formula takes into account only the estimate of the overall crude association between exposure and disease. It does not consider any potential

Table 10-8. Power calculation formula for
case-control studies using discrete data

$$z_{1-\beta} = \sqrt{\frac{n \times (p_1 - p_0)^2}{(p_0 q_0 + p_1 q_1)}} - z_{1-\alpha/2}$$

in which: $z_{1-\beta}$ = value of the standard normal
distribution corresponding to the power
of the study

p_1 = the proportion of exposure
among cases

p_0 = the proportion of exposure
among controls

$q_1 = 1 - p_1$

$q_0 = 1 - p_0$

n = the number of subjects in
each group

$z_{1-\alpha/2}$ = value of the standard normal
distribution corresponding to a
significance level of alpha

control of confounding through stratification, in which subgroups of the
data are evaluated and which consequently requires larger numbers.

Power Calculations

Under ideal conditions, every investigator would perform a sample size
determination and then design a study to collect data on the required
number of subjects. However, in actual practice, the number of available
subjects is often limited by factors such as the disease rate in the population of interest, logistic problems, or budgetary constraints. In such
circumstances, it is useful to calculate the power of the study given a
particular sample size and various postulated estimates of the magnitude
of the effect. This can be determined simply by solving the formula for
sample size in terms of power.

For example, in the case-control study of oral contraceptive use and
MI, the power of the study for a given sample size can be calculated from
the formula presented in Table 10-8. If the proportion of exposure in
the control group, the estimated relative risk, and the level of type I
error remain the same as in our initial sample size calculations but we
know that we can identify only 100 cases and 100 controls in a reason-

Table 10-9. Power associated with a study of OC use and risk of MI with a sample size of 100 cases and controls, with various postulated relative risks

Postulated relative risk	$z_{1-\beta}$*	Power
1.2	−1.51	0.066
1.3	−1.29	0.099
1.5	−0.89	0.187
1.8	−0.32	0.374
2.0	0.04	0.516
2.5	0.89	0.813
3.0	1.69	0.954

*When this number is ≤ 0.0, the power equals the area in one tail of the standard normal distribution corresponding to that value. When > 0.0, the power equals (1.0 − that area).

able time period, we can use this information to calculate what the power of the study would be in such a circumstance:

$$z_{1-\beta} = \sqrt{\frac{(100)(0.18 - 0.10)^2}{(0.10)(0.90) + (0.18)(0.82)}} - 1.96$$

$$= -0.32$$

Using the standard normal table (Appendix A, Table A-1), this value corresponds to a power of 0.374. Thus, the power of this study to detect a relative risk of MI associated with current OC use of 1.8 using a population of 100 cases and 100 controls would be only 37.4 percent.

Since the power of a study is dependent on both the magnitude of the effect and the size of the study population, varying either one will alter the power. For example, as shown in Table 10-9, for our sample size of 100 cases and 100 controls, the greatest power is associated with detecting relative risk estimates furthest from the null value. In this instance, the study would only have adequate power (i.e., ≥ 80%) to detect relative risks of 2.5 or greater.

STATISTICAL OVERVIEWS

As discussed in the previous section, the sample size of a study and its resultant statistical power are essential to an ability to evaluate the role of chance as an alternative explanation of study findings. If a study is of inadequate sample size, then a finding of no statistically significant association between exposure and disease, a so-called null finding, may well be uninformative, since a true lack of association will be difficult or impossible to distinguish from a true association that cannot be detected statistically because of inadequate power. Consequently, achieving adequate power is of paramount importance in the design and conduct of any epidemiologic study. Unfortunately, investigators often have difficulty assembling a sample size that is adequate to test the magnitude of effects that are most likely to occur. As a result, a number of studies may be available in the literature that all indicate a similar magnitude of effect of the exposure on disease but do not individually achieve statistical significance, primarily due to inadequate sample size. This problem of the effect of type II errors on the interpretation of randomized clinical trials was considered by reexamining the results of 71 null trials to determine whether, in fact, the studies had adequate statistical power to detect a 25 or 50 percent therapeutic improvement [8]. Of these 71 trials, 67 had a greater than 10 percent probability of failing to detect a 25 percent therapeutic improvement, and 50 could have missed a 50 percent improvement with the same probability.

In this circumstance, it would be useful to be able to consider the studies in aggregate in order to provide a more stable estimate of the most likely magnitude of the effect. This issue has been approached in a number of ways, from making a qualitative assessment of the trials that provide the "best" information, to combining the patients in all trials and reanalyzing as if the data had come from one single, large study. The problem with the latter approach is that patients admitted to one trial are likely to differ systematically from those enrolled in another with respect to factors that might affect their risk of the outcomes under study. Because of this, it is not valid to compare directly the experience of individual subjects in one trial with that of subjects in another. However, it is possible to compare the overall effect observed in one trial with that of another, since each is internally randomized. Thus, each trial can be considered as an individual stratum, and modifications of statistical methods for combining information from two-by-two tables can be used to combine the strata and obtain an overall estimate [19]. For example, for each trial, the observed number of events (O) in a treatment group can be contrasted with the number expected (E) under the null hypothesis [30]. If a treatment were of no benefit, the observed minus the expected number of events (O − E) would differ only randomly from zero. In contrast, if treatment were beneficial, then O − E would tend to be negative. Although in any one trial this tendency might be obscured or even reversed by the play of chance, it is far more likely to stand out clearly when the grand total of O − E from all individual trials is examined.

The use of this approach can be illustrated by considering an overview

Table 10-10. Mortality data from an overview of randomized trials of intravenous streptokinase in acute myocardial infarction

Study	Deaths		RR of mortality	P value (two-sided)
	Treated	Controls		
Fletcher 1959	1/12	4/11	0.2	NS
Dewar 1963	4/21	7/21	0.6	NS
First European 1969	20/83	15/84	1.3	NS
Heikenheimo 1971	22/219	17/207	1.2	NS
Italian 1971	19/164	18/157	1.0	NS
Second European 1971	69/373	94/357	0.7	< 0.02
Second Frankfurt 1973	13/102	29/104	0.5	< 0.01
NHLBI SMIT 1974	7/53	3/54	2.4	NS
Australian 1973, 1977	51/376	63/371	0.8	NS
Frank 1975	6/55	6/53	1.0	NS
Valere 1975	11/49	9/42	1.0	NS
UK Collaborative 1976	48/302	52/293	0.9	NS
Klein 1976	4/14	1/9	2.6	NS
North German Collab 1977	63/249	51/234	1.2	NS
Austrian 1977	37/352	65/376	0.6	< 0.01
Witchitz 1977	5/32	5/26	0.8	NS
Lasierra 1977	1/13	3/11	0.3	NS
Third European 1979	25/156	50/159	0.5	< 0.01
Olson 1984	5/28	5/24	0.9	NS
Schreiber 1984	1/19	4/19	0.3	NS
TOTAL	412/2672	501/2612		

"Typical" odds ratio = 0.76 (95% CI = 0.66–0.88)

Source: S. Yusuf, R. Collins, R. Peto, C. Furberg, M. J. Stampfer, S. K. Goldhaber, and C. H. Hennekens. Intravenous and intracoronary fibrinolytic therapy in acute myocardial infarction: Overview of results on mortality, reinfarction and side effects from 33 randomized controlled trials. *Eur. Heart J.* 6:556–585. 1985.

Table 10-11. Results of an overview of retrospective cohort studies of reproductive outcomes among female operating room personnel

	Spontaneous abortions		Congenital abnormalities	
	RR	95% CI	RR	95% CI
Physicians	1.4	(1.2–1.6)	1.4	(1.0–2.0)
Nurses	1.3	(1.1–1.4)	1.1	(0.9–1.4)
Total	1.3	(1.2–1.4)	1.2	(1.0–1.4)

Source: J. E. Buring, C. H. Hennekens, S. L. Mayrent, B. Rosner, E. R. Greenberg, and T. Colton. Health experiences of operating room personnel. *Anesthesiology* 62:325–330. 1985.

[30] of published randomized trials of intravenous (IV) streptokinase administered in the acute stage of MI. As shown in Table 10-10, with respect to mortality, while the majority of the relative risk estimates indicated a reduction in risk associated with the administration of streptokinase, the estimates of effect in the individual studies, most of which were of small sample size, varied widely, from a low of 0.2 to a high of 2.6, and only four of these results achieved statistical significance. The overview yielded a "typical" or pooled relative risk estimate of 0.76, a value that was highly statistically significant (95% confidence interval 0.66–0.88, $P < 0.001$). This indicates that patients treated with IV streptokinase experienced an approximate 24-percent reduction in subsequent mortality, a reduction that, based on all available data, is unlikely to be due to chance.

While a single well designed and conducted trial of sufficient sample size to detect the true effects of an intervention is always optimal, in the absence of a definitive study, overviews of data from several smaller trials can provide useful information [9]. Perhaps the chief utility of such overviews is to provide a reliable estimate of the most likely effect of an intervention, which can be used in planning a future trial with adequate power to detect that effect if it truly exists. For example, on the basis of the estimated 24-percent reduction in risk of mortality derived from the overview of trials of IV streptokinase presented in Table 10-10, the Second International Study of Infarct Survival (ISIS-2) [13] was designed to enroll a total of 20,000 subjects. This sample size is in marked contrast to the numbers of participants in all previous trials, which totalled 2672 in the treated group and 2612 in the comparison group. Similarly, the Physicians' Health Study [10] was designed to detect a 20-percent reduction in cardiovascular mortality due to aspirin based on an overview of six published trials of aspirin on risk of reinfarction and cardiovascular mortality among individuals with a history of MI [1], and enrolled 22,071 male U.S. physicians, aged 40 to 84, to address this issue adequately.

An overview can also be performed using data from observational studies. However, the results of such an analysis must be viewed with a greater degree of caution than an overview of randomized trials because of concerns related to uncontrolled confounding. For example, an overview of 17 published reports on the health experiences of operating room personnel [3] found that 6 of the studies, all using a retrospective cohort design, were sufficiently similar in terms of study population, end points, and exposures to permit combination of their data. The results of these overview analyses for reproductive outcomes among women are presented in Table 10-11.

As shown in Table 10-11, taken together, the data indicate that there were statistically significant increased risks of spontaneous abortion among both female physicians and female nurses, with an overall relative risk for all exposed women of 1.3 (95-percent confidence interval = 1.2–1.4). For congenital abnormalities, the data were less consistent. The increase was of borderline statistical significance and only for exposed physicians. While the narrow range of the confidence interval indicates that chance is an unlikely explanation of the findings, this result should be interpreted with particular caution because of the inadequacies of data from the individual studies. The authors concluded [3] that before firm decisions could be reached on health experiences of operating room personnel, it was necessary to conduct

prospective cohort studies . . . that permit the accurate recording, classifying, and quantifying of type, degree, and intensity of exposure; these studies should define rigorously the adverse outcomes of interest, and their occurrence should be confirmed by investigators unaware of the exposure status of the individual. If results of these prospective studies support the findings of the pooled analyses, they then could lead to the development of recommendations for special exposure groups such as pregnant women. . . .

In fact, the results of one such well designed and conducted prospective study have supported the findings of the overview on risk of spontaneous abortion among operating room personnel [16].

Thus, the use of a statistical overview or meta-analysis provides a quantitative method of obtaining an overall estimate of effect. However, the quality and usefulness of any overview is dependent on the quality of the component studies [26]. In particular, the studies combined should be similar with respect to the disease and the exposure or intervention being studied, and the characteristics of the subjects must be sufficiently similar to make combining the results of such studies reasonable. In addition, the magnitude of the effect of each of the studies must be sufficiently similar that their combination will not provide a distorted estimate. To the extent there is substantial heterogeneity, the information provided by any single overall estimate of effect will decrease.

CONCLUSION

The evaluation of the role of chance in epidemiologic research has traditionally involved the performance of a test of statistical significance and the calculation of a P value. Based on the P value, a decision is made as to whether an observed association is statistically significant at a specified level, usually 0.05. The interpretability of a P value, however, is limited because of its dependence on the estimate of the magnitude of the association as well as the size of the sample. Moreover, epidemiologic research, in addition to the assessment of whether statistical significance is achieved in a given study, should have as a paramount concern the estimation of parameters. In this regard, the confidence interval around an estimate of effect is of particular importance. The confidence interval provides information concerning the most precise estimate of the true effect. Finally, it is important to keep firmly in mind that hypothesis testing and calculation of the confidence interval, while necessary to evaluate the role of chance, are not sufficient to assess the validity of findings. Regardless of whether a statistically significant difference is found between the study groups, it is also essential to consider possible sources of bias as well as confounding, each or all of which could provide alternative explanations for the observed findings, either wholly or in part.

STUDY QUESTIONS

1. Define P value and confidence interval.
2. Why are confidence intervals preferable to P values in the interpretation of the role of chance as an alternative explanation for findings?
3. Discuss the interrelationships among size of the relative risk, size of a sample, and power of a study.
4. Define overviews of epidemiologic studies and list their chief uses.

REFERENCES

1. Aspirin for heart patients. *F.D.A. Drug Bull.* 15:34–136. 1985.
2. Bain, C., Willett, W., Hennekens, C. H., et al. Use of postmenopausal hormones and risk of myocardial infarction. *Circulation* 64:42–46, 1981.

3. Buring, J. E., Hennekens, C. H., Mayrent, S. L., et al. Health experiences of operating room personnel. *Anesthesiology* 62:325–330, 1985.
4. Casscells, W., Hennekens, C. H., Evans, D., et al. Retirement and coronary mortality. *Lancet* 1:1288–1289, 1980.
5. Colton, T. *Statistics in Medicine.* Boston: Little, Brown, 1974.
6. Conover, W. J. Some reasons for not using the Yates continuity correction on 2×2 contingency tables. *J. Am. Stat. Assoc.* 69:374–376, 1974.
7. Emerson, J. D., and Colditz, G. A. Use of statistical analysis in the *New England Journal of Medicine*. *N. Engl. J. Med.* 309:709–713, 1983.
8. Freiman, J. A., Chalmers, T. C., Smith, H., Jr., et al. The importance of beta, the type II error and sample size in the design and interpretation of the randomized controlled trial: Survey of 71 "negative" trials. *N. Engl. J. Med.* 299:690–694, 1978.
9. Hennekens, C. H., Buring, J. E., and Hebert, P. Implications of overviews for randomized trials. *Stat. Med.* 6:397–402, 1987.
10. Hennekens, C. H., and Eberlein, K. For the Physicians' Health Study Research Group. A randomized trial of aspirin and beta-carotene among U.S. physicians. *Prev. Med.* 14:165–168, 1985.
11. Hennekens, C. H., Drolette, M. E., Jesse, M. J., et al. Coffee drinking and death due to coronary heart disease. *N. Engl. J. Med.* 294:633–663, 1976.
12. Hennekens, C. H., Evans, D. A., Castelli, W. P., et al. Oral contraceptive use and fasting triglyceride, plasma cholesterol and HDL cholesterol. *Circulation* 60:486–489, 1979.
13. ISIS-2 Steering Committee (P. Sleight, Chairman; R. Collins, Coordinator; and R. Peto, Statistician). Personal communication, 1985.
14. Kelsey, J. L., Thompson, W. D., and Evans, A. S. *Methods in Observational Epidemiology.* New York: Oxford University Press, 1986.
15. Kleinbaum, D. G., Kupper, L. L., and Morgenstern, H. *Epidemiologic Research: Principles and Quantitative Methods.* Belmont, CA: Lifetime Learning Publications, 1982.
16. Knill-Jones, R. Personal communication, 1985.
17. MacMahon, B., Yen, S., Trichopoulos, D., et al. Coffee and cancer of the pancreas. *N. Engl. J. Med.* 304:630–633, 1981.
18. Mantel, N. Some reasons for not using the Yates continuity correction on 2×2 contingency tables: Comment and suggestion. *J. Am. Stat. Assoc.* 69:378–380, 1974.
19. Mantel, N., and Haenszel, W. Statistical aspects of the analysis of data from retrospective studies of disease. *J.N.C.I.* 22:719–748, 1959.
20. Miettinen, O. S. Some reasons for not using the Yates continuity correction on 2×2 contingency tables: Comment. *J. Am. Stat. Assoc.* 69:380–382, 1974.
21. Miettinen, O. S. Estimability and estimation in case-referent studies. *Am. J. Epidemiol.* 103:226–235, 1976.
22. Rosenberg, L., Hennekens, C. H., Rosner, B., et al. Oral contraceptive use in relation to nonfatal myocardial infarction. *Am. J. Epidemiol.* 111:59–66, 1980.
23. Rosner, B. *Fundamentals of Biostatistics.* Boston: Duxbury Press, 1982.
24. Rothman, K. J., and Boice, J. D., Jr. *Epidemiologic Analysis with a Programmable Calculator.* U.S. D.H.E.W. N.I.H. Publication No. 79-1649, 1979.

25. Rothman, K. J. *Modern Epidemiology.* Boston: Little, Brown, 1986.
26. Sacks, H. S., Berrier, J., Reitman, D., et al. Meta-analyses of randomized controlled trials. *N. Engl. J. Med.* 316:450–455, 1987.
27. Schlesselman, J. J. *Case-Control Studies: Design, Conduct, Analysis.* New York: Oxford University Press, 1982.
28. Woolf, B. On estimating the relation between blood group and disease. *Ann. Human Gen.* 19:251–253, 1955.
29. Yates, F. Contingency tables involving small numbers and the χ^2 test. *J. R. Stat. Soc.* [B] 1(Suppl.):217–235, 1934.
30. Yusuf, S., Collins, R., Peto, R., et al. Intravenous and intracoronary fibrinolytic therapy in acute myocardial infarction: Overview of results on mortality, reinfarction and side effects from 33 randomized controlled trials. *Eur. Heart J.* 6:556–585, 1985.

11

Analysis of Epidemiologic Studies: Evaluating the Role of Bias

Bias may be defined as any systematic error in an epidemiologic study that results in an incorrect estimate of the association between exposure and risk of disease. Since epidemiologic studies involve free-living human beings, even the most rigorously designed investigation will have the potential for one or more types of bias arising from a large number of specific sources including the manner in which subjects are selected into the study and the way in which information is obtained, reported, or interpreted. Consequently, evaluating the role of bias as an alternative explanation for an observed association is a necessary step in interpreting any study result. Unlike chance and confounding, which can be evaluated quantitatively, the effects of bias are far more difficult to evaluate and may even be impossible to take into account in the analysis. For this reason, it is of paramount importance to design and conduct each study in such a way that every possibility for introducing bias has been anticipated and that steps have been taken to minimize its occurrence. Since such errors may, nonetheless, occur, it is also important in the interpretation of findings to consider, at the very least, the types of bias that could have arisen in that particular study as well as the most likely direction and magnitude of their impact.

In this chapter, we provide a brief overview of various types of bias, some practical means to minimize their occurrence, as well as ways to evaluate their influence on the estimates of effect from a study. The reader should also refer to Chapters 6 to 8 for detailed discussions of the particular types of bias of most concern for each analytic study design.

TYPES OF BIAS

There are a number of ways of categorizing and naming the different types of bias that may distort the association between exposure and disease observed in a particular study [11]. One simple but useful approach involves two general classes of systematic error under which the specific types can fall. The first, selection bias, refers to any error that arises in the process of identifying the study populations. The second general category, observation or information bias, includes any systematic error in the measurement of information on exposure or outcome.

Selection Bias

Selection bias can occur whenever the identification of individual subjects for inclusion into the study on the basis of either exposure (cohort) or disease (case-control) status depends in some way on the other axis of interest. In other words, if in a case-control study, selection of cases and controls is based on different criteria and these, in turn, are related to exposure status, bias will result. Similarly, in a cohort study, if the choice of particular exposed and nonexposed individuals is related to their development of the outcome of interest, selection bias can occur. Selection bias is a particular problem in case-control and retrospective cohort studies, where both the exposure and outcome have occurred at the time individuals are selected into the study. Selection bias is unlikely to occur in a prospective cohort study because exposure is ascertained before the development of any outcomes of interest. In all instances where selection bias does occur the result is an observed relation between exposure and disease that is different among those who are entered into the study than among those who would have been eligible but were not chosen to participate.

Selection bias can result from a number of circumstances related to the way in which individuals are ascertained and selected for study. These include factors such as differential surveillance, diagnosis, or referral of individuals into the study. One classic example of this type of bias relates to case-control investigations of oral contraceptives (OC) and thromboembolism. When the first hospital-based case-control studies of OC use and thromboembolism were reported, there was some concern that since physicians were already aware of a possible relationship of these agents with thromboembolism, a proportion of the women in the case series had been hospitalized for evaluation of this disease because they were currently using OCs [12]. If so, any increased frequency of current OC use among women hospitalized for thromboembolism might actually be due, at least in part, to the fact that hospitalization and the determination of the diagnosis were both influenced by a history of OC use. Similarly, criticism concerning the increased risk of uterine cancer associated with use of exogenous estrogens observed in early case-control studies of this hypothesis was based on the argument that women who used estrogens experienced uterine bleeding and were, therefore, more likely to seek medical attention and have a diagnostic evaluation than women not on estrogens [5]. In such circumstances, further evidence supporting the validity of each of the observed associations could be derived from examination of the association among women who met certain objective diagnostic criteria and whose disease would consequently have come to medical attention regardless of exposure status [6].

Another source of selection bias in case-control studies derives from refusal or nonresponse among either study group. While neither low participation rates nor different rates of response between cases and controls necessarily indicates the presence of bias, if the rates of response are also related to exposure status, then bias will be a reasonable alternative explanation for any observed association between exposure and disease. For example, if controls are selected through household survey, it is very possible that nonresponse will be related to a large number of demographic and lifestyle variables associated with employment, some or all of which may also be risk factors for the outcome of interest. Under such circumstances, the possibility of selection bias will be a major problem in interpreting study results.

Observation (Information) Bias

Observation or information bias results from systematic differences in the way data on exposure or outcome are obtained from the various study groups. If data are inaccurate or incomplete, spurious associations may be introduced only if the inaccuracy or incompleteness affects the two groups to an unequal degree. There are several specific types of observation bias, depending on the source of noncomparability.

Recall bias arises when individuals with a particular adverse health outcome remember and report their previous exposure experience differently from those who are not similarly affected, or when those who have been exposed to a potential hazard report subsequent events with a different degree of completeness or accuracy than those nonexposed. This type of bias is especially problematic in case-control and retrospective cohort studies, since both exposure and disease have already occurred at the time participants enter into the study. One of the most common methods of gathering information, particularly in a case-control investigation, is by interviewing either the study subjects themselves or some surrogate, such as spouses of participants or mothers of affected children. Individuals who have experienced a disease or adverse health outcome tend to think about the possible "causes" of their illness and are likely to remember their exposure histories differently from those unaffected by the disease. This bias may also result from the selective recall of families of affected individuals as compared with healthy subjects. Recall bias can lead to either an over- or underestimate of the association between exposure and disease, depending on whether the cases recall their exposure to a greater or lesser extent than the controls.

A second type of systematic error in collecting information is interviewer bias. This refers to any systematic difference in the soliciting, recording, or interpreting of information from study participants and can affect every type of epidemiologic study. In case-control studies, this is a particular concern with respect to the ascertainment of exposure, since knowledge of a subject's disease status may result in differential probing for previous exposure history. Bias in ascertainment of exposure may, for the same reason, also be a problem in retrospective cohort studies. For prospective cohort studies, however, this will not be an issue because the outcome of interest has not yet occurred at the time exposure status is determined. On the other hand, there is particular potential for observation bias in the assessment of outcome for both retrospective and prospective cohort studies. Since information concerning a subject's exposure status is available at the time disease status is determined, investigators who are aware of the study hypothesis may be more (or less) likely to record the outcome of interest for individuals known to have the exposure under examination. This type of bias can also affect the ascertainment of outcome in intervention studies that do not utilize placebo control to maintain observer blindness. In all these circumstances, an association between the exposure and disease might result from or be obscured by this type of systematic error.

The major source of bias in cohort studies concerns the potential for loss of subjects to follow-up due to the necessity of following individuals for a period of time after exposure to determine whether they develop the outcome of interest. When persons lost to follow-up differ from those who remain with respect to both the exposure and the outcome, any observed association will be biased. For example, in a cohort study using mailed questionnaires to evaluate the relation between smoking and myocardial infarction (MI), to the extent that those who both smoke and develop MI are less (or more) likely to respond than nonsmokers who develop the disease, a biased estimate of the exposure and outcome will be obtained. The potential for bias due to losses to follow-up is present no matter how small the proportion of loss is, as long as such loss is related to both exposure and disease.

Another major type of observation or information bias is misclassification, which occurs whenever subjects are erroneously categorized with respect to either exposure or disease status. Since in any study some degree of inaccuracy in reporting or recording information is inevitable, misclassification is always a potential concern. The effect of such misclassification depends on whether the misclassification with respect to exposure (or disease) is dependent on the individual's disease (or exposure) status. When the misclassification is random or nondifferential, the proportions of subjects erroneously classified in the study groups are approximately equal. For example, in a case-control study of spermicides and birth defects [7], the investigators reported increased risks of several types of congenital malformations among women identified as having filled a prescription for these preparations within 600 days prior to the birth of the child. While defining exposure in this way will inevitably result in some degree of misclassification of the true exposure, the actual use of spermicides during a period relevant to teratogenicity, such misclassification is likely to be random, since recording of prescription data was made before the birth of the child. Because random misclassification increases the similarity between the exposed and nonexposed groups, any true association between the exposure and disease will be diluted.

Some degree of random misclassification of exposure and disease is present in almost all types of epidemiologic studies. Retrospective cohort studies of occupational exposures, for example, often obtain exposure information from records compiled many years prior to the initiation of the study. In addition, they frequently must use variables such as work assignment or membership in a union or professional society as a surrogate for exposure to a particular hazard. These proxy variables are, at best, only crude markers of actual exposure level, and at worst may bear little resemblance to any individual subject's true status. It is, however, unlikely that the accuracy or completeness of these records would be different for those who developed the outcome of interest and those who did not. Similarly, studies utilizing only self-reported exposure may be subject to substantial amounts of misclassification, depending on the nature of the study population and the particular exposures. Again, as long as the misclassification is random, it can only serve to dilute any true association between the exposure and outcome.

A more serious problem arises if the proportions of subjects misclassified differ between the study groups. The effect of such nonrandom or differential misclassification is that the observed estimate of effect can be biased in the direction of producing either an overestimate or underestimate of the true association, depending on the particular situation. It is even possible that the estimate will be correct due to the play of chance or the effect of an additional bias. Unfortunately, it is often difficult if not impossible to estimate the precise effect of differential misclassification.

CONTROL OF BIAS: STUDY DESIGN

The prevention and control of potential biases must be accomplished largely through careful study design. For some types of bias, an evaluation and control of their effects can be accomplished, at least to a partial degree, in the analysis. Others, however, such as selection bias, may not be rectifiable once they have occurred. Consequently, prevention of bias in the design phase of an investigation is crucial to the validity of the study results. There are a number of design features that can minimize the potential for bias in any study, ranging from general considerations, such as the choice of a study population and the sources of data to be utilized, to specific features of the data collection process.

Choice of Study Population

There are many ways in which the choice of study population can minimize potential biases. For example, the selection of hospitalized controls in a case-control study will increase comparability with the cases in terms of willingness to participate, the presence of selective factors that influenced the subjects' choice of a particular hospital, and awareness of antecedent exposures and events. This will decrease the likelihood of nonresponse, selection, and recall bias. For cohort studies and clinical trials, in which the ability to locate individuals over a period of time is crucial to minimizing bias due to losses to follow-up, investigators frequently choose populations that are well defined with respect to occupation, place of employment, area of residence, or some other characteristic that gains access to centralized sources of information, such as alumni of a particular institution, U.S. veterans, or members of a health maintenance organization. Another factor often considered in choosing a study population that will minimize biases related to nonresponse or losses to follow-up, particularly in intervention studies, is the selection of a population at above average risk of developing the outcome under investigation. Such individuals are likely to be more interested in taking part in health research than those at usual risk of the disease and thus are likely to maintain a higher level of compliance and commitment to the study.

Methods of Data Collection

In any analytic study, the actual means by which data are collected will have a major impact on the validity of results. There are usually many ways to obtain the same piece of information. The particular method implemented in any given investigation may mean the difference between obtaining useful and informative data or uninterpretable results. From a practical standpoint, two major aspects of the design of data collection procedures can minimize bias: (1) the construction of the specific instrument(s) to obtain information, including questionnaires, interviews, physical examinations, and forms for abstracting data from records; and (2) the administering of those instruments by study personnel. It is crucial to keep very clearly in mind that whatever the sources and methods of data collection utilized in a study, they should be similar for all study groups.

With respect to the data collection instruments, one of the most important ways to minimize bias is the use of highly objective, closed-ended questions. For example, if the variable of interest in a particular study were blood pressure level, information could be obtained through a variety of means ranging from a question about history of hypertension on a self-administered questionnaire to calculating the average of several blood pressure readings taken by a trained observer using a standardized protocol. A question about history of hypertension is clearly the most subjective and, therefore, has the greatest potential for introducing bias. Obtaining information on last recorded blood pressure, while not requiring a judgment about what constitutes hypertension, may be subject to recall bias if asked in an interview or questionnaire or, if the study is record-based, to differential availability of information. Obtaining an actual blood pressure reading eliminates all of these problems, but there may still remain errors due to variability of the measurement or to judgment on the part of the observer. In this instance, the most valid estimate would result from taking an average of several blood pressure readings, with trained observers following a detailed, standardized protocol [8, 9].

It is important to remember that for epidemiologic purposes, the less room there is for interpretation by either the investigator or the subject, the less likely it is that bias will occur. While the question "How do you feel?" may be clinically relevant in terms of eliciting information helpful to making a diagnosis, a more useful question epidemiologically would be "Have you experienced any of the following symptoms?" followed by a comprehensive list of specific conditions or reactions of interest.

With respect to the administration of the data collection instrument, the single most important way to minimize the potential for bias is to maintain blindness to the greatest extent possible. In practical terms, this means that study personnel who abstract records and interview or examine subjects should be unaware of an individual's exposure status when determining the outcome of interest in a cohort or intervention study, or an individual's disease status when assessing exposure in a case-control study. Furthermore, subjects should be kept as unaware of their own study status as well as of the specific hypotheses under investigation as is logistically feasible and ethical. For example, in a case-control study of alcohol consumption in relation to MI [2], the way in which the study was introduced to potential participants was as an investigation of risk factors for serious illness requiring hospitalization. Consequently, while the subjects certainly knew they had been hospitalized for MI, they were not aware that it was the diagnosis of MI rather than hospitalization per se that was the selection criterion used. Moreover, the investigators obtained information on a wide variety of factors, including demographic variables, medical history, family history, physical activity, personality type, medication use, smoking, coffee drinking, and an extensive dietary assessment, so that alcohol consumption was only one among dozens of variables mentioned. In these ways, the major hypothesis under investigation was masked to minimize the potential for bias in the recall of information by the subjects or the collection of the information by the interviewers.

While the effectiveness of blindness as a means to minimize bias is well recognized, it is not always possible to achieve. Studies of well-publicized hypotheses will often be difficult to disguise, and participants who are affected or unaffected by either the exposure or the outcome may respond differently according to their understanding of the aims of the study and their belief in the existence of the hypothesized association. Similarly, in case-control studies of serious illnesses, especially those that utilize community controls, it is inevitable that interviewers will know a participant's status as a case or control. Clinical trials testing interventions for which placebo control is either impossible or undesirable will also be unable to maintain blindness. When it is not possible to incorporate blinding of the subjects and/or investigators into the study design, it is especially important that other approaches known to minimize observation bias be utilized. For example, if those administering the treatment in a clinical trial that is not placebo-controlled are aware of the subject's exposure status, it would be most important for different study personnel who are blinded to exposure status to ascertain the endpoints of interest.

A second means to minimize the potential for bias in the administration of data collection instruments is the implementation of rigorous, standardized training of study personnel and the use of clearly written protocols. To decrease the likelihood of observation bias, it is important that any individuals who complete forms, examine subjects, or administer questionnaires follow very specific procedures that are identical for all subjects. Training in such procedures should include standardizing responses to questions about the study, adopting uniform ways of probing for additional information, and employing standard techniques for dealing with errors or missing information.

As a general check for observer bias, a number of items can be included in the data collection instrument that may alert the investigator to the presence of problems. First, study subjects may be compared with respect to their frequency of reporting (or other ascertainment) of dummy variables, which are factors believed to be either unrelated to the exposure or disease of interest or clearly related but in a known way. For example, in a case-control study of regular aspirin use in relation to risk of MI, information could be collected on a wide range of pharmacologic exposures, such as other analgesics, that are not known or suspected risk factors for MI. If cases and controls differ with respect to their reported use of aspirin but not in their use of other analgesics, these data would support the belief that the observed difference in reported aspirin use is real rather than a function of the study design or conduct. On the other hand, if reported use of both aspirin and other analgesics is higher in the cases than in the controls, the suspicion of some type of recall or interviewer bias must be raised. Similarly, information on a number of factors known to increase risk of MI could be obtained, such as history of hypertension or family history of coronary heart disease. The ability to reproduce these known associations using the study data would again add support to the belief in the validity of any findings regarding aspirin and MI. Second, it is possible to construct a questionnaire or interview that includes several items seeking the same information in different ways, in order to ascertain systematic differences in probing for specific responses. Third, the characteristics of the data collection procedures themselves can be examined, including recording the time an interview, examination, or form completion began and ended in order to check that study personnel are not systematically spending more or less time probing for information depending on an individual's exposure or disease status. Finally, it may be useful for the examiner to record a simple reliability score that reflects the interviewer's subjective assessment as to the participant's ability to understand the questions posed and respond reliably. Study subjects whose information is deemed unreliable may then be excluded from the study or analyzed separately.

Sources of Exposure and Disease Information

In addition to the means of collecting data, the number and nature of sources of exposure and disease information in a particular study will also affect the potential for bias. Information can be obtained from sources as varied as questioning the participants themselves, utilizing hospital or employment records or vital statistics data, or measuring variables directly. The use of preexisting records is the most unbiased source for such data, since the information was recorded prior to the onset of an outcome event. However, preexisting records may not have complete information on all factors of interest for each study subject, especially with respect to lifestyle variables such as smoking, exercise, or diet. Moreover, the amount of missing information may vary for different study groups. For example, in a case-control study of conjugated estrogen use in relation to uterine cancer [1], hospital records were used to identify exposure among the cases as well as a comparable group of women admitted for nonmalignant conditions. For each study participant, information on medication use was also obtained from her private gynecologist's records. With a positive notation of estrogen use from either the hospital or physician's records taken to indicate "true" use, 42 percent of current users among the controls would have been classified as nonusers on the basis of hospital charts alone, as compared with only 15 percent of women with uterine cancer. The most likely explanation for this differential recording of exposure information in these preexisting records is that knowledge or suspicion of a possible relationship between estrogen use and cancer caused staff members at the hospital to probe more thoroughly for details of drug use among women with cancer than among those with nonmalignant conditions.

As this example illustrates, one way to minimize this potential for bias is to use multiple sources of data whenever possible as a way to provide an independent verification of exposure or disease status. Record-based studies could use both hospital and physicians' records, for example, while interview or questionnaire data could be confirmed or supplemented through examination of medical records. Self-reported risk factors and diagnoses are frequently documented through examination of the relevant hospital discharge summaries, pathology reports, or other medical records. Diagnoses reported on a death certificate might be confirmed by abstracting information from hospital records if the subject died after admission, or by examining additional details about the death obtained from relatives. Similarly, in case-control studies, the identification of cases from hospital discharge summaries or pathology reports could be confirmed through a standardized, independent review of records and slides by a single study pathologist blinded to the exposure status of the subjects. In intervention studies, there is often an attempt to corroborate self-reports of compliance with the study regimen through the examination of biochemical or other objective markers of adherence. In all these instances, the goal is to provide evidence of exposure or disease status that is complete and unlikely to be subject to bias on the part of the study participants or observers.

The need for supplemental information will depend to a great extent on the nature of the particular outcome of interest [3]. All exposures and outcomes of interest should be carefully defined using standard, uniform criteria to minimize the need for interpretation on the part of study personnel. For example, many investigations of MI utilize criteria established by the World Health Organization [14]. It is also important that the individuals responsible for assigning such diagnoses be unaware of the subject's exposure status, since it is often difficult to eliminate completely the need for judgments on the part of the reviewer.

Finally, during the planning stages of any investigation, practical methods for minimizing losses to follow-up and obtaining complete ascertainment of outcome should be incorporated into the study design. Depending on the hypotheses being tested and the specific design features of the study, such methods might include, at a minimum, use of the National Death Index established by the National Center for Health Statistics [13], systematic searches of state vital statistics records, telephone calls to nonrespondents or dropouts, and brief written communications designed to ascertain vital status. For such strategies to minimize bias effectively, it is essential that they be implemented according to standardized protocols that apply equally to all participants, regardless of exposure or disease status.

EVALUATION OF THE ROLE OF BIAS

To the fullest extent possible, potential sources of bias should be eliminated or minimized through rigorous design and meticulous conduct of a study, as discussed in previous sections of this chapter. In practice, however, it is rarely possible to know with assurance that such efforts have been successful. Consequently, for any individual study it is always necessary to consider carefully what possible biases may have influenced the observed results; the direction of the likely effect, that is, whether the bias would have acted to mask a true association or to cause a spurious association where there truly is none; and, if possible, how great this distortion might be. This will involve consideration of the type of analytic study utilized (i.e., case-control, cohort, or intervention), specific aspects of the study design and conduct, and the nature of the findings (i.e., whether the results are reported as "null" or representing the presence of an association). Often when a study is published, a general criticism is raised that inaccuracies in the ascertainment of exposure or disease or the nature of the study participants themselves cast serious doubt on the validity of the findings. This criticism may be voiced despite the fact that sometimes the action of the putative bias is not even in a direction that could have accounted for the suggested result. For example, it would be inappropriate to suggest that the previously cited observed increased risk of congenital malformation among women who were identified as having filled a prescription for spermicides within 600 days before birth [7] is due to misclassification of exposure. While there is no doubt that such misclassification occurred and may even have been substantial, there is no reason to believe that the inaccuracies were differential between cases and controls, since the exposure information was recorded before the outcome was known. Such random misclassification could only have led to an observed underestimate of the effect of spermicide use on risk of congenital malformation. It could never have caused the observation of a spurious association.

In evaluating the likelihood that a potential bias may have affected the study results, investigators can sometimes take advantage of evidence from some aspect of the study itself. For example, in their early case-control study of smoking and lung cancer, Doll and Hill [4] found a higher frequency of those reporting heavy smoking among the cases than the controls. One concern in interpreting these findings was that the interviewers probed more deeply for a history of smoking among those with lung cancer than controls without the disease. Evidence to evaluate this possibility was provided by the fact that during the course of the same investigation, a number of patients were interviewed in the belief that they had lung cancer but were subsequently determined not to have this diagnosis. If observation bias were responsible for the increased proportion of smokers observed among the cases, then the subjects who were incorrectly diagnosed as having lung cancer should have had smoking histories similar to those of the actual lung cancer cases. In fact, the smoking histories of the incorrectly diagnosed patients more closely resembled those of the controls, suggesting that the observed difference in smoking habits was not the result of bias on the part of the patient or interviewer. Similarly, in the evaluation of the association between postmenopausal hormones and uterine cancer, the possibility was raised that subclinical cancers were being diagnosed more frequently in women using these agents as a result of closer medical surveillance and diagnostic evaluations that otherwise would not have been performed [5]. The fact that the association persisted even when such early in situ cases were excluded [6] supported the belief that such selection bias, although still a potential problem, could not have accounted for the entire increased risk observed.

In other circumstances, investigators may choose deliberately to build into the study design certain strategies to allow them to assess the extent to which a particular potential bias actually affects either their own or previously reported findings. For example, to address the issue of recall bias in studies of spermicide use and congenital malformation, a case-control study was conducted in which reported use of these preparations by mothers of children with Down's syndrome was compared with that of mothers of both healthy infants and children with congenital heart disease, a condition that in previous studies had not been associated with spermicide use [10]. This second control series was chosen specifically because the children were also ill and thus presumably the information provided by their mothers would be subject to the same recall bias as that from mothers of cases. In this manner, it was possible to evaluate the role of recall bias as an alternative explanation for the observed association between spermicides and Down's syndrome. Although the magnitude of the effect was somewhat smaller than the result using the nondiseased controls, the association between Down's syndrome and spermicide use persisted even when this second control series was examined.

In most circumstances, an evaluation of the role of bias as an alternative explanation of the study findings must involve considerations as to the type of study, its particular design, and the nature of the results.

While all analytic studies are subject to bias, each design has particular types to which it is inherently most vulnerable. For example, if a study uses the case-control approach, concern about the potential for bias would focus primarily upon two possibilities: (1) that knowledge of disease status influenced the determination of exposure status (recall bias), and (2) that knowledge of exposure status influenced the identification of diseased and nondiseased study subjects (selection bias). In a cohort study, the possibility for bias due to loss to follow-up would be a particular concern, as would selection bias if the study were retrospective. On the other hand, if the study were a prospective cohort investigation, selection bias would not be a major concern. In an intervention study, the degree of concern about the potential for observation bias would depend on the nature of the comparison group, the use of a placebo, and the degree of objectivity in the measurement of the outcome.

The potential for misclassification must also be considered in every type of epidemiologic study. The most important issue in this regard is whether the inaccuracies in classification of exposure or disease are differential or random. If differential, the misclassification could result in either an underestimate or overestimate of effect, depending on the direction of the error; for example, in a case-control study, whether the cases are more or less likely to report a positive exposure history than the controls. On the other hand, many inaccuracies in ascertainment of exposure or disease are inevitable in all epidemiologic research and are thus present to a similar degree in every study design. If the misclassification is likely to be random, that is, if there is no reason to believe that the level of error would be different in the different study groups, then such bias can only work in the direction of underestimating the study results. Therefore, in interpreting a particular study, if the results indicate the presence of an effect it is not possible to account for this result by any amount of random misclassification, no matter how substantial, since any estimate of the effect without the misclassification could only by more extreme. On the other hand, random misclassification could certainly be responsible, totally or in part, for a finding of no association between exposure and disease, depending on the size of the true effect and the magnitude of the misclassification, and must always be considered as a possible alternative explanation for a reported null finding.

CONCLUSION

Bias, like chance and confounding, should always be considered as a possible alternative explanation of any observed statistical association, whether positive, inverse, or null. Unlike chance and confounding, however, which can generally be taken into account in the analysis through the use of appropriate statistical techniques, bias is most effectively dealt with through careful design and meticulous conduct of a study. Once a potential source of bias is introduced, it is usually extremely difficult to correct for its effects analytically. It is, however, possible as well as necessary to identify likely sources of bias in a particular study and attempt to estimate both the direction in which the bias would have altered the estimate of effect and, when feasible, the magnitude of that influence. Investigators should discuss all these issues fully in published reports to provide readers with the maximum opportunity to judge for themselves whether bias is likely to account for observed findings. However, whether or not investigators follow this guideline, readers should always, to the extent possible, consider the potential role of bias as an explanation for reported results.

STUDY QUESTIONS

1. Compare and contrast the likelihood of occurrence of selection and observation bias in case-control and cohort studies.
2. Compare and contrast the effects of random and nonrandom misclassification in the estimate of relative risk.
3. What are the major options in the design of a study to minimize the occurrence of bias?

REFERENCES

1. Buring, J. E., Bain, C. J., and Hennekens, C. H. Alternative data sources in a case-control study of conjugated estrogens and cancer. *Am. J. Prev. Med.* 2:116–121, 1986.
2. Buring, J. E., Willett, W., Goldhaber, S. Z., et al. and the Boston Area Health Study Research Group. Alcohol and HDL in non-fatal myocardial infarction: Preliminary results from a case-control study. *Circulation* 68:227, 1983.
3. Colditz, G. A., Martin, P., Stampfer, J. J., et al. Validation of questionnaire information on risk factors and disease outcomes in a prospective cohort study of disease in women. *Am. J. Epidemiol.* 123:894–900, 1986.
4. Doll, R., and Hill, A. B. Smoking and carcinoma of the lung: Preliminary report. *Br. Med. J.* 2:739–748, 1950.
5. Feinstein, A. R., and Horwitz, R. I. A critique of the statistical evidence associating estrogens with endometrial cancer. *Cancer Research* 38:4001–4005, 1978.
6. Gordon, J., Reagan, J. W., Finkle, W. D., et al. Estrogen and endometrial carcinoma. An independent pathology review supporting original risk estimate. *N. Engl. J. Med.* 297:570–571, 1977.
7. Jick, H., Walker, A. M., Rothman, K. J., et al. Vaginal spermicides and congenital disorders. *J.A.M.A.* 245:1329–1332, 1981.

8. Rosner, B., and Polk, B. F. Predictive values of routine blood pressure measurements in screening for hypertension. *Am. J. Epidemiol.* 117:429–442, 1983.

9. Rosner, B., Cook, N. R., Evans, D. A., et al. Reproducibility and predictive values of routine blood pressure measurements in children: Comparison with adult values and implications for screening children for elevated blood pressure. *Am. J. Epidemiol.* In press, 1987.

10. Rothman, K. J. Spermicide use and Down's syndrome. *Am. J. Public Health* 72:399–401, 1982.

11. Sackett, D. L. Bias in analytic research. *J. Chronic Dis.* 32:51–63, 1979.

12. Sartwell, P. E., Masi, A. T., Arthes, F. G., et al. Thromboembolism and oral contraceptives: An epidemiologic case-control study. *Am. J. Epidemiol.* 90:365–380, 1969.

13. Stampfer, M. J., Willett, W. C., Speizer, F. E., et al. Test of the National Death Index. *Am. J. Epidemiol.* 119:837–893, 1984.

14. World Health Organization. *IHD Registers: Report of the Fifth Working Group.* Copenhagen: World Health Organization, 1971.

12

Analysis of Epidemiologic Studies: Evaluating the Role of Confounding

In Chapters 10 and 11, we discussed methods for evaluating the effects of two possible alternative explanations that must always be considered in assessing the presence of a valid statistical association in a given study—the role of chance and that of bias. The third alternative explanation, confounding, involves the possibility that the observed association is due, totally or in part, to the effects of differences between the study groups other than the exposure under study that could affect their risk of developing the outcome of interest. The concept of confounding is central to the interpretation of the findings of any epidemiologic study—most critically in observational studies but also for experimental investigations. Unlike bias, which is primarily introduced by the investigator or study participants, confounding is a function of the complex interrelationships between various exposures and disease.

THE NATURE OF CONFOUNDING

Intuitively, confounding can be thought of as a mixing of the effect of the exposure under study on the disease with that of a third factor. This third factor must be associated with the exposure and, independent of that exposure, be a risk factor for the disease. In such circumstances the observed relationship between the exposure and disease can be attributable, totally or in part, to the effect of the confounder. Confounding can lead to an overestimate or underestimate of the true association between exposure and disease and can even change the direction of the observed effect. For example, consider a study that showed a relationship between increased level of physical activity and decreased risk of myocardial infarction (MI). One additional variable that might affect the observed magnitude of this association is age. People who exercise heavily tend to be younger, as a group, than those who do not exercise. Moreover, independent of exercise, younger individuals have a lower risk of MI than older people. Thus, those who exercise could have a lower risk of MI quite apart from any effect of this habit simply as a consequence of the greater proportion of younger individuals in this group. In this circumstance, age would confound the observed association between exercise and MI and result in an overestimate of any inverse relationship. Similarly, differences in the proportions of men and women could also potentially affect the magnitude of the observed association between exercise and MI. A high level of exercise is likely to be more common in men, and, independent of exercise, men have a greater risk of MI than women. Thus, an inverse effect of exercise on risk of MI would be underestimated if differences in gender between exercisers and nonexercisers were not taken into account.

As can be seen from these examples, in the most general terms, for a variable to confound a relationship, it must be associated with both the exposure and the disease. If there is no association between the exposure and the potential confounder, or conversely, if the potential confounder has no relationship with risk of the disease, there can be no confounding by that factor. For example, those who exercise and those who do not are almost certain to differ with respect to their total daily consumption of fluids. Increased intake of fluids, however, has not in itself been shown to increase (or decrease) risk of MI. Thus, a difference in the level of this variable between those who are physically active and those who are not cannot be responsible for any decreased risk of MI observed among exercisers, and thus it is not a confounder of this association.

This general description of the characteristics of a confounder requires a number of refinements [16, 24]. First, while the potential confounding factor must, by definition, be predictive of the occurrence of disease, the association need not be causal. In fact, most frequently, confounding variables are only correlates of another causal factor. For example, age and sex are associated with virtually all diseases and are related to the presence or level of many exposures. Thus, they should always be considered as potential confounders of an association. These variables, however, may not be causally related to disease but rather act as surrogates for etiologic factors. The lower rates of coronary heart disease among women compared with men may not be due to gender, per se, but rather to correlates of sex, such as levels of endogenous hormones, that are more difficult to define and quantify.

Second, the potential confounding factor must be predictive of disease independently of its association with the exposure under study. In other words, the confounding factor cannot be related to risk of disease only through its association with the exposure. This means that there must be an association between the confounder and disease even among nonexposed individuals. In the previous example, if increased physical activity does, in fact, decrease risk of MI, then high levels of fluid consumption will also be associated with a decreased risk of MI, simply because fluid intake is associated with physical activity. However, fluid

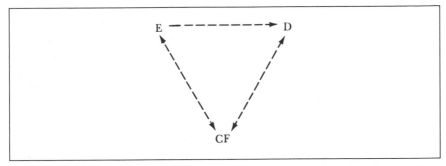

Fig. 12-1. Interrelationship between an exposure (E), confounding factor (CF), and disease (D).

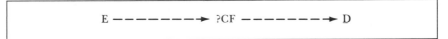

Fig. 12-2. Interrelationship between an exposure (E), disease (D), and a potential confounding factor (?CF) which is in the causal pathway and thus *not* a confounder.

consumption has not been shown to be associated with risk of MI among those who are physically inactive. Thus, this variable would not be a confounder of the association. This is clearly a different situation than for true potential confounders such as age, sex, and smoking, which not only are associated with physical activity, but, even among individuals who are not physically active, are risk factors for MI.

Finally, the potential confounder cannot merely be an intermediate link in the causal chain between the exposure and disease under study. This distinction is often not clear and requires knowledge or postulation of biologic mechanisms underlying the relationship of the exposure with disease. As shown in Figure 12-1, a confounder is a variable that is associated with the exposure and, independent of that exposure, is a risk factor for the disease. If, however, as shown in Figure 12-2, one mechanism of action of the exposure is to alter the level of the potential confounder, which in turn itself affects disease risk, then that factor is not a confounder but rather an intermediate step in the causal chain between the exposure and disease. For example, in evaluating the effect of moderate alcohol consumption on decreasing risk of MI, one variable that might at first glance be considered as a potential confounder is level of high-density lipoprotein (HDL) cholesterol. Studies have shown that alcohol raises HDL levels, and high levels of HDL are associated with reduced risk of MI independent of alcohol consumption [10]. However, it has also been postulated that one mechanism for the effect of moderate alcohol consumption on risk of MI may be that it is mediated totally or in part by changes in HDL. If such a mechanism is known or even assumed, then HDL would not be a confounder and should not be controlled for in the analysis. On the other hand, if it is of interest to assess the extent to which alcohol has an effect on MI by mechanisms other than by altering HDL levels, the analysis would need to control for HDL. Thus, level of HDL could be considered in different ways in separate analyses, depending on the specific research question as well as the known or postulated biologic mechanism.

As the foregoing discussion illustrates, the choice of the specific factors that should be considered as potential confounders of a particular association is often difficult. A practical means to determine whether a given factor is in fact an actual confounder in a study is to analyze the data, obtain a crude overall estimate of the association, control for the effect of the variable, and observe whether the estimate of the association between the exposure and disease is altered. A potential confounder would be an actual confounder if adjustment for the variable results in a change in the estimate of the association between the exposure and disease. It is important to note that in fact, the effect of any single confounder must be considered in the context of the effects of all other confounders in that study, since the ultimate concern is with the aggregate amount of confounding. However, long before that information is available, it is necessary in the design stage of the study to select variables that will be considered as potential confounders to ensure that adequate data are collected, since it is impossible to control later for the effects of a variable on which information was not obtained. The problem is that it is not logistically feasible to collect information on every variable that could possibly be related to either the exposure or the disease. Making a judicious choice about potential confounders depends on knowledge of the disease, previous evaluations of the same or related questions, and most importantly, the best judgment of the investigator at the time the study is initiated. Identification of a potential confounding factor is not a matter of determining the statistical significance of an association with the exposure or disease. As discussed in Chapter 10, statistical significance is a function of both the magnitude of an association and the sample size of the study. In a small sample, a confounding variable can certainly affect the magnitude of an observed association even if it does not achieve statistical significance in its relationship with either the exposure or disease. Conversely, in a very large study, a factor may be statistically significantly associated with exposure or disease even though it has only a small effect on the magnitude of the association. Thus, statistical significance is not the criterion on which to base the decision that a particular factor is or is not a potential confounder.

From a practical standpoint, since a confounder must be associated with both the exposure and the disease and it is often difficult to know what factors are correlated with the exposure, investigators may attempt to ensure that at the very least data are obtained on all available risk factors for the disease under study. For example, in a study of exercise and MI, it is not clear which demographic, medical, and life-style variables are associated with varying levels of physical activity. Since a number of specific factors have been shown consistently to affect risk of MI, at a minimum information on each of these could be collected. Moreover, the data collected need to be sufficiently detailed to permit adequate control of the effects of each variable. For example, to control the potential confounding effects of cigarette smoking on the association between exercise and MI, it would not be sufficient to define smoking status as simply ever versus never smoked, because risk of MI is associated with current rather than past habits. Since the group of ever smokers would include those who smoked currently, some control of confounding by this variable would be achieved; however, residual confounding due to this less than optimal categorization of smoking status would likely still affect the estimate of the magnitude of the association between exercise and MI. Since uncontrolled confounding is a major threat to the validity of results, it is imperative that the design features of the study permit the collection of adequate data to address this issue.

In assessing the effect of a potential confounding factor, it is important not merely to evaluate its presence or absence, but also to identify the direction and quantify the magnitude of its effect on the estimate of the association between the exposure and disease. The magnitude of the effect of the confounding present will depend on the magnitudes of the specific associations between the confounder and the exposure, as well as between the confounder and the disease. The direction of the effect of the confounding factor on the estimate of the observed association will depend on the nature of the interrelationships among the exposure, confounding factor, and disease. Positive confounding refers to the situation in which the effect of the confounding factor is to produce an observed estimate of the association between exposure and disease that is more extreme—either more positive or more negative—than the true association. For example, in a study of coffee consumption and MI, cigarette smoking would be a potential positive confounder since those who drink coffee are more likely to smoke and those who smoke are at an increased risk of MI. It therefore could appear that coffee drinkers have a higher risk of MI than they actually do, simply because they are also cigarette smokers, whose risk of MI is independently elevated. Analogously, smoking could also be a potential positive confounder of the protective association between physical activity and MI. Since those who exercise heavily tend to smoke less than those who do not and those who smoke less have a lower risk of MI than heavy smokers, it could appear that high levels of physical activity are even more protective than they actually are simply because of the lower proportion of smokers among those who are physically active. In contrast, negative confounding refers to the situation in which the effect of the confounding factor is to produce an observed estimate of the association between exposure and disease that is an underestimate of the true association. For physical activity and MI, for example, gender would be a potential negative confounder since being male is associated with increased level of physical activity but also with increased risk of MI. Consequently, a group of exercisers would contain a greater proportion of males than a comparison group of nonexercisers. This would result in a higher risk of MI among those who are physically active compared with those who are not due to the effect of the confounder. The observed magnitude of the association between physical activity and MI would therefore be closer to the null value than is actually true, thereby tending to underestimate any protective effect of physical activity on MI.

Note that the terms *positive* and *negative* in this context refer to the effects of the confounding factor on the direction of the observed risk estimate relative to the true parameter, regardless of the direction of the true effect of exposure on disease. Failure to control for negative confounding results in an observed estimate of effect that is diluted towards the null, meaning that any true increased or true decreased risk will be underestimated and appear as less of an association than is actually the case. Similarly, failure to control for positive confounding results in a more extreme estimate of effect observed than is actually the case. This can be in the direction of either an apparently stronger increased risk or an apparently more protective effect, depending on the direction of the true association.

An understanding of the direction in which a potential confounder is likely to affect the association between an exposure and disease can be very informative in situations where the factor was not or could not be controlled. For example, in one of the earliest analytic studies evaluating the relationship of smoking with lung cancer, Doll and Hill [6] found a highly significant difference in the percentage of smokers between cases of lung cancer and controls of the same age and sex with diseases other than cancer. One concern in interpreting those results was that the cases and controls differed with respect to place of residence. Specifically, a higher proportion of the lung cancer patients resided in rural areas outside of London at the time of their admission to the hospital. Since there were also urban/rural differences with respect to smoking patterns, place of residence fulfilled the requirements for being a potential confounder. The real question, however, is whether the uncontrolled effect of differences in place of residence between cases and controls could have accounted for the observed increased risk of lung cancer associated with smoking. The relationship of place of residence with smoking was such that rural areas had a lower smoking rate than urban areas. Rural place of residence would therefore be a negative confounder in these data, since cases had a higher proportion of those from rural areas, those from the rural areas were less likely to smoke, and those less likely to smoke were less likely to develop lung cancer. Thus, in these data, urban/rural differences could only act to underestimate any true association between smoking and lung cancer and could not have been responsible for the observed increased risk.

There are a number of methods that can be employed, singly or in combination, to control for the effects of confounding in analytic epidemiologic studies. These include randomization and restriction, which are features adopted in the design phase of a study; matching, which involves both study design and analysis; and two specific analytic techniques, stratification and multivariate analysis. The basic strategy underlying all of these methods derives directly from the definition of confounding. A factor can confound an association only if it differs between the study groups. As mentioned in the example of exercise and risk of MI, gender would be a confounder only if there were different proportions of men and women among those who exercise and those who do not and if, in addition, gender were an independent risk factor for the disease. If gender did not vary between exercisers and nonexercisers, it could not be a confounder of the association between exercise and MI. Thus, if through the way we design or analyze the study, we make comparisons only among individuals with the same level of the confounding variable, then the confounding effect of that factor will be controlled. If we examine the association between exercise and MI among only men, or among only women, or among both men and women but separately, then gender will not vary within each of these groups of subjects, and the resultant estimate of the association will not be confounded by this variable.

METHODS TO CONTROL CONFOUNDING IN THE DESIGN

There are three methods that can be used to control confounding in the design of analytic epidemiologic studies: randomization, restriction, and matching. Randomization is applicable only to intervention studies, while restriction and matching can be considered for all analytic study designs.

Randomization

Randomization, as discussed in detail in Chapter 8, is for many reasons the procedure of choice in an intervention study for the allocation of study subjects to the various exposure categories. The unique strength of randomization relates to its ability to control confounding. With a sufficient sample size, randomization will virtually ensure that all potential confounding factors—those known to the investigator and, even more importantly, those currently unknown or even as yet unsuspected—are evenly distributed among the treatment groups. This ability of randomization to control for unknown confounders cannot be achieved by any other approach in the design or analysis of an epidemiologic study. If there are imbalances in known or suspected risk factors due to small sample size, or to the play of chance even in a large sample, these can be controlled in the analysis using the techniques that will be discussed below. Of course, imbalances with respect to unknown risk factors can never be controlled in the analysis. Thus, when using randomization to control confounding, it is important that the sample size of the study be sufficiently large.

Restriction

As stated earlier, confounding cannot occur if the potential confounding factors do not vary across either the exposure or the disease categories. One way to achieve this is to restrict the admissibility criteria for subjects and limit entrance into the study to individuals who fall within a specified category or categories of the confounder. For example, if sex and race are potential confounding factors, the study could include only nonwhite men or only white women. Similarly, control of age could be achieved by restricting admissibility to those within a narrow range that corresponds to a relatively homogeneous rate of disease incidence. To the extent that variation in the confounding factor can be either eliminated (as in the case of race and sex) or substantially reduced (as in the case of age) by restricting the study population, the confounding effect of that variable is correspondingly eliminated or minimized.

Restriction is a straightforward, convenient, and inexpensive means to control confounding. If the range of permissible values of a potential confounder is sufficiently narrow, restriction offers virtually complete control. There are, however, a number of limitations to the use of restriction that should be considered. First, the use of restriction may substantially reduce the number of subjects eligible to participate in the study, which may present difficulties in achieving the sample size necessary for adequate statistical power in a reasonable period of time. Second, the use of restriction involves the potential for residual confounding if the criteria are not sufficiently narrow. For example, in a study of physical activity and MI, one important potential confounding factor that might be dealt with by restriction would be age. If, however, the study population were restricted to the category of those aged 40 to 65, it is certain that there would be residual confounding, because the rates of both MI and physical activity vary widely within that broad age range. Similarly, restricting the study population to individuals who had ever smoked cigarettes would not be sufficient to control adequately for the effects of smoking because risk of MI is most strongly associated with current, not past smoking.

Finally, perhaps the most serious potential disadvantage is that while restriction can deal effectively with the effects of a confounding variable, it does not permit evaluation of the association between exposure and disease for varying levels of the factor. For example, in assessing the association between exercise and risk of MI, restricting the study population to either men or women would certainly eliminate any effect of sex as a confounding factor. On the other hand, it might also be of interest to know whether the existence or magnitude of the association between exercise and MI differs between men and women. Clearly, this question could not be evaluated directly in a study that restricted the population to only one sex. It must be kept in mind that restriction may limit generalizability but in no way affects the validity of any observed association between the groups that were included in the study. Indeed, restriction enhances validity by providing an estimate that is unconfounded by the restriction factors.

Matching

Unlike randomization and restriction, which are used to control confounding in the design stage of a study, matching is a strategy that must include elements of both design and analysis. With restriction, the control of confounding is achieved by selecting into the study only individuals with certain homogeneous levels of the potential confounders. With matching, all levels of these factors are allowable for inclusion in the study, but the particular subjects are selected in such a way that the potential confounders are distributed in an identical manner among each of the study groups. For example, in a case-control study of exercise and risk of MI in which age, sex, and smoking are potential confounders, for each case of MI a control would be selected of the same age, sex, and level of smoking. Specifically, a 65-year-old female MI patient who was currently a heavy cigarette smoker would be matched to a woman of the same age and smoking status who had never suffered an MI. In this way, matching forces the distribution of these potential confounders to be identical in both study groups. When matching in the design is combined with the appropriate analysis, as discussed below, control of confounding by the matching factors is achieved.

Matching as a technique for the control of confounding has great intuitive appeal and has been widely used over the years; however, it also has a number of logistic and scientific disadvantages. These disadvantages, coupled with the more recent development of alternative techniques for the control of confounding in the analysis, have lessened the desirability of and necessity for matching except in certain clearly defined circumstances. The first disadvantage of matching is that it can be difficult, expensive, and time-consuming to find a comparison subject with the right set of characteristics with respect to every matching variable for each individual enrolled in a study. Thus, although in principle matching can be used in any analytic study design, it is rarely used in large-scale cohort studies. In such studies it is usually more cost-effective simply to admit a large pool of comparison subjects and use other methods for controlling confounding, such as stratification or multivariate analysis. One exception to this rule is when there are a very large number of comparison subjects available and their data are easily and cheaply accessible, such as by computer tape. In this circumstance, the costs with respect to time and money in identifying matched controls will be negligible.

Thus, matching is primarily utilized in case-control studies, which in general tend to be smaller in sample size. Even here, the cost of obtaining information on potential confounders and selecting matched controls must be taken into account. It can often be expensive and time-consuming to assemble a suitable study population if matching is employed. For example, even if there are only three factors that are to be matched on—age (in five categories), sex (in two categories), and race (in three categories)—there are already 30 ($5 \times 2 \times 3$) possible combinations that may have to be considered in finding an appropriate control. A number of potential controls may have to be excluded before finding one with the particular set of characteristics of the case. When there are sufficient numbers of cases available for study, a 1 : 1 match (one control per case) provides the most statistically efficient design. When the number of cases is limited or fixed, however, the statistical power of the study to detect an association if one truly exists can be increased by selecting more than one control per case (referred to as R : 1 matching). This is an especially attractive alternative when the cost of obtaining information from cases and controls is similar. In general, however, as the ratio of controls to cases increases beyond 4 : 1, the additional gain in statistical power for the crude comparison may be small compared with the costs in terms of both time and money [18].

In addition to these disadvantages in terms of time, money, and loss of potential study subjects, as was the case with restriction, another limitation of matching is the inability to evaluate the effect of a factor that has been matched on the risk of the outcome. Thus, the effect of the confounding factor itself on risk of disease, such as the effect of smoking on risk of MI in a case-control evaluation of exercise and MI where smoking levels have been matched, cannot be explored because the distribution of that factor has been forced to be identical between cases and controls. Moreover, the use of matching does not control potential confounding by factors other than those for which matching was done, except indirectly for factors highly correlated with the matching variables. Matching may, in fact, result in greater difficulty in controlling for additional confounders. Stratified analysis cannot easily be used with matched data to control for additional confounders that were not included as matching factors. Although they can be controlled using specialized multivariate techniques, including matched-pair conditional logistic regression [21, 22], the effective sample size is reduced because the analyses are based on only discordant pairs, as will be discussed below. This can add both inefficiency and complexity that would not have been necessary if matching had not been utilized and the effects of all potential confounders had been controlled in the analysis.

Despite these substantial scientific limitations and logistic difficulties, there are some circumstances in which matching is desirable and even necessary. First, for certain variables, if matching were not employed in the design phase of the study, there would not be a sufficient number of individuals in the study groups who were alike with respect to these confounding factors to allow for any type of control in the analysis. In other words, matching is necessary for any factors for which there would otherwise be insufficient overlap between the study groups. Complex nominal variables such as neighborhood or sibship, which represent a wide and undefinable range of environmental and genetic factors, are especially difficult, if not impossible, to quantify and thus control by other means. By matching each case to a sibling control, for example, the investigator attempts to control for a number of general characteristics highly correlated with membership in a particular family, including genetic factors, early environmental exposures, dietary habits, socioeconomic status, and utilization of health care resources. In the same way, individuals from the same neighborhood are likely to have experienced similar environmental exposures and be more alike with respect to individual life-style variables as well as correlates of social class and ethnic group. If controls were selected at random from the general population and the association between the exposure and disease among those living in the same neighborhood were examined afterward, it is very likely that only one or two individuals would come from each neighborhood, making an analysis impossible. A control from that neighborhood would therefore need to be specially selected or matched to each case to ensure that the necessary comparable information is available. This would be true of any such variable with a number of possible values on a nominal scale.

A second circumstance in which matching may be useful is when the case series is very small. In this situation, baseline characteristics are very likely to differ between the study groups due to chance variability, and yet the sample size will simply not be sufficient to form adequate subgroups of the confounders to control such variables in the analysis.

Matching a number of controls to each case with respect to the potential confounders will ensure an adequate number of cases and controls for each of the subgroups so that it will be possible to evaluate efficiently the association between exposure and disease.

Taking these disadvantages and advantages into account, we believe that matching should not be used routinely, but only after careful consideration of its appropriateness for a particular study. The wide availability of alternative techniques for the control of confounding in the analysis has markedly decreased the necessity and desirability of matching except in certain clearly defined circumstances. In most situations, it seems far preferable to choose an adequate sample of the comparison group and control for confounding through stratification and/or multivariate analysis.

In considering the analysis of data from case-control studies that have utilized matching, it is important to understand the role of matching in the design on the control of confounding. By matching cases and controls for a number of potential confounders, the groups have been selected to be more alike with respect to these factors than would have occurred had two independent series of cases and controls been chosen. If the matching factors are true confounders, the matching will result in a greater similarity between cases and controls with respect to their exposure histories than would otherwise be the case. If this similarity produced by the matching is not taken into account in the analysis by utilizing statistical techniques that make explicit provision for the matched nature of the data, an underestimate of the true association between exposure and disease will result. Thus, matching in the design of a case-control study does not by itself control confounding. Rather, control of confounding results from matching in the design coupled with stratification in the analysis. The true utility of matching in the control of confounding relates primarily to considerations of analytic efficiency or the ability to test a hypothesis with adequate statistical power and thereby produce a precise estimate of effect. By ensuring an adequate number of cases and controls for each level of a given confounding factor, matching permits effective control in the analysis through the use of stratification or multivariate analytic techniques.

Figure 12-3 illustrates the presentation of data for the analysis of a matched-pair case-control study. Unlike the two-by-two table for unmatched data, in which each cell represents the number of individuals with a certain exposure and disease status, the cells for a matched study denote the number of pairs that fall into each category. In this table, the rows indicate the exposure status of the case, and the columns indicate the corresponding status of the control member of the matched pair. Thus, cell *a* indicates the number of pairs in which both the case and control are exposed, *b* the pairs in which the case is exposed but the control nonexposed, *c* those where the control is exposed but not the

	Control		
	Exposed	Nonexposed	
Case			
Exposed	a	b	$a + b$
Nonexposed	c	d	$c + d$
	$a + c$	$b + d$	T

Fig. 12-3. Presentation of Data From a Matched Pair Case-Control Study in a 2×2 Table

case, and d the pairs in which neither the case nor the control is exposed. The margins indicate the total number of pairs in which the case was exposed $(a + b)$ or nonexposed $(c + d)$, the total pairs in which the control was exposed $(a + c)$ or nonexposed $(b + d)$, and the total number of case-control pairs in the study $(a + b + c + d = T)$.

This presentation of matched-pair data can be illustrated using data from a study of postmenopausal estrogens and endometrial cancer [28]. As shown in Table 12-1, 317 cases of endometrial cancer were identified and matched to an equal number of women with other gynecologic neoplasms on the basis of age at diagnosis (within 4 years) and year of diagnosis (within 2 years). Exposure was defined as at least 6 months of estrogen use recorded before the diagnosis of the cancer. There were 39 pairs in which both the case and her matching control used estrogens, as well as 150 pairs in which neither the case nor her matching control used estrogens. Since for these concordant pairs there was no difference between cases and controls with respect to their exposure, they provide no information on the magnitude of the association between estrogen use and risk of endometrial cancer. All such information is provided by the discordant pairs, that is, those in which one member was exposed and the other was not. In this study, there were 128 pairs discordant for estrogen use: 113 in which the case was exposed but not the control, and 15 in which the control reported estrogen use while the case did not.

In a matched-pair analysis, the estimate of the magnitude of the association between the exposure and disease is based entirely on the ratio of the discordant pairs. Specifically, the relative risk of disease associated with exposure is calculated as the ratio of the number of pairs in which the case is exposed and the control nonexposed to the number of pairs

Table 12-1. Data from a matched-pair case-control study of exogenous estrogens and endometrial carcinoma

| | Control | | Total |
	Exposed	Nonexposed	Total
Case			
Exposed	39	113	152
Nonexposed	15	150	165
Total	54	263	317

$$RR = \frac{b}{c} = \frac{113}{15} = 7.5$$

$$\chi^2_{(1)} = \frac{(b - c)^2}{(b + c)}$$

$$= \frac{(113 - 15)^2}{(113 + 15)}$$

$$= 75.03$$

$$95\% \ CI = RR^{(1 \pm 1.96/\chi)}$$

$$= 7.5^{(1 \pm 1.96/8.66)}$$

$$= (4.72, 11.92)$$

Source: Data from D. C. Smith et al., Association of exogenous estrogen and endometrial carcinoma. *N. Engl. J. Med.* 293:1164, 1975.

in which the control is exposed but not the case. This calculation can be represented as follows:

$$RR = \frac{b}{c}$$

Cells a and d, which represent the concordant pairs in which case and control are similar with respect to the exposure of interest, provide no information for this calculation. The estimate of the relative risk of endometrial cancer for those who used postmenopausal estrogens is therefore as follows:

$$RR = \frac{b}{c}$$

$$= \frac{113}{15}$$

$$= 7.5$$

This indicates that compared with women who did not use estrogens, those who used these agents were seven and a half times more likely to develop endometrial cancer. This estimate of effect can then be tested for statistical significance using the McNemar test or chi-square test for matched-pair data [7]:

$$\chi^2_{(1)} = \frac{(b-c)^2}{(b+c)}$$

$$= \frac{(113-15)^2}{(113+15)}$$

$$= 75.03, P = 4.8 \times 10^{-18}$$

Corresponding confidence intervals can also be calculated from the standard formulas presented in Chapter 10. For example, using a test-based approach, the matched-pair estimates of the relative risk and chi-square can be utilized. Thus, for the example above:

$$95\% \ CI = RR^{(1 \pm 1.96/\sqrt{\chi^2})}$$

$$= 7.5^{(1 \pm 1.96/8.66)}$$

$$= 7.5^{(1 \pm 0.23)}$$

$$= (4.72, 11.92)$$

In this example, the estimate of the relative risk calculated from the matched-pair analysis differs appreciably from that which would have been calculated from the same data with the matched pairs not retained in the analysis. As shown in Table 12-2, the information on the cases and controls can be considered as if derived from totally independent samples by inserting the numbers from the margins of the matched table, which represent the total numbers of subjects in each exposure and disease category, into the appropriate cells of the unmatched table. Thus, there were a total of 634 (317 times 2) individuals in the original study: 317 cases and 317 controls. Of the 317 cases, 152 used estrogens (ignoring the status of the matched control) and 165 were nonusers. Similarly, of the 317 controls, a total of 54 used estrogens and 263 did not. The unmatched relative risk would then be calculated:

$$RR = \frac{ad}{bc}$$

$$= \frac{(152)(263)}{(54)(165)}$$

$$= 4.5$$

Table 12-2. Unmatched analysis of data from a matched-pair
case-control study of exogenous estrogens and endometrial cancer

	Cases	Controls	Total
Case			
Exposed	152	54	206
Nonexposed	165	263	428
Total	317	317	634

$$RR = \frac{ad}{bc} = \frac{(152)(263)}{(54)(165)} = 4.5$$

Source: Data from D. C. Smith et al., Association of exogenous estrogen and
endometrial carcinoma. *N. Engl. J. Med.* 293:1164, 1975.

The unmatched estimate of effect is different from that of the matched,
reflecting the fact that the matching variables were in fact confounders
of the association between exogenous estrogens and endometrial cancer.
Thus, the matching must be taken into account in the analysis to provide
a valid estimate of the association between estrogen use and risk of this
disease.

On the other hand, if the relative risk estimates from the matched and
unmatched data had been similar, then the matching did not introduce
a similarity between the cases and controls with respect to exposure history, and the analyses can be reported using unmatched data. Tables 12-
3 and 12-4 present findings from the Boston Area Health Study [3], a
case-control study of risk factors for MI. Cases of first MI from six Boston area hospitals were matched to controls of the same age (within 5
years), sex, and neighborhood of residence. One hypothesis of interest
was the relationship of level of physical activity, represented by an index
that measures total kilocalories of energy expended from stairs climbed,
blocks walked, and recreational/leisure-time activities, with risk of MI.
High-level exercise was defined as a physical activity index of 2500 kcal
or more per day.

Table 12-3 presents the results of the matched-pair analysis. The relative risk estimate calculated from these data is 0.60, indicating that compared with individuals who do not exercise, those who have a high level
of physical activity had a statistically significant 40-percent decreased
risk of MI. When the matching was ignored (Table 12-4), the relative
risk estimate calculated was virtually identical, indicating that there was
no material confounding of the association between physical activity and
MI by the matching factors. Consequently, the matching need not be
retained in the analysis. As a result, the analyses did not have to be limited to the cases and controls for whom a suitable match was available.
The entire sample, in this instance a total of 366 cases and 423 controls,

Table 12-3. Data from a case-control study of physical activity and myocardial infarction: matched-pair analysis

	Control		
	Exposed*	Nonexposed	Total
Case			
Exposed*	115	59	174
Nonexposed	99	67	166
Total	214	126	340

$$RR = \frac{b}{c} = \frac{59}{99} = 0.60$$

$$\chi^2_{(1)} = \frac{(b-c)^2}{b+c}$$

$$= \frac{(59-99)^2}{59+99}$$

$$= 10.13, P - 0.0015$$

$$95\% \; CI = RR^{(1 \pm 1.96/x)}$$

$$= 0.60^{(1 \pm 1.96/3.18)}$$

$$= (0.44, 0.82)$$

*Exposed = physical activity index $\geq$ 2500/kcal/day.

Table 12-4. Data from a case-control study of physical activity and myocardial infarction: unmatched analysis

	Cases	Controls	Total
Exposure*			
Yes	174	214	388
No	166	126	292
Total	340	340	680

$$RR = \frac{ad}{bc} = \frac{(174)(126)}{(214)(166)} = 0.62$$

$$\chi^2_{(1)} = \frac{\left[a - \frac{(a+b)(a+c)}{T}\right]^2}{\frac{(a+b)(c+d)(a+c)(b+d)}{T^2(T-1)}} = \frac{\left[174 - \frac{(388)(340)}{680}\right]^2}{\frac{(388)(292)(340)(340)}{680^2(679)}}$$

$$= 9.59, P = 0.002$$

$$95\% \; CI = RR^{(1 \pm 1.96/\sqrt{\chi^2})} = 0.62^{(1 \pm 1.96/3.1)}$$

$$= (0.46, 0.84)$$

*Exposed = physical activity index $\geq$ 2500/kcal/day.

could be included in subsequent analyses, potentially increasing the statistical power of the study.

The magnitude of the underestimate of effect that may be introduced by analyzing matched data as if they were unmatched relates to the degree of confounding by matching factors in the study. When there is little or no confounding by the matching factors, as in the above example; when the data have been frequency matched (in which the matching is done in groups so that the same proportions of cases and controls are in each stratum of the confounder); or when matching has been used primarily for convenience, as is often the case with age and sex, the matched and unmatched relative risk estimates will be virtually identical, and an unmatched analysis can be done. The advantage of doing this is that it will more easily permit control in the analysis of the matching factors as well as other confounding variables that were not considered in the matching process by using stratification or multivariate analysis techniques as described below. Unnecessary matching may, in fact, result in a loss of statistical efficiency relative to having selected an unmatched comparison series, especially in a case-control study [12, 17]. The magnitude of the loss in efficiency will depend on the interrelationships among the exposure, the disease, and the confounder. Matching on variables that are either weak risk factors for the disease or not risk factors at all will, in fact, result in a substantial reduction of information in the analysis.

The formulas provided in this section pertain to individual 1 : 1 matching. Analogous formulas for parameter estimation and testing of matched data with more than one control per case (R : 1 matching) with a variable control to case ratio, and with multiple exposure levels are also available [19, 24].

METHODS TO CONTROL CONFOUNDING IN THE ANALYSIS

Stratified Analysis

Stratification is a technique to control confounding in the analysis of a study that involves the evaluation of the association within homogeneous categories or strata of the confounding variable. If, for example, sex were a potential confounder, an estimate of the association between the exposure and disease would be calculated for men and for women separately. Each of these stratum-specific estimates is, by definition, unconfounded by sex, since there is no variability of the confounding variable within the stratum. Similarly, if race (defined as black, white, and other) were also a potential confounder, to control for both race and sex simultaneously, stratum-specific estimates would be calculated separately

Table 12-5. Data from a case-control study of physical
activity and risk of MI, stratified by history of cigarette smoking

Smoking history	Physical activity index	Cases	Controls	Total	
Never smoker	2500+ kcals	41	84	125	
	< 2500 kcals	46	52	98	RR = 0.55
	Total	87	134	223	
Exsmoker 10+	2500+ kcals	41	80	121	
years	< 2500 kcals	30	39	69	RR = 0.67
	Total	71	119	190	
Exsmoker < 10	2500+ kcals	22	34	56	
years	< 2500 kcals	21	26	47	RR = 0.80
	Total	43	60	103	
Current smoker	2500+ kcals	86	68	154	
	< 2500 kcals	79	40	119	RR = 0.64
	Total	165	108	273	
Total	2500+ kcals	190	266	456	
	< 2500 kcals	176	157	333	RR = 0.64
	Total	366	423	789	

for six categories: black men, black women, white men, white women,
and men and women of "other" race. Each of these estimates would
similarly be unconfounded by sex and race. It is possible simply to report
the unconfounded relative risk estimate for each stratum and calculate
a confidence interval around each estimate. It is also useful, however, to
calculate a single overall estimate of the association between exposure
and disease, once the effect of the confounding factor (or factors) has
been taken into account. A number of statistical methods are available
to combine the results of the unconfounded stratum-specific values into
a single overall unconfounded estimate, all of which calculate a weighted
average of the stratum-specific estimates of effect. The choice of the
particular weights depends on the characteristics of the data.

The use of stratified analysis to control confounding can be illustrated
by the earlier example concerning the association between level of physical activity and risk of MI. Cigarette smoking might potentially confound the association, since it is an independent risk factor for MI, and
may be related to level of physical activity. To control for this variable,
the overall association between physical activity level and MI is first considered separately for each stratum of cigarette smoking. As seen in Table 12-5, increased level of physical activity is protective for each of the

four levels of smoking, with an estimated relative risk of MI associated with physical activity of 0.55 for those who never smoked, and 0.67, 0.80, and 0.64 for exsmokers of 10+ years, exsmokers of less than 10 years, and current smokers, respectively. Each of these stratum-specific relative risks is an estimate of the association between physical activity and risk of MI that is unconfounded within that defined range of cigarette smoking.

A single summary estimate of the association between physical activity and risk of MI that is unconfounded by smoking can then be derived from the stratified data by calculating a weighted average of the stratum-specific estimates. When, as in the example above, the stratum-specific relative risk estimates appear to be similar or uniform over the range of the confounding variable, they can each be considered as providing a separate estimate of the same value of the magnitude of the overall association, with the individual estimates varying merely because of sampling variability or random error. The similarity of the estimates can be judged either by "eyeballing" the data or by performing an appropriate test of statistical significance. In this circumstance, to calculate a weighted average, the most precise estimate of the overall effect will derive from giving the greatest weight to the stratum-specific estimates with the largest sample sizes and thus the smallest variability. Specifically, this can be accomplished by assigning weights to the stratum-specific values that are inversely proportional to the variance of each estimate. This method of calculating the most precise overall estimate of effect, assuming uniformity of the stratum-specific estimates, is often referred to as pooling.

A simple method for calculating a pooled summary relative risk estimate from a series of two-by-two tables was proposed by Mantel and Haenszel [15]. Using standard notation as reviewed in Table 12-6, the formula for the pooled estimate of the relative risk for a case-control study can be expressed as follows:

$$\mathrm{RR}_{\mathrm{MH}} = \frac{\sum \dfrac{ad}{T}}{\sum \dfrac{bc}{T}}$$

where the quantities in the numerator and denominator are summed separately over each of the individual strata. Analogous formulas for the pooled estimators of the relative risk for cohort studies with count and person-year denominators are provided in Table 12-7 [25]. Analogous formulas for the pooled estimate of the attributable risk are considered elsewhere [9].

Calculating a pooled estimate of the association between physical ac-

Table 12-6. Notation of a two-by-two table

CASE-CONTROL OR COHORT STUDY WITH COUNT DENOMINATORS

	Cases	Controls	Total
Exposed	a	b	$a + b$
Nonexposed	c	d	$c + d$
Total	$a + c$	$b + d$	$a + b + c + d = T$

Case-control: $\text{RR} = \text{OR} = \dfrac{ad}{bc}$

Cohort: $\text{RR} = \dfrac{I_e}{I_0} = \dfrac{a/(a+b)}{c/(c+d)}$

COHORT STUDY WITH PERSON-YEARS DENOMINATORS

	Cases	Controls	
Exposed	a	—	PY_1
Nonexposed	c	—	PY_0
Total	$a + c$		T

$\text{RR} = \dfrac{I_e}{I_0} = \dfrac{a/PY_1}{c/PY_0}$

Table 12-7. Formulas for the calculation of the Mantel-Haenszel pooled relative risk estimate or its analogues, assuming uniform stratum-specific estimates

CASE-CONTROL STUDY:

$$\text{RR}_{\text{MH}} = \frac{\Sigma ad/T}{\Sigma bc/T}$$

COHORT STUDY WITH COUNT DENOMINATORS:

$$\text{RR}_{\text{MH}} = \frac{\Sigma a(c + d)/T}{\Sigma c(a + b)/T}$$

COHORT STUDY WITH PERSON-YEARS DENOMINATORS:

$$\text{RR}_{\text{MH}} = \frac{\Sigma a(PY_0)/T}{\Sigma c(PY_1)/T}$$

tivity and MI, stratified by cigarette smoking (Table 12-5), yields the following:

$$RR_{MH} = \frac{\sum \frac{ad}{T}}{\sum \frac{bc}{T}}$$

$$= \frac{\frac{(41)\,(52)}{223} + \frac{(41)\,(39)}{190} + \frac{(22)\,(26)}{103} + \frac{(86)\,(40)}{273}}{\frac{(84)\,(46)}{223} + \frac{(80)\,(30)}{190} + \frac{(34)\,(21)}{103} + \frac{(68)\,(79)}{273}}$$

$$= 0.64$$

This value means that, once differences in cigarette smoking have been taken into account, the relative risk of MI associated with high levels of physical activity is 0.64. This estimate is adjusted for, or unconfounded by, cigarette smoking.

The magnitude of confounding in any study is evaluated by observing the degree of discrepancy between the crude and adjusted estimates. The fact that the crude and adjusted relative risk estimates in the example above are identical indicates that there was no confounding of the association between physical activity and MI by cigarette smoking as categorized in these data.

As discussed earlier in this chapter, the presence or absence of confounding should never be assessed by using a statistical test of significance. A large sample size could easily result in a statistically significant association between the confounder and the exposure or disease, even though the magnitude may be too small to result in any material amount of confounding. On the other hand, even strong associations that could produce confounding of substantial epidemiologic importance may fail to reach statistical significance with a small sample size. Significance testing can be used, however, to evaluate whether the unconfounded estimate of effect differs from the null value of no association. Hypothesis testing for stratified data is a straightforward extension of the tests applied to crude data. The components of the test statistic are now derived not from a single table, but as a sum of the relevant components in each of the strata. The Mantel-Haenszel test statistic with one degree of freedom is a simple extension of the chi-square formula for a series of two-by-two tables of either case-control or cohort data with count denominators. This can be expressed as

$$\chi^2_{MH} = \frac{\left[\sum a - \sum\frac{(a+b)\,(a+c)}{T}\right]^2}{\sum\frac{(a+b)\,(c+d)\,(a+c)\,(b+d)}{T^2(T-1)}}$$

Analogously, the formula for a cohort study with person-year denominators is

$$\chi^2_{MH} = \frac{\left[\sum a - \sum\frac{(a+c)\,(PY_1)}{T}\right]^2}{\sum\frac{(a+c)\,(PY_1)\,(PY_0)}{T^2}}$$

Thus, to evaluate the likelihood that the association between physical activity and risk of MI, after adjustment for cigarette smoking, is due to chance, the Mantel-Haenszel chi-square statistic can be calculated as follows:

χ^2_{MH}

$$= \frac{\left[190 - \left(\frac{(125)\,(87)}{223} + \frac{(121)\,(71)}{190} + \frac{(56)\,(43)}{103} + \frac{(154)\,(165)}{273}\right)\right]^2}{\frac{(125)\,(98)\,(87)\,(134)}{223^2\,(222)} + \frac{(121)\,(69)\,(71)\,(119)}{190^2\,(189)} + \frac{(56)\,(47)\,(43)\,(60)}{103^2\,(102)} + \frac{(154)\,(119)\,(165)\,(108)}{273^2\,(272)}}$$

$= 9.16, P = 0.0023$

This means that in these data, there is a statistically significant association between level of physical activity and risk of MI, once the effect of cigarette smoking has been taken into account. It should be noted that in such a circumstance, where the stratified analysis demonstrated no confounding by a given variable, hypothesis testing could have been performed on the crude rather than the stratified data. Again, as with the analysis of crude data, exact confidence intervals can be calculated [8], as can a number of forms of approximate confidence limits [12, 24, 27]. The test-based confidence interval [20] is particularly easy to compute by substituting into the general formula the pooled estimate of the relative risk, as well as the value from the Mantel-Haenszel chi-square statistic. In the example above of physical activity and MI, this calculation would be as follows:

$$95\% \text{ CI} = RR_{MH}^{(1 \,\pm\, 1.96/\sqrt{\chi^2_{MH}})}$$

$$= 0.64^{(1 \,\pm\, 1.96/\sqrt{9.16})}$$

$$= (0.48, 0.85)$$

In summary, these data indicate a statistically significant inverse association between level of physical activity and risk of MI once the effect of cigarette smoking has been taken into account. The overall estimate of effect is 0.64 and, with 95-percent confidence, the true relative risk lies between 0.48 and 0.85. Cigarette smoking is not a confounder of the association in these data. Moreover, the magnitude of the observed reduction in risk of MI associated with increased levels of physical activity is the same regardless of whether an individual is a lifelong nonsmoker, an exsmoker, or a current smoker.

The fact that the stratum-specific estimates were similar or uniform indicates that the magnitude of association between physical activity and MI did not change according to the level of a third variable, cigarette smoking. This suggests that there was no modification by cigarette smoking of the effect of physical activity on risk of MI. In other words, regardless of a person's smoking history, there was a similar protective effect on risk of MI observed with increased level of physical activity. A different situation exists with respect to the interrelationship between physical activity, MI, and gender. As with cigarette smoking, gender is a potential confounder, since it may be associated with degree of physical activity and is independently associated with risk of MI. As seen in Table 12-8, however, when the data are stratified by gender, the association between physical activity and MI appears markedly different for men and women.

Specifically, among men, there is a statistically significant protective effect of physical activity on risk of MI (RR = 0.53, 95% CI = 0.38–0.72). In contrast, for women there was no evidence of an inverse association between physical activity and MI, and in fact, the data are compatible with the possibility of a small increased risk (RR = 1.19, 95% CI = 0.65–2.16). There are a number of possible explanations for this finding, including a true physiologic difference between men and women concerning the effect of physical activity on risk of MI. The relatively wide confidence interval, however, suggests that the sample size of women available may simply have been too small to estimate the magnitude of the association in this subgroup with any precision. The important point is that any such possible effect modification of the association between physical activity and MI by gender is best reported and explored. The nature of the relationship between physical activity and MI can be explored in the pattern of the stratum-specific estimates. If only a single summary estimate were reported, the fact that there was effect modification—that is, that the magnitude or, even more extreme, the direction of the association under study differs for varying levels of another factor—would be completely obscured.

When there is effect modification—that is, when the association between the exposure and disease under study varies by levels of a third factor—the emphasis in the analysis of the data and the presentation of

Table 12-8. Data from a case-control study of
physical activity and risk of MI, stratified by gender

Gender	Physical activity index	Cases	Controls	Total	RR, 95% CI
Men	2500+ kcals	141	208	349	
	< 2500 kcals	144	112	256	0.53, (0.38–0.73)
	Total	285	320	605	
Women	2500+ kcals	49	58	107	
	< 2500 kcals	32	45	77	1.19, (0.65–2.16)
	Total	81	103	184	
Total	2500+ kcals	190	266	456	
	< 2500 kcals	176	157	333	0.64
	Total	366	423	789	

the study results should be on describing how the association of interest is modified by the stratification factor. The first step in any stratified analysis, therefore, is the determination of whether effect modification is present in the data. In most circumstances, this decision should be based on simply "eyeballing" the data to judge the observed patterns of variation. This should be performed in the context of evidence from other investigations to achieve a biologic understanding of the nature of the association under study. If a more formal statistical evaluation of the uniformity of the stratum-specific estimates is desired, a variety of chi-square tests for homogeneity are available that test the null hypothesis that the degree of variability in the series of stratum-specific estimates is consistent with random variation [29]. Again, however, statistical testing to determine the presence or absence of effect modification should only be used as a guide, since statistical significance is so heavily influenced by sample size.

When the stratum-specific estimates vary sufficiently to indicate that there is likely to be variation in the underlying magnitude of the association between exposure and disease, the primary and most informative approach to the presentation of the data is to report separately for each stratum the estimate of effect as well as the confidence interval. The calculation of a summary unconfounded measure is possible but much less important because it does not represent the nature of the association observed in all of the groups. If, however, it seems desirable to calculate, in addition to the stratum-specific estimates, a single unconfounded measure of effect, it would not be appropriate to use a pooled estimate since the weights for the pooled estimate have been chosen to provide the most precise estimate of a uniform value of effect. When there is effect modification, specific weights are selected to standardize the stra-

Table 12-9. Formulas for the calculation
of a relative risk estimate standardized to the exposed
population, assuming stratum-specific relative risks to be non-uniform

CASE-CONTROL STUDY:

$$RR_{STD} = \frac{\Sigma a}{\Sigma \frac{bc}{d}}$$

COHORT STUDY WITH COUNT DENOMINATORS:

$$RR_{STD} = \frac{\Sigma a}{\Sigma \frac{(c)(a + b)}{(c + d)}}$$

COHORT STUDY WITH PERSON-YEARS DENOMINATORS:

$$RR_{STD} = \frac{\Sigma a}{\Sigma \frac{(c)(PY_1)}{PY_0}}$$

tum-specific values to standard distributions such as those of the exposed or nonexposed populations. As summarized in Table 12-9, formulas for the calculation of the standardized relative risk estimate are available for case-control studies, cohort studies with count denominators, and cohort studies with person-years.

Applying these formulas to the case-control data in Table 12-8 would lead to a standardized relative risk estimate of the association between level of physical activity and MI, adjusted for gender, as follows:

$$RR_{STD} = \frac{\Sigma a}{\Sigma \frac{bc}{d}}$$

$$= \frac{190}{\frac{(208)\,(144)}{112} + \frac{(58)\,(32)}{45}}$$

$$= 0.62$$

The crude (RR = 0.64) and adjusted (RR = 0.62) relative risk estimates are similar, indicating that, as with cigarette smoking, there was virtually no confounding of the association under study by gender. Unlike cigarette smoking, however, gender is a possible effect modifier of the association between physical activity and risk of MI.

For any association under study, a given factor can be both a confounder and an effect modifier, a confounder but not an effect modifier, an effect modifier but not a confounder, or neither. Confounding and effect modification are very different in both the information each provides and what is done with that information. Whether a factor is a confounder or not depends solely on whether it is distributed unevenly between the study groups and may thus in itself have accounted, totally or in part, for the observed association between exposure and disease. Confounding is a nuisance effect, resulting in a distortion of the true relationship between the exposure and risk of disease due solely to the particular mix of subjects included in the study. In another investigation, with a different group of subjects or a different design, the same variable may not be a confounder of the same association [16]. Thus, the aim is to control confounding and eliminate its effects. Effect modification is assessed by determining whether the magnitude or even direction of the association under study varies according to the presence or level of a third factor. This reflects a characteristic of nature that exists independently of any particular study design or subjects. Whether the association between physical activity and MI is different for men and women (effect modification) is in no way influenced by whether men and women in the study sample are likely to have different physical activity levels (confounding). Effect modification answers the question of whether the relationship between the exposure and disease appears to be the same or different for varying levels of a factor after baseline differences in that factor are controlled. Effect modification is to be described and reported, not controlled. Exploring the nature of the interaction, whether qualitative or quantitative, multiplicative or additive, may provide tremendous insight into the interrelationships between, and mechanisms of action of, the exposures and disease [13, 23, 26].

The process of stratification is used to evaluate both confounding and effect modification, to control the former, and to describe the latter. As summarized in Table 12-10, the approach to a stratified analysis involves a number of steps. First, the data representing the overall crude association between exposure and disease is stratified by levels of the potential confounding factor. Stratum-specific relative risk estimates are then calculated, each of which is unconfounded. To decide how best to present the data, the stratum-specific relative risk estimates are then evaluated for similarity, either by "eyeballing" or by performing a test of statistical significance. If the effects are thought to be uniform, a single summary unconfounded relative risk estimate can be calculated by pooling the stratum-specific values, using a Mantel-Haenszel relative risk estimator. Hypothesis testing is then performed on the unconfounded estimate using the appropriate Mantel-Haenszel chi-square, and the confidence interval is computed. If the stratum-specific estimates are not uniform, effect modification may be present, and the stratum-specific values should be reported and described. In addition, a single summary esti-

Table 12-10. Steps for the control of confounding and the evaluation of effect modification through stratified analysis

1. Stratify by levels of the potential confounding factor.

2. Compute stratum-specific unconfounded relative risk estimates.

3. Evaluate similarity of the stratum-specific estimates by either eyeballing or performing test of statistical significance.

4. If effect is thought to be uniform, calculate a pooled unconfounded summary estimate using RR_{MH}.

5. Perform hypothesis testing on the unconfounded estimate, using Mantel-Haenszel chi-square and compute confidence interval.

6. If effect is not thought to be uniform (i.e., if effect modification is present):
   a. Report stratum-specific estimates, results of hypothesis testing, and confidence intervals for each estimate
   b. If desired, calculate a summary unconfounded estimate using a standardized formula.

mate that is unconfounded can be calculated using a standardized measure.

Multivariate Analysis

As illustrated in the previous section, stratification in the analysis as a technique to control confounding has a number of advantages. It is easy to carry out; it permits the evaluation of effect modification; and, perhaps more importantly, it allows both the investigators and the readers to achieve a clear understanding of the interrelationships among the exposure, disease, and additional confounding and effect modifying variables. A fundamental problem with stratified analysis, however, is its inability to control simultaneously for even a moderate number of potential confounders. For example, in the study of physical activity and MI, suppose that the investigators chose to consider only four potential confounding factors: sex (male, female), age (less than 50, 50–59, 60–69, 70+), smoking status (never smoker, past smoker, current smoker), and Quetelet's index, a measure of obesity defined as weight in pounds divided by height in inches squared (lowest, second, third, highest quartiles). These variables would require a total of $2 \times 4 \times 3 \times 4 = 96$ strata to represent the possible combinations of sex, age, smoking, and obesity. Even with a relatively large study, it is very likely that many of these strata would contain few, if any, individuals, making analysis unreliable or even impossible. The control of an additional variable would necessitate multiplying the 96 strata by the number of values of still another factor, and the total number of individuals in the sample would very quickly become inadequate.

Multivariate analysis allows for the efficient estimation of measures of association while controlling for a number of confounding factors simultaneously, even in situations where stratification would fail because of insufficient numbers. In general, a multivariate technique refers to any analysis of data that takes into account a number of variables simultaneously. All types of multivariate analysis involve the construction of a mathematical model to describe most efficiently the association between exposure and disease as well as other variables that may confound or modify the effect of exposure. A large number of multivariate models have been developed for specialized purposes, each with a particular set of assumptions underlying its applicability. The choice of the appropriate model is complex and is based on the underlying design of the study, the nature of the variables, as well as assumptions regarding the interrelationship between the exposures and outcomes under investigation. Multivariate analysis is the subject of many advanced textbooks [1, 2, 5, 11, 12]. The application of the techniques, especially the selection and form of the categorization of the variables for inclusion into the model, requires expert guidance. It is beyond the scope of this textbook to provide a full discussion of each multivariate technique and its underlying theory and applications. What we wish to do here, however, is to describe intuitively the rationale for the use of multivariate analysis in epidemiologic research, a few of the strategies that are most often encountered, and a brief discussion of their strengths and limitations.

The most common way that many factors are controlled for simultaneously is through the use of a multiple regression model. Multiple regression is an extension of the most fundamental model describing the relationship between two variables, namely a straight line. In simple linear regression, the relationship between the mean of the dependent, or outcome, variable (Y) and an independent, or predictor, variable (X) can be simply expressed as $Y = a + bX$. In this equation, a is the linear regression intercept or constant, that is, the average value of the dependent variable when $X = 0$, and the coefficient b is the slope of the line representing the association between X and Y, that is, the estimated mean change in the expected value of the dependent variable for each unit change of the independent variable. For example, in evaluating the relationship between the independent variable age and systolic blood pressure, the coefficient b would indicate the mean change in systolic blood pressure for every unit change (e.g., year) of age. Multiple linear regression involves expanding this equation to include a number of independent variables:

$$Y = a + b_1 X_1 + b_2 X_2 + \ldots b_n X_n$$

where:

n = the number of independent predictor variables

$X_1 . . . X_n$ = an individual's particular set of values for the independent variables

$b_1 . . . b_n$ = the respective coefficients for each of the independent variables

As with every type of mathematical model, linear regression involves assumptions about the characteristics of and relationship between the dependent and independent variables. Specifically, both simple and multiple regression assume a linear function of the variables included in the model. While few relationships between variables are strictly linear, often the true association is close enough to allow reasonable inferences to be made from such a model. The adequacy of a linear fit can be tested by a number of statistical techniques [4, 14]. If the relationship between variables is inherently nonlinear, some type of transformation can often be performed to accommodate the situation. For example, the incidence of many diseases, such as cancer, increases with age, but as a curved or exponential rather than linear relationship. A linear regression that utilized the square of age rather than age itself would result in a better representation of the true association between age and incidence of disease and enable a linear model to accommodate a basically nonlinear relationship.

The coefficients in the model result from a method that calculates the "best fitting" line, that is, the unique line that best describes the population that gave rise to the observed data. The common method of calculating these coefficients is that of least squares, which minimizes the sum of the squared deviations of each observation from the fitted line. The coefficient of each independent variable can be interpreted as the magnitude of the increase (or, if negative, the decrease) in the value of the mean of the dependent variable for every unit increase in that predictor variable, taking into account the effect of all other variables in the model. For example, with respect to evaluating the relationship of age and systolic blood pressure, a number of potential confounders such as sex, obesity, smoking, exercise, and dietary factors could also be entered into the model. The coefficient for age in such a model would indicate the mean change in systolic blood pressure for every unit change in age, controlling for the effects of all these other variables. It is just this conditional interpretation of the coefficients of multivariate analysis that makes this analytic technique so useful for epidemiologic studies, because the effect of any variable unconfounded by all other factors in the model can be assessed.

Multiple linear regression is most appropriately used when the dependent outcome variable is continuously distributed, as with levels of blood pressure or serum cholesterol. In many epidemiologic studies, the outcome of interest is a binary variable such as diseased versus nondiseased or dead versus alive. In such circumstances, it is possible to use a specialized type of multiple regression called logistic regression analysis, which is a powerful statistical tool for estimating the magnitude of the association between an exposure and a binary outcome after adjusting simultaneously for a number of potential confounding factors. This model is a simple variant of the multiple regression equation, in which the risk of developing an outcome is expressed as a function of independent predictor variables. Specifically, the dependent variable is defined as the natural logarithm (ln) of the odds of disease, or the logit. If Y is the probability of disease, then $Y/(1-Y)$ represents the "odds" of developing the outcome, and the log odds of disease, or the logit, can be written as $\ln[Y/(1-Y)]$. The log odds of disease as the dependent variable can then be expressed as a simple linear function of the independent predictor variables using the following formula:

$$\ln\left[\frac{Y}{1-Y}\right] = a + b_1 X_1 + \ldots + b_n X_n$$

This equation can be rewritten to represent the probability of disease as:

$$Y = \frac{1}{1 + e^{-(a + b_1 X_1 + \ldots + b_n X_n)}}$$

As with multiple linear regression, the specific set of values for the intercept a and for $b_1, \ldots, b_n$ in logistic regression are calculated to represent those that provide the most likely estimate of the population from which the observed data arose. Since the logistic model for the probability of disease yields values that are always between zero and one, its use has important implications for the interpretation of the coefficients. The coefficients obtained through logistic regression by definition denote the magnitude of the increase or decrease in the log odds produced by one unit of change in the value of the independent variable and thus indicate the effect of an individual factor on the log odds of the outcome with all remaining variables held constant. One very practical advantage of logistic regression over multiple linear regression in epidemiologic research is that these coefficients can be directly converted to an odds ratio that provides an estimate of the relative risk that is adjusted for confounding. If the independent variable is binary, the antilogarithm of the coefficient for that variable in a logistic regression is the odds ratio representing the magnitude of the association between the factor and the outcome, controlling for the effects of all other variables in the model [30]:

$$RR\ (x_i) = e^{b_i}$$

Confidence limits around this estimate of relative risk can then be obtained using the coefficient and its related standard error:

$$95\%\ CI = e^{(b_i \pm 1.96 SE_{b_i})}$$

Relative risk estimates for increments of independent variables that are ordinal or continuous can also be obtained [12, 25]. Alternatively, such variables can be redefined and entered into the model as a series of binary variables, and the above formula can be used to calculate the odds ratio of developing the disease at a given level of exposure relative to the specified referent group.

The use and interpretation of logistic regression can be illustrated with the previous example of level of physical activity and risk of MI. Because the univariate stratified analyses suggested possible effect modification of the association by gender, separate multivariate analyses were performed for men and women. Variables entered into the model included demographic factors (age, educational level), medical history (diastolic blood pressure, treatment of hypertension, family history of MI, obesity, diabetes, cholesterol level), and life-style factors (cigarette smoking, personality type, alcohol consumption, total daily calories, daily saturated fat intake). The coefficient associated with a Physical Activity Index of 2500 kcal per day, controlling for the simultaneous effects of the above variables, was −0.766, with a standard error of 0.266. Thus, the relative risk estimate for physical activity and MI among men, controlling for confounding by these factors, is as follows:

$$RR = e^{(-0.766)}$$
$$= 0.46$$

This compares with the calculated crude value of 0.53, indicating that there was little confounding of the association between physical activity and MI by the combined effect of these factors. The 95-percent confidence interval around the adjusted estimate can be calculated as

$$95\%\ CI = e^{[-0.766 \pm 1.96(0.266)]}$$
$$= (0.28, 0.78)$$

This model for logistic regression assumes that the estimate of effect is uniform across the different levels of the confounding variables, that is, there is no effect modification by the variables included in the model. If that assumption cannot be made, a product term representing a combination of the exposure and potential effect modifier can also be added to the model to allow for the assessment of interactions. Thus, to evaluate, for example, possible effect modification of the association among men between physical activity and MI by family history of the disease, the logistic regression model could be set up as follows:

$$\ln\left[\frac{Y}{1-Y}\right] = a + b_1X_1 + b_2X_2 + b_3(X_1X_2) + \ldots + b_nX_n$$

where:

Y = probability of MI

X_1 = physical activity level (1 = high, 0 = low)

X_2 = family history of MI (1 = present, 0 = absent)

X_1X_2 = status on both physical activity and family history of MI

$X_3 \ldots X_n$ = other independent variables

$b_1 \ldots b_n$ = the respective coefficients of each of the independent variables or combination of variables

The coefficient of the product term (b_3) permits assessment of whether the magnitude of the contribution of physical activity to the log odds of MI varies according to family history of the disease, that is, whether there is evidence of effect modification. The calculation of the effect of physical activity on risk of MI will then involve information from b_1, the coefficient for physical activity, as well as b_3 [12].

In studies where participants have not all been followed for an equal period of time to determine the development of the outcomes of interest, the multivariate techniques that have been described are not applicable. A specialized type of multivariate analysis, called the proportional hazards model, was developed by Cox [5] to take into account the unequal lengths of time that each cohort member is observed for the occurrence of the outcome of interest. The proportional hazards model describes the relation of the independent variable to the natural logarithm of the incidence rate of disease rather than to the odds of disease. The form of this model is similar to that of multiple logistic regression but slightly more complicated since the components must be dependent on time. Specifically:

$$\ln[\text{incidence rate } (t)] = a(t) + b_1X_1 + \ldots + b_nX_n$$

where:

$a(t)$ = the baseline incidence rate expressed as a function of time

$X_1, \ldots X_n$ = a person's particular set of values for the independent variables

$b_1, \ldots b_n$ = the respective coefficients for each independent variable

The construction and interpretation of coefficients from the proportional hazards model as estimates of the incidence density ratio is analogous to that of the coefficients from the logistic regression model.

Multivariate modeling can be used in epidemiologic research for both explanatory and predictive purposes. With respect to explanatory uses, as in the examples above, the interrelationships between the exposure, disease, and other factors can be described. With respect to predictive purposes, the estimated coefficients can be used to calculate the probability that an individual having a specific set of values for the predictor variables will experience the outcome of interest. This can be accomplished in a straightforward manner in a cohort study. In a case-control study, on the other hand, because the relative numbers of cases and controls in the sample are determined by the investigator and not by the incidence of disease in the population, the intercept term for the prediction equation is simply an artifact of the study design. Thus, as with case-control studies in general, it is not possible using multivariate modeling to calculate absolute rates or risks for an individual with a particular set of values for the predictor variables unless information on the absolute rate of disease is available from sources outside the study. The study results can, however, provide the relative magnitudes of the rates of disease for subjects having various sets of values for the predictor variables.

Perhaps the main disadvantage of all multivariate techniques is that the process of efficient mathematical modeling can often occur at the expense of a clear understanding of the data by either the investigator or the reader. In many ways, the use of multivariate analysis can appear like a "black box" strategy, in which all of the variables are entered into a specialized computer program, and the net result is a single value representing the magnitude of the association between the exposure and disease after the effects of all confounders have been taken into account. As discussed in the beginning of this section, the selection of the appropriate model and variables, as well as the way in which these variables are entered into the model, is a complex issue that should be accomplished in consultation with someone experienced in the use of these techniques. It can be difficult for the investigator to both understand and communicate the results of this process to the reader, as well as to keep clearly in mind the limitations of the data from which the results arose. Thus, while multivariate analysis is undeniably useful for the control of confounding when stratified analysis is impractical, it is important that it be performed and interpreted carefully and that the control of confounding by this method not be achieved at the expense of lack of familiarity with the basic data. A stratified analysis should always be examined prior to performing multivariate procedures and presented in conjunction with the multivariate results. This will help ensure an understanding of the nature of the individual confounding variables as well as the interactions between the factors under study, assist in choosing the particular variables to be included in the multivariate analysis, and provide information concerning the degree to which the data conform to the assumptions of the particular multivariate model chosen. This thorough exploration of the basic data prior to the more complex analyses can be easily accomplished with available programs suitable for hand-held programmable calculators [25] and personal computers.

CONCLUSION

In all analytic studies, particularly observational case-control and cohort designs, confounding must always be considered as an alternative explanation for study findings. There are a number of methods available for the control of confounding in the design or analysis of any study. These include restriction, matching, or randomization (in clinical trials) in the design as well as stratification and multivariate techniques in the analysis. No single method can be considered optimal in every situation. Each has its strengths and limitations, which must be carefully considered at the beginning of the study. In most situations, a combination of strategies will provide better insights into the nature of the data and more efficient control of confounding than any single approach.

STUDY QUESTIONS

1. In matched-pair designs, why is it always necessary first to conduct a matched analysis? In what circumstances can the matching safely be disregarded?
2. In stratified analyses, compare and contrast the evaluation of confounding and effect modification.
3. What are the chief strengths and limitations of multivariate analysis?

REFERENCES

1. Bishop, Y. M. M., Fienberg, S. E., and Holland, P. W. *Discrete Multivariate Analysis: Theory and Practice.* Cambridge, MA: MIT Press, 1975.
2. Breslow, N. E., and Day, N. E. *Statistical Methods in Cancer Research: Vol. I. The Analysis of Case-Control Studies.* Lyon, France: IARC Scientific Publications, 1981.

3. Buring, J. E., Willett, W., Goldhaber, S. Z., et al. Alcohol and HDL in non-fatal myocardial infarction: Preliminary results from a case-control study. *Circulation* 68:227, 1983.
4. Colton, T. *Statistics in Medicine.* Boston: Little, Brown, 1974.
5. Cox, D. R. *Analysis of Binary Data.* London: Methuen, 1970.
6. Doll, R., and Hill, A. B. Smoking and carcinoma of the lung: Preliminary report. *Br. Med. J.* 2:739–748, 1950.
7. Fleiss, J. L. *Statistical Methods for Rates and Proportions.* New York: Wiley-Interscience, 1973.
8. Gart, J. J. Point and interval estimation of the common odds ratio in the combination of 2 × 2 tables with fixed margins. *Biometrika* 57:471–475, 1970.
9. Greenland, S., and Robins, J. M. Estimation of a common effect parameter from sparse follow-up data. *Biometrics* 41:55, 1985.
10. Hennekens, C. H. Alcohol. In N. Kaplan and J. Stamler (eds.), *Prevention of Coronary Heart Disease.* Philadelphia: Saunders, 1983. Pp. 130–138.
11. Kleinbaum, D. G., and Kupper, L. L. *Applied Regression Analysis and Other Multivariable Methods.* Boston: Duxbury Press, 1978.
12. Kleinbaum, D. G., Kupper, L. L., and Morgenstern, H. *Epidemiologic Research: Principles and Quantitative Methods.* Belmont, CA: Lifetime Learning Publications, 1982.
13. Kupper, L., and Hogan, M. D. Interaction in epidemiologic studies. *Am. J. Epidemiol.* 108:447–453, 1978.
14. Lemenstrow, S., and Hosmer, D. W. A review of goodness of fit statistics for use in development of logistic regression models. *Am. J. Epidemiol.* 115:92–106, 1982.
15. Mantel, N., and Haenszel, W. Statistical aspects of the analysis of data from retrospective studies of disease. *J.N.C.I.* 22:719–748, 1959.
16. Miettinen, O. S. Confounding and effect modification. *Am. J. Epidemiol.* 100:350, 1974.
17. Miettinen, O. S. Matching and design efficiency in retrospective studies. *Am. J. Epidemiol.* 91:111, 1970.
18. Miettinen, O. S. Individual matching with multiple controls in the case of all or none responses. *Biometrics* 22:339–355, 1969.
19. Miettinen, O. S. Estimation of relative risk from individually matched series. *Biometrics* 26:75–86, 1970.
20. Miettinen, O. S. Estimability and estimation in case-referent studies. *Am. J. Epidemiol.* 103:226–235, 1976.
21. Prentice, R. Use of the logistic model in retrospective studies. *Biometrics* 32:599–606, 1976.
22. Rosner, B., and Hennekens, C. H. Analytic methods in matched pair epidemiologic studies. *Int. J. Epidemiol.* 7:367–372, 1978.
23. Rothman, K. J. Synergy and antagonism in cause-effect relationships. *Am. J. Epidemiol.* 103:506–511, 1976.
24. Rothman, K. J. *Modern Epidemiology.* Boston: Little, Brown, 1986.
25. Rothman, K. J., and Boice, J. D., Jr. *Epidemiologic Analysis with a Programmable Calculator.* U.S. D.H.E.W. N.I.H. Publication No. 79-1649, 1979.
26. Rothman, K. J., Greenland, S., and Walker, A. M. K. Concepts of interaction. *Am. J. Epidemiol.* 112:467–470, 1980.

27. Schlesselman, J. J. *Case-Control Studies: Design, Conduct, Analysis.* New York: Oxford University Press, 1982.
28. Smith, D. C., Prentice, R., Thompson, D. J., et al. Association of exogenous estrogen and endometrial carcinoma. *N. Engl. J. Med.* 293:1164–1167, 1975.
29. Snedecor, G. W., and Cochrane, W. G. *Statistical Methods* (6th ed.). Ames, IA: Iowa State University Press, 1967.
30. Truett, J., Cornfield, J., and Kannel, W. A multivariate analysis of the risk of coronary heart disease in Framingham. *J. Chronic Dis.* 20:511–524, 1967.

IV. EPIDEMIOLOGY IN DISEASE CONTROL

13

Screening

The preceding sections of this textbook have focused on principles and methods of epidemiology, with a primary emphasis on increased understanding of distributions and determinants of disease. Regarding determinants, the ultimate goal is to prevent the development of disease in healthy persons. The same principles and methods can also be applied to the question of whether it is possible to improve the outcome of illness among affected individuals by reducing the number or severity of various clinical manifestations or the rate of recurrence, with a primary aim for fatal diseases being to reduce mortality. One particularly attractive option to achieve these objectives is screening for early detection of disease. In this context, screening refers to the application of a test to people who are as yet asymptomatic for the purpose of classifying them with respect to their likelihood of having a particular disease. The screening procedure itself does not diagnose illness. Those who test positive are sent on for further evaluation by a subsequent diagnostic test or procedure to determine whether they do in fact have the disease.

An implicit assumption underlying the concept of screening is that early detection, before the development of symptoms, will lead to a more favorable prognosis because treatment begun before the disease becomes clinically manifest will be more effective than later treatment. This assumption has intuitive appeal, and screening has played an important role in improving public health over the years. In some circumstances, the search for early asymptomatic disease is now considered a routine and important aspect of good medical care, yet the concept of screening, including its appropriateness and evaluation, is not as straightforward as it may at first appear. Even the basic assumption that early treatment will improve prognosis is not true in all circumstances. Moreover, even if the assumption is justifiable in a particular situation, there are often risks or costs associated with the screening and/or consequent diagnostic procedures that must be weighed against the benefits. All these considerations emphasize that the value of screening for disease control is never self-evident. Indeed, a new screening procedure should always be considered a promising but as yet unproved prospect for disease control until risks and benefits have been rigorously evaluated. Optimally, such evaluations ought to be completed before widespread screening for a disease is undertaken or even recommended.

The evaluation of a screening program will involve using all of the epidemiologic principles and methods that we have discussed in this book, including measures of disease frequency, the choice of various design strategies considering their inherent strengths and limitations, and issues in interpretation, particularly types of bias.

A number of comprehensive articles and books [4, 6, 7, 14, 28, 30, 40, 43] have considered in detail the issues involved in screening for diseases with long latent periods, the diseases toward which screening programs for early diagnosis and treatment are primarily directed. In this chapter, we will provide a general discussion of the concept of screening, including the types of diseases that are most suitable for such a program, as well as factors that need to be considered in the evaluation of a screening program, including the validity of the test itself, feasibility of the program, and whether its implementation actually achieves a reduction in morbidity and mortality from the disease.

DISEASES APPROPRIATE FOR SCREENING

Some diseases are not suitable candidates for the application of a screening program. To be appropriate for screening, a disease should be serious; treatment given before symptoms develop should be more beneficial in terms of reducing morbidity or mortality than that given after they develop; and the prevalence of preclinical disease should be high among the population screened. The criterion of seriousness relates primarily to issues of cost-effectiveness and ethics. The expenditure of resources on screening must be justifiable in terms of eliminating or ameliorating adverse health consequences. Similarly, with respect to ethics, the consequences of failing to diagnose and treat early must be sufficiently grave to warrant undergoing the risks and discomforts of the screening procedure itself. Life-threatening diseases, such as breast cancer, and those known to have serious and irreversible consequences if not treated early, such as congenital hypothyroidism and phenylketonuria, clearly meet the criterion of seriousness. On the other hand, medical problems such as gallstones, which are usually not life-threatening and may, in fact, never become symptomatic, may not be suitable for screening.

One question of importance is whether treatment of preclinical disease is more effective than treatment begun after the development of symptoms. To evaluate this, it is necessary to consider the natural history

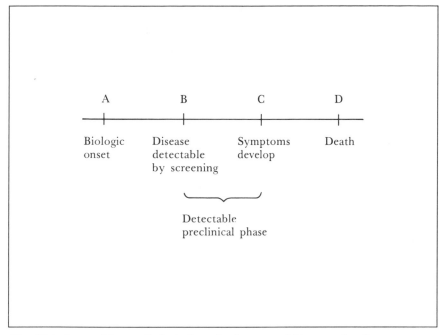

Fig. 13-1. Detectable preclinical phase in the natural history of a disease.

of a disease. As shown in Figure 13-1, there is a period after biologic onset during which the disease is asymptomatic but detectable by screening. The interval of time between the point at which the disease can be detected by screening and the point at which the individual becomes symptomatic and seeks medical attention has been termed the detectable preclinical phase (DPCP) [4].

For screening to be of benefit, treatment given during the detectable preclinical phase must result in a better prognosis than therapy given after symptoms develop. For example, cancer of the uterine cervix develops slowly, taking perhaps more than a decade for the cancer cells, which are initially confined to the outer layer of the cervix, to progress to a phase of invasiveness. During this preinvasive stage, the cancer is usually asymptomatic but can be detected by screening using the Papanicolaou smear. It is far preferable to begin treatment during this stage than when the cancer has become invasive. On the other hand, if early treatment makes no difference because the prognosis is equally good (or equally bad) whether treatment is begun before or after symptoms develop, then the application of a screening test will be neither necessary nor effective. For example, lung cancer has a very poor prognosis regardless of when treatment is initiated. Since earlier diagnosis and treatment appear to prolong life little more than therapy after symptoms have developed [1, 36], screening to detect asymptomatic lung cancer using currently available techniques would not be beneficial. Analogously, screening for nonmelanotic skin cancer would not be a high priority compared with screening for other conditions, since this disease is virtually completely curable even after it becomes symptomatic and is brought to medical attention [12].

Finally, the requirement that the prevalence of the detectable preclinical phase of disease is high among the population screened relates to the issue of the costs of the screening program relative to the numbers of cases detected. The prevalence of the detectable preclinical phase of disease and thus the number of cases detected by screening can be increased by screening high-risk groups, such as targeting bladder cancer screening to those with relevant occupational exposures or breast cancer screening to women with a family history of the disease.

Hypertension meets all the criteria of suitability for screening. First, it is a serious disease, in that greater mortality in hypertensive individuals is well documented, with the risk of death increasing with higher levels of either diastolic or systolic blood pressure [20, 21]. Second, early treatment of hypertension has been shown to reduce the risk of subsequent morbidity and mortality from all vascular diseases combined, and from stroke [16, 38, 39]. For example, the Hypertension Detection and Follow-Up Program [16, 35] compared aggressive pharmacologic treatment (stepped care) with usual care for hypertension diagnosed by community-based screening. At the end of 5 years, for those with initial mild elevations of blood pressure, there were 20 percent fewer deaths in the stepped-care group. Third, the prevalence of hypertension in a screened population is likely to be high, since approximately 20 to 25 percent of adults in the U.S. have diastolic pressures of 90 mm Hg or greater [21].

While all these criteria should be considered in deciding whether a disease is suitable for screening, not all are necessary in a particular situation. For example, phenylketonuria (PKU) is a rare disease but has very serious long-term consequences if left untreated. In this congenital metabolic disorder, there is an absence of phenylalanine hydroxylase activity in the liver. When a newborn with PKU ingests proteins containing the amino acid phenylalanine, accumulation of certain metabolites affects the developing brain and results in severe mental retardation [23, 31]. Dietary intervention (restriction of phenylalanine) begun soon after birth can prevent mental retardation [11, 13, 19]. Although PKU occurs in only 1 out of every approximately 15,000 births [29], the serious and irreversible consequences of an undetected case combined with the availability of a simple, accurate, and inexpensive test have led public health officials in a number of states to require PKU screening for all newborns.

SCREENING TESTS

For a screening program to be successful, not only must it be applied to a disease with characteristics appropriate for screening, but in addition, a suitable screening test must be available. A screening test should ideally be inexpensive, easy to administer, and impose minimal discomfort on the patients. In addition, the results of the screening test must be valid, reliable, and reproducible.

The validity of a screening test is measured by its ability to do what it is supposed to do, that is, correctly categorize persons who have preclinical disease as test-positive and those without preclinical disease as test-negative. Table 13-1 summarizes the relationship between the results of a screening test and the actual presence of disease as determined by the results of an appropriate subsequent diagnostic test. In this table,

a = The number of individuals for whom the screening test is positive and the individual actually has the disease (true positive).
b = The number for whom the screening test is positive but the individual does not have the disease (false positive).
c = The number for whom the screening test is negative but the individual does have the disease (false negative).
d = The number for whom the screening test is negative and the individual does not have the disease (true negative).

Table 13-1. Results of a screening test

	Disease status (Dx) ("truth")		
	Positive	Negative	Total
Results of screening test (T)			
Positive	a	b	$a + b$
Negative	c	d	$c + d$
Total	$a + c$	$b + d$	

$$\text{Sensitivity} = \text{Probability } (T^+|Dx^+) = \frac{a}{a+c}$$

$$\text{Specificity} = \text{Probability } (T^-|Dx^-) = \frac{d}{b+d}$$

$$PV^+ = \text{Probability } (Dx^+|T^+) = \frac{a}{a+b}$$

$$PV^- = \text{Probability } (Dx^-|T^-) = \frac{d}{c+d}$$

Sensitivity and specificity are two measures of the validity of a screening test. Sensitivity is defined as the probability of testing positive if the disease is truly present and is calculated by $a/(a + c)$. As the sensitivity of a test increases, the number of persons with the disease who are missed by being incorrectly classified as test-negative (false negatives) will decrease. Specificity is defined as the probability of screening negative if the disease is truly absent and is calculated by $d/(b + d)$. A highly specific test will rarely be positive in the absence of disease and will therefore result in a lower proportion of persons without disease who are incorrectly classified as test-positive (false positives).

The calculation of the sensitivity and specificity of a screening test can be illustrated using data from the Breast Cancer Screening Project of the Health Insurance Plan of Greater New York (HIP) [15, 32, 33, 34]. A total of 62,000 women aged 40 to 64 years who had been members of HIP for at least 1 year were identified for study. The women were assigned alternately, based on identification number, to a study (screened) or comparison (usual care) group. The women in the screened group were offered an initial screening examination for breast cancer (consisting of a combination of mammography and physical examination) followed by three follow-up examinations at yearly intervals. The women in the comparison group were not offered the screening examination but rather continued to receive their usual health care. As shown in Table 13-2, a total of 64,810 screening examinations were performed among the study population. During the first 5 years of observation, 132 breast cancers were diagnosed among the 1,115 biopsies or aspirations that were recommended on the basis of the results of the screening procedures [15]. In addition, 45 cases of breast cancer were detected among women who screened negative but were diagnosed with the disease during the subsequent year. These women were assumed to have been false negatives, that is, they were assumed to have had the disease at the time of the screening test. Thus, the sensitivity of mammography plus physical examination in these data would be 132/177 or 74.6 percent. This means that of those diagnosed with breast cancer during the study period, approximately 75 percent tested positive on the screening procedure. The specificity of the screening program would equal 63,650/64,633 or 98.5 percent, indicating that virtually all women who did not have the disease tested negative.

Obviously, it would be desirable to have a screening test that was both highly sensitive and highly specific. Usually that is not possible, and there is generally a tradeoff between the sensitivity and specificity of a given screening test. This tradeoff has to do with the fact that for many clinical tests, there are some people who are clearly normal, some clearly abnormal, and some who fall into the grey zone between the two. In these situations, the cutoff between normal and abnormal is an arbitrary

Table 13-2. Sensitivity and specificity of breast cancer screening examination (HIP program)

	Breast cancer		
	Cancer confirmed	Cancer not confirmed	Total
Screening test (physical examination and mammography)			
Positive	132	983	1115
Negative	45	63,650	63,695
Total	177	64,633	64,810

$$\text{Sensitivity} = \frac{a}{a+c} = \frac{132}{177} = 74.6\%$$

$$\text{Specificity} = \frac{d}{b+d} = \frac{63,650}{64,633} = 98.5\%$$

$$\text{PV}^+ = \frac{a}{a+b} = \frac{132}{1115} = 11.8\%$$

$$\text{PV}^- = \frac{d}{c+d} = \frac{63,650}{63,695} = 99.9\%$$

Data from S. Shapiro, J. D. Goldberg, and G. B. Hutchison. Lead time in breast cancer detection and implications for periodicity of screening. *Am. J. Epidemiol.* 100:357–366, 1974; and G. B. Hutchison. Personal communication, 1987.

decision. Because of this, any screening test result based on such a scale will of necessity have an increased ability to avoid missing a true case (sensitivity) only at the expense of an increase in the number of individuals without the disease who will erroneously be picked up by the screening program (specificity).

Thus, altering the criterion of positivity or abnormality will influence both the sensitivity and specificity of the test. Lowering or making less stringent the criterion of positivity will mean that more people who actually have the disease will be test-positive (increased sensitivity), but so will a number of people who do not have the disease (decreased specificity). Conversely, making the criterion more stringent will mean that a greater proportion of those who test negative will actually not have the disease (increased specificity), but a larger number of true cases will also be missed (decreased sensitivity). For example, if in a hypertension screening program the criterion of positivity for diastolic blood pressure were set low, at 88 mm Hg, very few people with actual hypertension would be missed but many normotensive individuals would be falsely labeled as hypertensive. Thus, the test would be very sensitive but non-specific. If, on the other hand, the criterion of positivity were set higher, at 100 mm Hg for example, exactly the opposite would occur, in that a higher proportion of those without hypertension would test negative, but so would a greater proportion of persons with the disease.

Any decision regarding specific criteria for acceptable levels of sensitivity and specificity in a given situation involves weighing the consequences of leaving cases undetected (false negatives) against erroneously classifying healthy persons as diseased (false positives). Sensitivity should be increased at the expense of specificity when the penalty associated with missing a case is high, such as when the disease is serious and definitive treatment exists (PKU), when the disease can be spread (syphilis or gonorrhea), or when subsequent diagnostic evaluations of positive screening tests are associated with minimal cost and risk, such as a further series of blood pressure readings to ascertain hypertension. On the other hand, specificity should be increased relative to sensitivity when the costs or risks associated with further diagnostic techniques are substantial, such as with breast cancer, for which the definitive diagnostic evaluation of a positive screening test is a biopsy. In this circumstance, however, it must be made quite clear to those screened that a negative screening test is not a guarantee of being disease-free, but rather that the likelihood of having the disease is low so that the individual will not be lulled into a false sense of security and ignore any symptoms of the disease that subsequently develop.

One way of addressing the problem of the trade-off between sensitivity and specificity is to use the results of several screening tests together, with these tests administered either in parallel or in series. When screening tests are given in parallel, all are administered at the same time, and persons with positive results on any test are considered positive. In general, parallel testing results in increased sensitivity compared with that of each individual test, since disease is less likely to be missed, but lower specificity because false positive diagnoses are also more likely. For example, the diagnosis of deep vein thrombosis is often made by using, in parallel, impedance plethysmography and leg scanning after injection with ^{125}I fibrinogen. The sensitivity of these two diagnostic procedures together is far greater than that of either test alone [24]. When screening tests are given in series, an initial screening test is administered, and only persons with a positive test are reevaluated with an additional screening procedure. In general, serial testing results in an increase in specificity compared with a single test, because a positive series is more likely to represent true disease. For example, series testing has been used for mass screening for syphilis [2, 17]. Initially, a Rapid Plasmin Reagin (RPR) card test or a Venereal Disease Research Laboratory (VDRL) slide test is administered. These screening tests are relatively simple and economical. They are also quite sensitive but not very specific and therefore result in large numbers of false positive tests. Persons positive for the RPR or VDRL test are then given a Fluorescent Treponemal Antibody Absorption (FTA-ABS) test, which has a high specificity as well as sensitivity; however, it requires greater laboratory proficiency and is costly. The FTA-ABS test serves to weed out false positives as designated by the RPR or VDRL tests. Because it is given only if the RPR card or VDRL slide test is positive, screening is more economical, and diagnostic laboratories are not deluged with requests for the more difficult test.

After the validity of the screening test has been evaluated, it is necessary to consider its reliability, which refers to the consistency of results when repeat examinations are performed on the same persons under the same conditions. There are four sources of variability that can affect the reproducibility of results of a screening test. The first relates to the biological variation inherent in the actual manifestation being measured, such as blood pressure, which varies considerably for a given individual with time and other circumstances. The second, variation due to the test method or measurement, relates to the reliability of the instrument itself, such as a standard mercury sphygmomanometer for blood pressure. The third, intraobserver variability, refers to differences in repeated measurements by the same screener. The fourth source, interobserver variation, refers to inconsistencies attributable to differences in the way different screeners apply or interpret test results. Interobserver variability is minimized when end points are well defined and quantifiable, as in tonometry for glaucoma screening, and is greater when the criteria are vague and subjective, as in the interpretation of chest x-rays. Agreement between observers also tends to increase when the categories of test results are few and straightforward (i.e., positive or negative) and to decrease when more categories, which inevitably require a greater degree of interpretation, are incorporated into the classification scheme.

EVALUATION OF SCREENING PROGRAMS: FEASIBILITY AND EFFICACY

Even after a disease is determined to be appropriate for screening and a valid test becomes available, it remains unclear whether a widespread screening program for that disease should be implemented. Evaluation of a potential screening program involves consideration of two issues: first, whether the proposed program is feasible, and second, whether it is effective. Both must be considered carefully. No matter how effective a screening procedure is in reducing subsequent morbidity and mortality, it will not be accepted if it cannot be conducted efficiently, with minimal inconvenience and discomfort, and at a reasonable cost. Conversely, the implementation of a screening program, no matter how cost-effective, will not be warranted if it does not accomplish its goal of reducing morbidity and mortality.

Feasibility

The feasibility of a screening program is determined by a number of factors related to program performance, which measure the acceptability of the program to the potential screenees, cost effectiveness, the subsequent diagnosis and treatment of individuals who test positive, and the yield of cases. The screening program must be acceptable to the population being screened, which generally means that it must be quickly and easily administered, with a minimum of discomfort. For example, the Papanicolaou smear for cervical cancer is relatively quick and painless and is widely accepted by women. In contrast, sigmoidoscopy to detect colon cancer is a more lengthy procedure, which may involve considerable discomfort. In part due to this situation, it has not been widely accepted as a screening procedure either by the general public or even by clinicians who perform the examination. The acceptability of the program can be measured by factors such as the number of persons examined and the proportion of the target population that is screened. In addition, the costs of the potential screening program must be considered, in terms of total costs as well as with regard to resources expended per detected case of the disease. The costs of a screening test include not only those related to the procedure itself, but also those arising from subsequent evaluations of individuals who test positive. A successful screening program must also include provision for follow-up of persons whose screening tests are positive. This can be measured by considering the proportions of those with positive tests who are followed, diagnosed, and treated.

With respect to the yield, or number of cases detected by a screening program, one measure that is commonly considered is the predictive value of the screening test [37]. Predictive value measures whether or not an individual actually has the disease, given the results of the screening test. Predictive value positive (PV^+) is the probability that a person actually has the disease given that he or she tests positive and is calculated (using the notation in Table 13-1) as:

$$PV^+ = \frac{a}{a + b}$$

Analogously, predictive value negative (PV^-) is the probability that an individual is truly disease-free given a negative screening test and is calculated as follows:

$$PV^- = \frac{d}{c + d}$$

The calculation of these measures can be illustrated using data from the HIP Breast Cancer Screening Project presented in Table 13-2. The predictive value positive, or the probability that a woman who tested positive on the screen actually had breast cancer, is 132/1115 or 11.8 percent. This indicates that approximately 1 out of every 8 women who were referred for diagnostic evaluation after testing positive on mammography and physical examination actually did have breast cancer. The predictive value negative, or the probability that a woman who tested negative truly did not have breast cancer, is 63,650/63,695 or 99.9 percent. Thus, virtually all women who tested negative were in fact free from the disease. A high predictive value negative is to be expected in any screening program for a rare disease because the vast majority of those screened will by definition be disease-free.

The predictive value of a screening test is determined not only by factors that determine validity of the test itself (i.e., sensitivity and specificity), but also by the characteristics of the population to which the test is applied, in particular the prevalence of preclinical disease. The more sensitive a test, the less likely it is that an individual with a negative test will have the disease, and thus the greater the predictive value negative. The more specific the test, the less likely an individual with a positive test will be to be free from the disease and the greater the predictive value positive. For rare diseases, however, the major determinant of the predictive value positive is the prevalence of the preclinical disease in the screened population. No matter how specific the test, if the population is at low risk of having the disease, results that are positive will mostly be false positives.

The interrelationships of sensitivity, specificity, and prevalence with predictive value can be illustrated using hypothetical data on a group of 100,000 screened persons. As shown in Table 13-3, where the disease is rare (prevalence = 0.01), the sensitivity of the screening test is 90 percent and the specificity 95 percent, the PV^+ would be 15.4 percent. If the specificity of the screening test were raised from 95 percent to 98 percent (Table 13-4), the predictive value positive increases to 31.3 percent, about twice the original value, while the negative predictive value remains the same. It is not possible to bring about the same increase in the predictive value positive by raising the sensitivity. With a specificity of 95 percent, even if the sensitivity were raised to 100 percent, the re-

Table 13-3. Hypothetical results of a screening program
with 90 percent sensitivity and 95 percent specificity

	Disease		Total
	Present	Absent	
Screening test			
Positive	900	4950	5850
Negative	100	94,050	94,150
Total	1000	99,000	100,000

$$\text{Sensitivity} = \frac{a}{a+c} = \frac{900}{1000} = 90\%$$

$$\text{Specificity} = \frac{d}{b+d} = \frac{94,050}{99,000} = 95\%$$

$$PV^+ = \frac{a}{a+b} = \frac{900}{5850} = 15.4\%$$

$$PV^- = \frac{d}{c+d} = \frac{94,050}{94,150} = 99.9\%$$

Table 13-4. Hypothetical results of a screening program
with 90 percent sensitivity and 98 percent specificity

	Disease		Total
	Present	Absent	
Screening test			
Positive	900	1980	2880
Negative	100	97,020	97,120
Total	1000	99,000	100,000

$$\text{Sensitivity} = \frac{a}{a+c} = \frac{900}{1000} = 90\%$$

$$\text{Specificity} = \frac{d}{b+d} = \frac{97,020}{99,000} = 98\%$$

$$PV^+ = \frac{a}{a+b} = \frac{900}{2880} = 31.3\%$$

$$PV^- = \frac{d}{c+d} = \frac{97,020}{97,120} = 99.9\%$$

Table 13-5. Effect of prevalence on predictive
value positive with constant sensitivity and specificity

Prevalence (%)	PV$^+$ (%)	Sensitivity (%)	Specificity (%)
0.1	1.8	90	95
1.0	15.4	90	95
5.0	48.6	90	95
50.0	94.7	90	95

sulting predictive value positive would be only 16.8 percent. Thus, for a rare disease such as cancer, an increase in the specificity of a screening test will have a much greater effect on predictive value positive than an increase in sensitivity.

The effect of prevalence on predictive value positive for a test with a given sensitivity and specificity is illustrated in Table 13-5.

As can be seen, when the prevalence of preclinical disease is low, the predictive value positive will be low even using a test with high sensitivity and specificity. Thus, for rare diseases, which in this respect means those chronic diseases most likely to be screened for in the United States, a large proportion of those with positive screening tests will inevitably be found not to have the disease upon further diagnostic testing.

The predictive value positive, or yield, of a screening test can thus be increased by either increasing the specificity of the test (by changing the criterion of positivity) or by increasing the prevalence of preclinical disease in the screened population. This can be accomplished by targetting the screening program to groups of individuals who are at high risk of developing the disease of interest on the basis of considerations such as demographic factors, medical history, or occupation. For example, clearly, a sickle cell screening test among blacks or screening for Tay-Sachs disease among Jews of Eastern European origin would result in a far higher predictive value positive, and thus be more cost-effective, than comparable programs applied to the general population. Similarly, in screening for breast cancer, targeting the program to women with a positive family history will detect more cases than screening among the general population.

Effectiveness

The second, and ultimately most important, aspect of evaluating a screening program is whether it is effective in reducing morbidity and mortality from the disease. Even if a screening program will accurately and inexpensively identify large numbers of individuals with preclinical disease, it will have little public health value if early diagnosis and treatment do not have an impact on the ultimate outcome of those cases.

Thus, the evaluation of the effectiveness of a screening program must be based on measures that reflect the impact of the program on the course of the disease. A number of factors can be evaluated within a short period of time after initiation of a screening program, such as the severity of the disease at the time of diagnosis. For example, an observed shift in the stage distribution of cervical cancer toward less advanced disease among screen-detected relative to symptom-diagnosed cases might seem to suggest that the screening program will result in lower mortality from cervical cancer. However, such measures are very difficult to evaluate because this shift could also be due to the fact that participants in a screening program may be, as a group, more health conscious and thus more likely to have their disease diagnosed at an early stage than those whose disease was diagnosed because of symptoms, regardless of the screening test itself [4]. The most definitive measure of the efficacy of a screening program is a comparison of the cause-specific mortality rates among those whose disease was picked up by screening and those whose diagnosis was related to the development of symptoms.

In determining the efficacy of screening, the groups must be comparable with regard to all factors affecting the end point under evaluation, with the exception of the screening experience, as well as equally scrutinized for ascertainment of the outcomes. In addition, there are three sources of bias of particular importance in the evaluation of a screening program: patient self-selection bias (volunteer bias), lead time bias, and length bias. Each of these sources may result in an erroneous appraisal of the mortality experience of screened as compared with symptom-diagnosed cases.

People who choose to participate in screening programs are likely to be different from those who do not volunteer in a number of ways that affect survival [9, 42]. In general, volunteers tend to have better health and lower mortality rates than the general population and are more likely to adhere to prescribed medical regimens. Consequently, if one were to use an observational study design to compare mortality rates of screenees with those of the general population or an unscreened group, it is likely that those screened voluntarily would have lower mortality rates regardless of any effect of screening. On the other hand, those who volunteer for a screening program may represent the "worried well," that is, asymptomatic individuals who are at higher risk of developing the disease because of medical or family history, or any number of lifestyle characteristics. Such individuals might have an increased risk of mortality regardless of the efficacy of the screening program. The direction of the potential patient selection bias may be difficult to predict and the magnitude of such effects even more difficult to quantify.

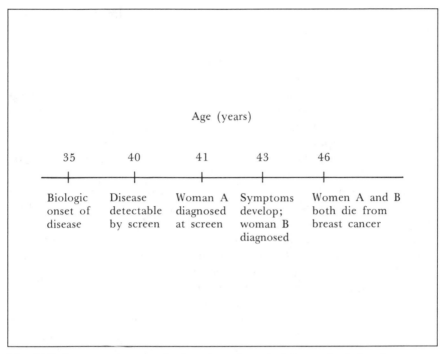

Fig. 13-2. Apparent increase in duration of survival due to lead time in hypothetical screened and symptom-diagnosed cases of breast cancer.

Lead time is defined as the interval between the diagnosis of a disease at screening and when it would have been detected due to development of symptoms. It therefore represents the amount of time by which the diagnosis has been advanced as a result of screening. Since screening is applied to asymptomatic individuals, by definition every case detected by screening will have had its diagnosis advanced by some amount of time. Whether that lead time is a matter of days, months, or years, however, will vary by the disease, the individual, and the screening procedure. Cases progressing rapidly from preclinical to clinical disease will gain less lead time from screening than those that develop slowly, with a long preclinical phase. The amount of lead time will also depend on how soon the screening is performed after the preclinical disease becomes detectable. If an estimate of lead time is not taken into account when comparing mortality among screened and unscreened groups, survival may erroneously appear to be increased among screen-detected cases simply because the diagnosis was made earlier in the course of disease (lead time bias) [14, 27, 33].

For example, Figure 13-2 illustrates the hypothetical histories of two women who developed breast cancer. For both, the biologic onset of the disease was at age 35, and the disease was detectable by screening at age 40. One of the women (A) was screened at age 41, and her breast cancer was detected at that time. The other woman (B) was not screened and at age 43 detected a breast lump, which was consequently diagnosed. Both women died from breast cancer at age 46. From the time of diagnosis, woman A survived a total of 5 years, or 2 years longer than woman B. However, although an examination of length of survival following diagnosis would appear to indicate that screening was beneficial, in fact it only pushed forward the time of diagnosis; both women died at exactly the same age.

There are two ways that the effect of lead time on the evaluation of the efficacy of a screening program can be taken into account. The first is to compare not the length of survival from diagnosis to death, but rather the age-specific death rates in the screened and nonscreened groups. In the example above, the death rates at age 46 for both women were identical, indicating that the screening in fact had no effect on mortality. Alternatively, if the lead time for a given disease can be estimated, it can be taken into account and thus allow a comparison of the survival experience of screen- and symptom-detected cases. For example, the HIP study findings were used to determine the average lead time for breast cancer, which was calculated as approximately 1 year [14, 33]. Consequently, to evaluate the efficacy of a breast cancer screening program, the 6-year case-fatality rate of the screenees should be compared with the 5-year case-fatality rate of symptom-diagnosed cases.

Length bias refers to the overrepresentation among screen-detected cases of those with a long preclinical phase of disease and thus a more favorable prognosis [43]. This occurs because diseases tend to be heterogeneous with respect to their natural history, and the prevalence of preclinical disease is dependent on its duration. Thus, those with a long preclinical phase are more readily detectable by screening than more rapidly progressing cases with a short preclinical phase. An assumption underlying the concept of length bias is that cases with long preclinical phases would have a more favorable prognosis than those with shorter preclinical phases that progress more rapidly to symptoms, regardless of any effect of the screening program itself. Thus, length bias could lead to an erroneous conclusion that screening was beneficial when, in fact, observed differences in mortality were a result merely of the detection of less rapidly fatal cases through screening, while those more rapidly fatal are diagnosed after the development of symptoms. Length bias is very difficult to quantify. Since its effect, however, would be greatest for cases detected at the initial screen, one approach that has been used to control for this bias is to compare the experience of screened and symptom-detected cases at subsequent screening examinations [4].

Study Designs Used to Evaluate Screening Programs

A number of epidemiologic design strategies are utilized to evaluate the efficacy of a screening program, including correlational and observational studies, as well as randomized trials. The same strengths and limitations of each approach that were discussed with respect to the testing of etiologic hypotheses are applicable to the choice of a particular study design and the interpretation of the results from the evaluation of a screening program.

Correlational studies have been used to examine trends in disease rates in relation to screening frequencies within a population, or to compare the relationship between the frequencies of screening and disease rates for different populations. Such descriptive studies are very useful in suggesting that a relationship exists between screening and a decline in morbidity or mortality. However, the limitations inherent in correlational studies must be borne in mind. First, since the information from such studies concerns populations rather than individuals, it is not possible to establish that those experiencing the decreased mortality are in fact the same persons who received the screening. Moreover, such studies cannot allow for control of potential confounding factors. Finally, the measure of screening frequency employed is usually an average value for the population, so that it is not possible to determine an optimal screening strategy for an individual. Thus, correlational studies can suggest the possibility of a benefit of a screening program, but they cannot test that hypothesis.

For example, a number of correlational studies have shown an inverse relationship between the frequency of use of the Pap smear and the rate of cervical cancer mortality [5, 8, 10, 18, 25]. Some of the findings, however, have been very difficult to interpret because the decline in cervical cancer mortality in most developed countries began before Pap smears were widely used, raising the question of whether other factors might have been responsible. Moreover, most studies have not been able to take into account the effect of potential confounding by factors such as socioeconomic status. Socioeconomic status is of particular importance, since it is strongly and inversely related to the incidence of cervical cancer, and women at the greater risk of developing cervical cancer are less likely to have had a Pap smear [22]. Thus, it is difficult to know, using this design, whether the women who experienced the decline in cervical cancer mortality were in fact those who underwent the screening procedure.

Observational analytic studies, both case-control and cohort, are often utilized to evaluate the efficacy of screening programs. In the case-control design, individuals with and without the disease are compared with respect to their past exposure (screening). For example, in a case-control study in which history of Pap smear was examined in newly diagnosed cases of invasive cervical cancer and controls [3], significantly fewer cases than controls had received a Pap smear during the 5 years prior to the year of diagnosis. The risk of invasive cervical cancer among women who had not had a Pap smear was over three times that of women who had, even after the effects of several potential confounding factors, including socioeconomic status, were controlled. As with any case-control study, the definition and selection of the cases and controls are of crucial importance to the validity of the findings [26, 41].

Using a cohort design, the case-fatality rate of those who chose to be screened is compared with the comparable rate among those whose diagnoses were symptom-related. This is the most frequently used approach to the evaluation of a screening program. However, in interpreting the results of such studies, the potential effects of the self-selection of participants as well as lead-time and length bias must be taken into account [27].

Since noncomparability of screened and symptom-diagnosed cases is the chief threat to validity, the optimal assessment of the efficacy of a screening program derives from randomized trials. When the sample size is sufficiently large, the control of confounding is virtually assured by the process of randomization. Patient self-selection or volunteer bias, which is problematic for the comparison of screened and nonscreened groups in observational studies, cannot influence the validity of the results of randomized trials, since the screening program is allocated at random by the investigators after individuals have agreed to participate in the trial. Lead time bias can be taken into account by adjusting for the average lead time when comparing survival of screened versus symptom-detected cases or, preferably, by comparing the age-specific mortality rates for the screened and nonscreened groups. Trials also can address the potential for length bias by comparing the mortality experience of the groups after repeated screening.

As discussed earlier, the HIP Breast Cancer Screening Project [32] was a randomized trial designed to evaluate whether periodic breast cancer screening with mammography and physical examination would result in reduced breast cancer mortality among women aged 40 to 64 years. After 9 years of follow-up, there was an overall statistically significant reduction in breast cancer mortality among women who were offered screening compared with women assigned to continuing to receive their usual medical care. This effect was due almost exclusively to a reduction among the subgroup of women over 50 years of age; there was no apparent reduction in breast cancer mortality among screened women between the ages of 40 and 49.

While randomized trials can provide the best and most valid evidence concerning the efficacy of a screening program, as with the evaluation of etiologic hypotheses, because of the inherent problems related to costs, ethics, and feasibility most evidence on the effects of screening programs will come from the nonexperimental study designs. Especially in the numerous situations where randomized trials are not possible, such as with well-established procedures like the Pap smear, observational approaches can provide useful and necessary information.

CONCLUSION

The primary objective of screening is to reduce morbidity and mortality from disease through early detection and treatment. Given a disease with characteristics appropriate for screening and a valid screening test, both the feasibility and the effectiveness of screening must be evaluated. The same epidemiologic principles and methods that apply to primary prevention of diseases apply to the evaluation of screening programs as a means of disease control.

STUDY QUESTIONS

1. Discuss the criteria of suitability of a disease for screening.
2. What factors can increase the positive predictive value of a screening test?
3. Define the two major potential biases in the evaluation of screening programs.
4. Discuss the various issues that must be considered in the evaluation of a screening program.

REFERENCES

1. Boucot, K. R., and Weiss, W. Is curable lung cancer detected by semiannual screening? *J.A.M.A.* 224:1362–1365, 1973.
2. Centers for Disease Control. Current trends: Technical problems with the FTA-ABS test for syphilis—Virginia. *M.M.W.R.* 22:102, 107, 1973.
3. Clarke, E. A., and Anderson, T. W. Does screening by "Pap" smears help prevent cervical cancer? A case-control study. *Lancet* 2:1–4, 1979.
4. Cole, P., and Morrison, A. S. Basic issues in population screening for cancer. *J.N.C.I.* 64:1263–1272, 1980.
5. Cramer, D. W. The role of cervical cytology in the declining morbidity and mortality of cervical cancer. *Cancer* 34:2018–2027, 1974.
6. Eddy, D. M. *Screening for Cancer: Theory, Analysis and Design.* New Jersey: Prentice-Hall, 1980.
7. Fletcher, R. H., Fletcher, S. W., and Wagner, E. H. *Clinical Epidemiology—the Essentials.* Baltimore: Williams & Wilkins, 1982.

8. Gardner, J. W., and Lyon, J. L. Efficacy of cervical cytological screening in the control of cervical cancer. *Prev. Med.* 6:487, 1977.
9. Greenlick, M. R., Bailey, J. W., Wild, J., et al. Characteristics of men most likely to respond to an invitation to be screened. *Am. J. Public Health* 69:1011, 1979.
10. Guzick, D. S. Efficacy of screening for cervical cancer: A review. *Am. J. Public Health* 68:125–134, 1978.
11. Hanley, W. B., Linsao, L. S., and Netley, C. The efficacy of dietary therapy for phenylketonuria. *Can. Med. Assoc. J.* 104:1089–1091, 1971.
12. Helem, F. Basal Cell Carcinoma. In S. Madden (ed.), *Current Dermatologic Management.* St. Louis: Mosby, 1975. Pp. 90–95.
13. Hudson, F. P., Mordaunt, V. L., and Leahy, I. Evaluation of treatment begun in the first three months of life in 184 cases of phenylketonuria. *Arch. Dis. Child.* 45:5–12, 1970.
14. Hutchison, G. B., and Shapiro, S. Lead time gained by diagnostic screening for breast cancer. *J.N.C.I.* 41:665–681, 1968.
15. Hutchison, G. B. Personal communication, 1987.
16. Hypertension Detection and Follow-up Program Cooperative Group. Five-year findings of the Hypertension Detection and Follow-up Program: I. Reduction in mortality of persons with high blood pressure, including mild hypertension. *J.A.M.A.* 242:2562–2571, 1979.
17. Jaffe, H. W. The laboratory diagnosis of syphilis: New concepts. *Ann. Intern. Med.* 83:846–850, 1975.
18. Johannesson, G., Geirsson, G., and Day, N. The effect of mass screening in Iceland, 1965–1974, on the incidence and mortality of cervical cancer. *Int. J. Cancer* 21:418–425, 1978.
19. Kang, E. S., Sollee, N. D., and Gerald, P. S. Results of treatment and termination of the diet in phenylketonuria (PKU). *Pediatrics* 46:83–92, 1970.
20. Kannel, W. B., Dawber, T. R., and McGee, D. L. Perspectives on systolic hypertension: The Framingham Study. *Circulation* 61:1183–1187, 1980.
21. Kaplan, N. M. Hypertension. In N. M. Kaplan and J. Stamler (eds.), *Prevention of Coronary Heart Disease.* Philadelphia: Saunders, 1983. Pp. 61–72.
22. Kleinman, J. C. Who is being screened for cervical cancer? *Am. J. Public Health* 71:73–76, 1981.
23. MacCready, R. A. Admissions of phenylketonuric patients to residential institutions before and after screening programs of the newborn infant. *J. Pediatr.* 85:383–385, 1974.
24. Markisz, J. A. Radiologic and nuclear medicine diagnoses. In S. Z. Goldhaber (ed.), *Pulmonary Embolism and Deep Vein Thrombosis.* Philadelphia: Saunders, 1985. Pp. 41–75.
25. Miller, A. B., Lindsay, J., and Hill, G. B. Mortality from cancer of the uterus in Canada and its relationship to screening for cancer of the cervix. *Int. J. Cancer* 17:602–612, 1976.
26. Morrison, A. S. Case definition in case-control studies of the efficacy of screening. *Am. J. Epidemiol.* 115:6–8, 1982.
27. Morrison, A. S. The effects of early treatment, lead time, and length bias on the mortality experienced by cases detected by screening. *Int. J. Epidemiol.* 111:261–267, 1982.

28. Morrison, A. S. Screening in chronic disease. *Monographs in Epidemiology and Biostatistics,* Vol. 7. Oxford: Oxford University Press, 1985.
29. Poskanzer, D. C. Neurological disorders. In D. W. Clark and B. MacMahon (eds.), *Preventive and Community Medicine.* Boston: Little, Brown, 1981. Pp. 265–291.
30. Sackett, D. L., Haynes, R. B., and Tugwell, P. *Clinical Epidemiology: A Basic Science for Clinical Medicine.* Boston: Little, Brown, 1985.
31. Scriver, C. R., and Clow, C. L. Phenylketonuria: Epitome of human biochemical genetics. *N. Engl. J. Med.* 303:1394–1400, 1980.
32. Shapiro, S. Evidence on screening for breast cancer from a randomized trial. *Cancer* 39:2772–2782, 1977.
33. Shapiro, S., Goldberg, J. D., and Hutchison, G. B. Lead time in breast cancer detection and implications for periodicity of screening. *Am. J. Epidemiol.* 100:357–366, 1974.
34. Shapiro, S., Strax, P., and Venet, L. Periodic breast cancer screening—the first two years of screening. *Arch. Environ. Health* 15:547–553, 1967.
35. Taylor, J. The Hypertension Detection and Follow-up Program: a progress report. *Circ. Res.* 40(Suppl. I):106–109, 1977.
36. Taylor, W. F., Fontana, R. S., Uhlenhopp, M. A., et al. Some results of screening for early lung cancer. *Cancer* 47:1114–1120, 1981.
37. Vecchio, T. J. Predictive value of a single diagnostic test in unselected populations. *N. Engl. J. Med.* 271:1171–1173, 1966.
38. Veterans Administration Cooperative Study Group on Antihypertensive Agents. Effects of treatment on morbidity in hypertension: I. Results in patients with diastolic blood pressures averaging 115 through 129 mm Hg. *J.A.M.A.* 202:1028–1034, 1967.
39. Veterans Administration Cooperative Study Group on Antihypertensive Agents. Effects of treatment on morbidity in hypertension: II. Results in patients with diastolic blood pressure averaging 90 through 114 mm Hg. *J.A.M.A.* 213:1143–1152, 1970.
40. Weiss, N. S. *Clinical Epidemiology: The Study of the Outcome of Illness.* New York: Oxford University Press, 1986.
41. Weiss, N. S. Control definition in case-control studies of the efficacy of screening and diagnostic testing. *Am. J. Epidemiol.* 116:457–460, 1983.
42. Wilhelmsen, L., Ljungberg, S., Wedel, H., et al. A comparison between participants and non-participants in a primary preventive trial. *J. Chronic Dis.* 29:331–339, 1976.
43. Zelen, M. Theory of early detection of breast cancer in the general population. In J. C. Heuson, W. H. Mattheim, and M. Rozencweig (eds.), *Breast Cancer: Trends in Research and Treatment.* New York: Raven Press, 1976. Pp. 287–300.

APPENDIXES

A

Standard Statistical Tables

Table A-1. Areas in one tail of the standard normal curve

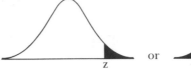

This table shows the shaded area ———— z —— or —— − z ————

z	.00	.01	.02	.03	.04	.05	.06	.07	.08	.09
0.0	.500	.496	.492	.488	.484	.480	.476	.472	.468	.464
0.1	.460	.456	.452	.448	.444	.440	.436	.433	.429	.425
0.2	.421	.417	.413	.409	.405	.401	.397	.394	.390	.386
0.3	.382	.378	.374	.371	.367	.363	.359	.356	.352	.348
0.4	.345	.341	.337	.334	.330	.326	.323	.319	.316	.312
0.5	.309	.305	.302	.298	.295	.291	.288	.284	.281	.278
0.6	.274	.271	.268	.264	.261	.258	.255	.251	.248	.245
0.7	.242	.239	.236	.233	.230	.227	.224	.221	.218	.215
0.8	.212	.209	.206	.203	.200	.198	.195	.192	.189	.187
0.9	.184	.181	.179	.176	.174	.171	.169	.166	.164	.161
1.0	.159	.156	.154	.152	.149	.147	.145	.142	.140	.138
1.1	.136	.133	.131	.129	.127	.125	.123	.121	.119	.117
1.2	.115	.113	.111	.109	.107	.106	.104	.102	.100	.099
1.3	.097	.095	.093	.092	.090	.089	.087	.085	.084	.082
1.4	.081	.079	.078	.076	.075	.074	.072	.071	.069	.068
1.5	.067	.066	.064	.063	.062	.061	.059	.058	.057	.056
1.6	.055	.054	.053	.052	.051	.049	.048	.048	.046	.046
1.7	.045	.044	.043	.042	.041	.040	.039	.038	.038	.037
1.8	.036	.035	.034	.034	.033	.032	.031	.031	.030	.029
1.9	.029	.028	.027	.027	.026	.026	.025	.024	.024	.023
2.0	.023	.022	.022	.021	.021	.020	.020	.019	.019	.018
2.1	.018	.017	.017	.017	.016	.016	.015	.015	.015	.014
2.2	.014	.014	.013	.013	.013	.012	.012	.012	.011	.011
2.3	.011	.010	.010	.010	.010	.009	.009	.009	.009	.008
2.4	.008	.008	.008	.008	.007	.007	.007	.007	.007	.006
2.5	.006	.006	.006	.006	.006	.005	.005	.005	.005	.005
2.6	.005	.005	.004	.004	.004	.004	.004	.004	.004	.004
2.7	.003	.003	.003	.003	.003	.003	.003	.003	.003	.003
2.8	.003	.002	.002	.002	.002	.002	.002	.002	.002	.002
2.9	.002	.002	.002	.002	.002	.002	.002	.001	.001	.001
3.0	.001									

Table A-2. Areas in two tails of the standard normal curve

This table shows
the shaded areas

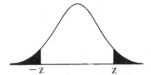

z	.00	.01	.02	.03	.04	.05	.06	.07	.08	.09
0.0	1.000	.992	.984	.976	.968	.960	.952	.944	.936	.928
0.1	.920	.912	.904	.897	.889	.881	.873	.865	.857	.849
0.2	.841	.834	.826	.818	.810	.803	.795	.787	.779	.772
0.3	.764	.757	.749	.741	.734	.726	.719	.711	.704	.697
0.4	.689	.682	.674	.667	.660	.653	.646	.638	.631	.624
0.5	.617	.610	.603	.596	.589	.582	.575	.569	.562	.555
0.6	.549	.542	.535	.529	.522	.516	.509	.503	.497	.490
0.7	.484	.478	.472	.465	.459	.453	.447	.441	.435	.430
0.8	.424	.418	.412	.407	.401	.395	.390	.384	.379	.373
0.9	.368	.363	.358	.352	.347	.342	.337	.332	.327	.322
1.0	.317	.312	.308	.303	.298	.294	.289	.285	.280	.276
1.1	.271	.267	.263	.258	.254	.250	.246	.242	.238	.234
1.2	.230	.226	.222	.219	.215	.211	.208	.204	.201	.197
1.3	.194	.190	.187	.184	.180	.177	.174	.171	.168	.165
1.4	.162	.159	.156	.153	.150	.147	.144	.142	.139	.136
1.5	.134	.131	.129	.126	.124	.121	.119	.116	.114	.112
1.6	.110	.107	.105	.103	.101	.099	.097	.095	.093	.091
1.7	.089	.087	.085	.084	.082	.080	.078	.077	.075	.073
1.8	.072	.070	.069	.067	.066	.064	.063	.061	.060	.059
1.9	.057	.056	.055	.054	.052	.051	.050	.049	.048	.047
2.0	.046	.044	.043	.042	.041	.040	.039	.038	.038	.037
2.1	.036	.035	.034	.033	.032	.032	.031	.030	.029	.029
2.2	.028	.027	.026	.026	.025	.024	.024	.023	.023	.022
2.3	.021	.021	.020	.020	.019	.019	.018	.018	.017	.017
2.4	.016	.016	.016	.015	.015	.014	.014	.014	.013	.013
2.5	.012	.012	.012	.011	.011	.011	.010	.010	.010	.010
2.6	.009	.009	.009	.009	.008	.008	.008	.008	.007	.007
2.7	.007	.007	.007	.006	.006	.006	.006	.006	.005	.005
2.8	.005	.005	.005	.005	.005	.004	.004	.004	.004	.004
2.9	.004	.004	.004	.003	.003	.003	.003	.003	.003	.003
3.0	.003									

Table A-3. Percentage points of the *t* distribution (this table gives the values of *t* for differing df that cut off specified proportions of the area in one and in two tails of the *t* distribution)

df	Area in two tails				
	.10	.05	.02	.01	.001
	Area in one tail				
	.05	.025	.01	.005	.0005
1	6.314	12.706	31.821	63.657	636.619
2	2.920	4.303	6.965	9.925	31.598
3	2.353	3.182	4.541	5.841	12.941
4	2.132	2.776	3.747	4.604	8.610
5	2.015	2.571	3.365	4.032	6.859
6	1.943	2.447	3.143	3.707	5.959
7	1.895	2.365	2.998	3.499	5.405
8	1.860	2.306	2.896	3.355	5.041
9	1.833	2.262	2.821	3.250	4.781
10	1.812	2.228	2.764	3.169	4.587
11	1.796	2.201	2.718	3.106	4.437
12	1.782	2.179	2.681	3.055	4.318
13	1.771	2.160	2.650	3.012	4.221
14	1.761	2.145	2.624	2.977	4.140
15	1.753	2.131	2.602	2.947	4.073
16	1.746	2.120	2.583	2.921	4.015
17	1.740	2.110	2.567	2.898	3.965
18	1.734	2.101	2.552	2.878	3.922
19	1.729	2.093	2.539	2.861	3.883
20	1.725	2.086	2.528	2.845	3.850
21	1.721	2.080	2.518	2.831	3.819
22	1.717	2.074	2.508	2.819	3.792
23	1.714	2.069	2.500	2.807	3.767
24	1.711	2.064	2.492	2.797	3.745
25	1.708	2.060	2.485	2.787	3.725
26	1.706	2.056	2.479	2.779	3.707
27	1.703	2.052	2.473	2.771	3.690
28	1.701	2.048	2.467	2.763	3.674
29	1.699	2.045	2.462	2.756	3.659
30	1.697	2.042	2.457	2.750	3.646
40	1.684	2.021	2.423	2.704	3.551
60	1.671	2.000	2.390	2.660	3.460
120	1.658	1.980	2.358	2.617	3.373
∞	1.645	1.960	2.326	2.576	3.291

Table A-4. Percentage points of the chi-square distribution (this table gives the values of χ^2 for differing df that cut off specified proportions of the upper tail of the chi-square distribution)

df	Area in upper tail			
	.10	.05	.01	.001
1	2.71	3.84	6.63	10.83
2	4.61	5.99	9.21	13.82
3	6.25	7.81	11.34	16.27
4	7.78	9.49	13.28	18.47
5	9.24	11.07	15.09	20.52
6	10.64	12.59	16.81	22.46
7	12.02	14.07	18.48	24.32
8	13.36	15.51	20.09	26.13
9	14.68	16.92	21.67	27.88
10	15.99	18.31	23.21	29.59
11	17.28	19.68	24.73	31.26
12	18.55	21.03	26.22	32.91
13	19.81	22.36	27.69	34.53
14	21.06	23.68	29.14	36.12
15	22.31	25.00	30.58	37.70
16	23.54	26.30	32.00	39.25
17	24.77	27.59	33.41	40.79
18	25.99	28.87	34.81	42.31
19	27.20	30.14	36.19	43.82
20	28.41	31.41	37.57	45.32
21	29.62	32.67	38.93	46.80
22	30.81	33.92	40.29	48.27
23	32.01	35.17	41.64	49.73
24	33.20	36.42	42.98	51.18
25	34.38	37.65	44.31	52.62

B

Selection of an Appropriate
Test of Statistical Significance

As discussed in Chapter 10, there is a wide variety of tests of statistical significance available. At first glance, this array of possible tests can appear daunting, and the method for selecting the appropriate procedure for a particular analysis may seem unclear. However, an understanding of the details of the study, such as the type of data collected, the size of the sample and the specific research questions being asked, makes the choice of the appropriate test of statistical significance relatively straightforward.

A discussion of every available statistical procedure is beyond the scope of this book and can be found in textbooks of biostatistics [1, 3]. In fact, over two-thirds of the tests of statistical significance encountered in the medical literature relate to comparing proportions of individuals falling into various categories (discrete data) or comparing means (continuous data) [2]. In this appendix, therefore, we present two flow diagrams to facilitate the choice of the most appropriate statistical procedure for testing hypotheses concerning proportions (Fig. B-1) and means (Fig. B-2).

When considering discrete data, the principal research question relates to how the proportion of individuals in a particular category compares with one or more other proportions. The statistical procedures that address these questions can be broadly categorized into two groups: tests that utilize the underlying distribution of the variable (so-called exact tests), and those that approximate it by the chi-square distribution. The suitability of each of these two approaches depends on the size of the sample. Thus, as shown in Figure B-1, the first question to ask in determining an appropriate statistical procedure for testing proportions is whether the sample size is small (less than five individuals expected under the null hypothesis in any cell of the contingency table) or large (five or more individuals expected in every cell). If the sample size is small, the statistical test chosen should involve either calculating the probability of the observed event based on knowledge of the underlying distribution to address whether the observed proportion differs from a specified theoretical value, or utilizing one of a number of specific tests designed to address whether two or more independent or paired proportions differ from each other. On the other hand, if the sample size is

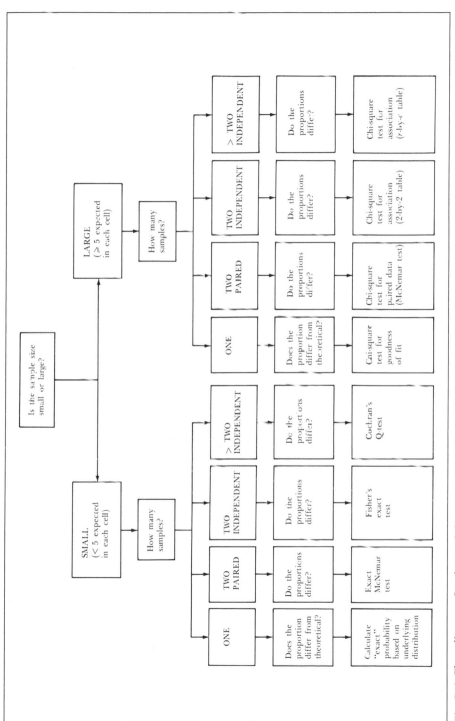

Fig. B-1. Flow diagram for determining an appropriate statistical procedure for discrete data: Inferences on proportions.

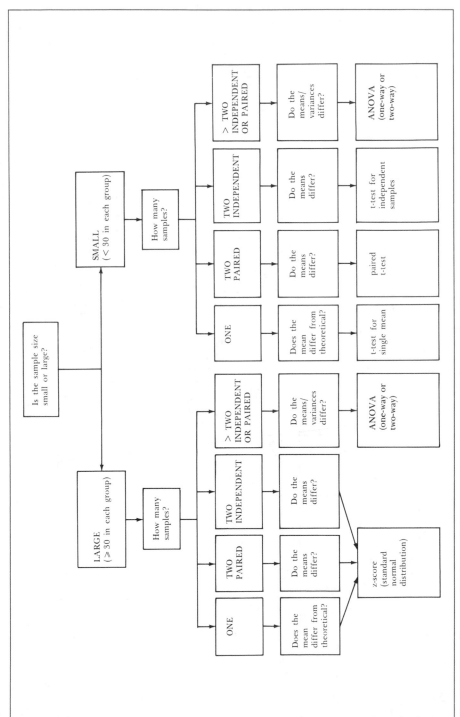

Fig. B-2. Flow diagram for determining an appropriate statistical procedure for continuous data: Inferences on means.

large, one of the various chi-square tests should be used. The form of the chi-square test statistic will depend on the particular research question: specifically, whether the observed proportion differs from a specified theoretical value (chi-square test for goodness of fit), whether two proportions from paired samples differ (chi-square test for paired data), whether two proportions from independent samples differ (chi-square test for association in a two-by-two table), or whether more than two proportions from independent samples differ (chi-square test for association, r-by-c table).

With continuous data, the most common situation involves testing differences between means. The particular statistical tests that address this question utilize either the standard normal distribution or the t distribution. The basic difference between these two sets of tests relates to the fact that all formulas for the testing of means require information on the variance of the underlying distribution(s) of the variables. If the true variance is known (which is rarely the case) or, more commonly, the sample size is large enough that the variance calculated from the sample is a stable estimate of the value for the underlying population, then the test statistic is based on a standard normal distribution. On the other hand, if the sample size is small, then the variability inherent in having to estimate the population variance from the sample must be taken into account by basing the test statistic on the t distribution. Of course, as the sample size gets larger, the values for the normal and t test statistics will approach each other. Thus, as shown in Figure B-2, the first question to ask in determining an appropriate test of statistical significance based on means is whether the sample size is small (less than 30 individuals in any group) or large (30 or more in each group). If small, the appropriate test will be either a t test for a single mean (to address whether an observed and theoretical mean differ), t test for the difference in means of two paired or two independent samples, or a one-way analysis of variance (ANOVA) (to test the difference in means/variances of more than two independent or paired samples). If the sample size is large, the statistical tests will involve calculating a z score for the standard normal distribution, with the particular form of the z score depending on whether the specific research question relates to whether an observed mean differs from a theoretical mean, or whether two or more means from paired or independent samples differ. For more than two independent or paired samples, the one-way ANOVA is performed.

REFERENCES

1. Colton, T. *Statistics in Medicine*. Boston: Little, Brown, 1974.
2. Emerson, J. D., and Colditz, G. A. The use of statistical analysis in the *New England Journal of Medicine*. *N. Engl. J. Med.* 309:709, 1983.
3. Rosner, B. *Fundamentals of Biostatistics*. Boston: Duxbury Press, 1982.

C

Answers to Study Questions

Chapter 1

1-1. The chief causes of death in the U.S. in 1900 were infectious diseases, which are characterized by relatively short latency periods between exposure and the onset of illness. The average life expectancy at that time was about 50 years. Advances in the prevention of such diseases through improved living conditions brought about by industrialization, as well as the development of antibiotics to treat them, have resulted in a dramatic decline in the mortality rates from infectious diseases. Consequently, people are now living longer, with an average life expectancy of about 74 years, and the current leading causes of death are chronic diseases, which are characterized by long latency periods. These include vascular diseases of the heart, accounting for about one-third of deaths, vascular disease of the brain, which accounts for about one-sixth, as well as cancer, which is responsible for about one-sixth of all deaths in the U.S. In addition, up to 1970, most gains were due to improved survival of mothers and infants. In contrast, since 1970 there have been improvements in the lifespans of middle-aged adults, due largely to the 25- to 30-percent decline in mortality from vascular diseases of the heart and brain.

1-2. Laboratory studies on experimental animals are capable of providing definitive answers about mechanisms of disease because they have the possibility of achieving complete control of exposures, environment, and sometimes even genetics. However, the applicability of these findings to human populations is uncertain, since mechanisms of disease in animals vary from species to species. Furthermore, the doses and routes of administration of exposures in animal studies are often very different from those in humans. Thus, while these studies are unlikely to provide any reliable quantitative estimate of human risk, they do provide information that can be used to set priorities for research in humans. Epidemiologic studies are far less well controlled, but their unique contribution is that their findings allow quantification of the magnitude of exposure-disease relationships in humans. Although they cannot, in general, elucidate mechanisms, well-designed and conducted epidemiologic studies can provide evidence on which to base public health policy to alter the frequency of human disease through intervention.

Chapter 2

2-1. The investigators first collected data on cases with keratoconus and, as the exposure, quantified the frequency of use of hard contact lenses prior to diagnosis. For this to have been a case-control study, the investigators would have needed to assemble a control group of comparable subjects without keratoconus and assess their use of hard lenses. Instead, they identified a nonexposed group of soft contact lens wearers and ascertained their development of the disease. Since it is impossible to compare either the rate of the exposure among diseased and nondiseased individuals (as in a case-control study) or the rate of disease among exposed and nonexposed individuals (as in a cohort study), the results of this study are uninterpretable.

2-2. There is no one analytic study design that is uniformly optimal for the evaluation of every hypothesis. The choice depends on the specific research question under investigation as well as issues of cost and feasibility. For example, case-control studies are generally preferable for the evaluation of rare diseases or to explore the roles of a number of different risk factors for a single outcome. They can often be conducted at a fraction of the cost and time of a prospective cohort study. A cohort study, on the other hand, is optimal for the evaluation of a rare exposure or for multiple outcomes of a single exposure. The (mistaken) belief in the inate superiority of the prospective cohort over the case control design is a result of two problems inherent in the latter: (1), that the temporal sequence between cause and effect is more difficult to establish in a case-control study, and (2) that because both exposure and disease have occurred at the time the groups are selected for study, there is a greater potential for bias. While these problems are certainly real, they simply mean that more care must be taken in the design and conduct of a case-control study to ensure that valid results are obtained. However desirable theoretically, a prospective cohort study can also result in uninterpretable findings if potential confounding factors are not taken into account and complete follow-up of study participants is not achieved. The goal in designing any study is to obtain a valid result, and this can be accomplished using either a case-control or a cohort study, so long as each is well-designed and carefully conducted.

Chapter 3

3-1. These studies provide little support for an association between exposure to hair dyes and an increased risk of cancer. The first study, which was reported to show an increased risk of lung cancer, utilized data from death certificates and was therefore unable to control for the potential effects of cigarette smoking, the strongest known determinant of lung cancer, accounting for a 20-fold increased risk. In the second study, the investigators again did not have information available on smoking but were able to control for the effects of social class, and the observed risk decreased from sixfold to twofold. Since social class may be related to smoking behavior, the decrease in risk may have been attributable, at least in part, to smoking. A study that controls for the effects of a single variable such as social class and observes such a large decrease in the estimate of effect suggests that control for the more powerful determinant of lung cancer risk, cigarette smoking, if more common among beauticians, would result in a finding of no association. These data illustrate the necessity of controlling for confounding variables before concluding the presence of a valid statistical association.

3-2. The judgment of a cause-effect relationship involves assessing the validity of a given study, as well as viewing that study in the context of all available data. Although the cohort study cited observed a 2½-fold increased risk, the confidence interval was very wide, indicating that the sample size was small and the estimate unstable. Moreover, the results of previous investigations, including three case-control and one cohort, had been inconsistent and inconclusive. At the time it was made, the public health recommendation concerning coffee consumption was unfounded based on the totality of evidence.

3-3. The presence of a valid statistical association in a particular study can be concluded after the exclusion of chance, bias, and confounding as alternative explanations for a finding. Causation, on the other hand, is a judgment that can only in the rarest of circumstances be made on the basis of the findings from any one study. Such results must be viewed in the context of all available information, using positive criteria such as the strength of association, the consistency of findings from study to study, and compatibility with a known or postulated biologic mechanism.

Chapter 4

4-1. a.

| | Myocardial infarction | | |
	CASES	CONTROLS	TOTAL
Current smoker			
Yes	157	110	267
No	209	313	522
Total	366	423	789

The relative risk is estimated in a case-control study by calculating the odds ratio:

$$RR = OR = \frac{ad}{bc} = \frac{(157)\,(313)}{(209)\,(110)}$$

$$= 2.14$$

These data indicate that current cigarette smokers were 2.14 times as likely to develop a myocardial infarction than those who were not current smokers.

b. The attributable-risk percent can be calculated from these data as a measure of the excess risk of myocardial infarction among cigarette smokers that is due to cigarette smoking.

$$AR\% = \frac{RR - 1}{RR} \times 100\%$$

$$= \frac{2.14 - 1}{2.14} \times 100\%$$

$$= 53\%$$

These data suggest that 53 percent of the myocardial infarctions among current cigarette smokers could be eliminated if they were to stop smoking. In order to make this calculation, we assumed that cigarette smoking is causally related to myocardial infarction. The attributable risk cannot be calculated, since additional information on the incidence rate of the disease is not provided.

4-2. These data indicate that the rate of development of breast cancer in the U.S. in 1985 was greater than that of lung cancer but that the mortality rate from lung cancer was higher. Thus, at any point in time, the prevalence (or proportion of existing cases) must be greater for breast than lung cancer, as will be the duration of disease from diagnosis to death. The case fatality rate would correspondingly be greater for lung than breast cancer. Parenthetically, in 1985 there were 500,000 prevalent cases of breast cancer compared with 20,000 cases of lung cancer. Moreover, the average duration of disease for breast cancer was five years, while for lung cancer it was 6 months. The case-fatality rate was 35 percent for breast cancer and 90 percent for lung cancer.

Chapter 5

5-1. Since exposure and disease are assessed at the same point in time, cross-sectional surveys may not be able to discern the temporal relationship between exposure and disease. When exposure variables are unaltered over time, such as eye color or blood group, valid tests of hypotheses can be done. However, when the risk factors under study can change over time and, in particular, as a consequence of the disease process itself, then cross-sectional data can only suggest the presence of an association.

5-2. Correlational studies of populations cannot link exposure with disease in individuals, cannot control the potential effects of confounding, and can evaluate only average levels of an exposure rather than actual values. Thus, the presence of a correlation does not necessarily indicate the existence of a valid statistical association, nor does the absence of a correlation preclude the possibility of such an association.

5-3. a. The death rate from this episode was very high and was inversely related to socioeconomic class. In addition, it was highest in adult males and lowest in adult females. Among adult males, the social class gradient is less marked, while among females it is striking. Among children, only those of low social class died. There was a very large proportion for whom social class was unknown. Virtually all those of unknown social class who died were adult males.

b. A disaster causing a high death rate occurred, which predominantly affected men of all social classes, women of low social class, and children only of low social class. The sinking of the Titanic conforms to these epidemiologic features, taking into account the positioning of the lifeboats and the priorities for their use, as well as the fact that many male immigrants gained passage below decks on this voyage and their social class was not recorded.

Chapter 6

6-1. The strengths of case-control studies include the ability to study rare diseases efficiently, their usefulness in the early stages of knowledge about an exposure-disease relationship, and their ability to investigate multiple exposures simultaneously. In addition, they are in general less costly and time-consuming than other analytic epidemiologic study designs.

   Their main disadvantages include the fact that the temporal relationship between exposure and disease may be more difficult to establish and the increased susceptibility to bias.

6-2. The advantages of using hospital controls include the fact that they are easily identified and readily available in sufficient numbers. For these reasons, their use is usually less costly than that of community controls. In addition, they are more likely than healthy individuals to be comparable to cases with respect to awareness of previous exposure and are generally more willing to cooperate. On the other hand, the use of hospital controls may lead to bias since they may be hospitalized for reasons that are also related to the exposure of interest. As a result, their exposure history may not be comparable with that of the source population that gave rise to the cases.

While the use of neighborhood controls offers the potential for a more generalizable result, there are the serious disadvantages of being more difficult to gain cooperation, being more costly and time-consuming, and having a greater potential for recall bias.

6-3. The potential for bias is of particular concern in case-control studies because both exposure and disease have already occurred at the time information on study subjects is obtained. Thus, it is possible that knowledge of exposure status could influence the way in which diseased or nondiseased individuals are selected into the study (selection bias) or that knowledge of disease status could influence the way in which information on exposure is reported by the study participants (recall bias) or collected or interpreted by the investigators (observation or information bias).

6-4. Selection and information bias are of most concern in case-control studies. Selection bias may arise when cases and controls are selected into the study differentially, based on exposure status. Information bias results from data being reported, collected, or interpreted differently for cases and controls. Two main types of information bias are recall bias and observer bias. The potential for recall bias comes from the fact that people who are sick tend to remember events differently from those who are well. Observer bias arises when those responsible for obtaining study information do so in a noncomparable manner for cases and controls.

Chapter 7

7-1. The chief strengths of cohort studies are their usefulness in studying rare exposures and multiple effects of a single exposure, as well as their ability to minimize selection bias (if prospective). Their limitations include the need to study very large sample sizes for rare diseases, their high costs, and the potential for bias due to losses to follow-up.

7-2. All cohort studies classify individuals on the basis of their exposure status. In retrospective cohort studies, all events of interest, both exposure and disease, have already occurred at the time the study is initiated. In prospective cohort studies, the outcomes of interest have not yet occurred at the beginning of the study, and individuals must be followed forward in time for the development of disease. Since disease has not yet occurred at their initiation, prospective cohort studies are more expensive and time-consuming than retrospective investigations but minimize the potential for bias in the ascertainment of outcomes.

7-3. Loss to follow-up is a particular concern for cohort studies. An investigation that has a low follow-up rate or even a high follow-up rate that is noncomparable for exposed and nonexposed individuals, cannot provide interpretable results. Random misclassification is also a problem in the ascertainment of exposure, especially in retrospective cohort studies that must use job titles or other surrogate measures to define exposure status.

Chapter 8

8-1. a. The investigators expected that the mortality of participants in the Physicians' Health Study would be lower than that of the general U.S. male population of the same age, based on the healthy volunteer effect, the fact that physicians as a group are very health-conscious and of a relatively high socioeconomic status, and the impact of the exclusion criteria in eliminating prevalent cases of cancer or heart disease. The fact that the mortality rate was far lower even than expected was probably due to the generally excellent health of these participants as well as their strikingly low rate of smoking.

b. Extending the length of the follow-up period would allow the observation of an adequate number of end points, since they accumulate more than arithmetically with increasing age.

8-2. The major advantage would be the ability to assess the relationships of aspirin with cardiovascular mortality and beta-carotene with cancer incidence in women as well as in men. The disadvantages are based on the fact that there are far fewer female than male physicians in that age group and that women in general experience fewer coronary events than men. In particular, in the U.S., fewer than 10 percent of physicians over age 40 are women. Furthermore, in the Framingham Heart Study data, by the age of 60, 1 in 5 men but only 1 in 17 women have suffered a coronary event. Thus, while 1000 coronary deaths would be anticipated in men, only 33 would be expected in women. Thus, there would be insufficient power to detect a 20-percent decrease in cardiovascular mortality, let alone to assess whether the effect in women differed from that in men.

8-3. a. There were two major factors that contributed to the inability of the trial to detect a statistically significant reduction in risk associated with the intervention. First, there was a 25- to 30-percent decline in cardiovascular mortality rates for the general U.S. population during the study period. In addition, participants in the usual care group also reduced their cardiovascular risk through smoking cessation, hypertension control, and cholesterol reduction. Consequently, the intervention and comparison groups became more similar, resulting in an observed underestimate of any true effects of the intervention itself. Together, these two factors reduced the number of end points in the trial, resulting in a study with inadequate power to detect the most reasonable alternative hypotheses.

b. The power of the trial to detect the hypothesized effect could have been increased by extending the length of follow-up to allow observation of additional end points.

Chapter 9

9-1. Discrete variables are those having values that can fall into only a limited number of separate categories with no possible intermediate levels. These include variables that are dichotomous (e.g., male or female), multichotomous (e.g., blood groups A, B, AB, and O), ordinal (e.g., nonsmoker; exsmoker; current smoker of light, moderate, or heavy amounts), and numerical discrete (e.g., parity). The basic analysis of discrete data involves comparison of the proportion of subjects falling into each of the various categories. Discrete data are most frequently presented in the form of frequency distributions or contingency tables.

Continuous variables are those that theoretically can assume all possible values within a specified range along a continuum. These include many clinical measurements, such as weight, age, white blood count, or blood pressure. Groups are most often compared in terms of average values of the variables. Continuous data are presented in frequency distributions or polygons, or can be degraded into a number of discrete categories.

9-2. Presenting the raw or actual data provides the maximum information about the findings of a study. However, this can be cumbersome and even unintelligible because of the large amount of information usually involved. Descriptive statistics are useful to summarize data in a form that permits the clearest and most efficient presentation of the most information. Since this summarization by definition involves a reduction in the amount of data presented, there is inevitably a loss of information involved. For each individual situation, the amount and nature of the data presented must be a judgment made by the investigator after consideration of the various advantages and disadvantages of the different approaches.

9-3. Frequency distributions provide the most complete and convenient way to summarize quantitative variables. As the data increase in terms of number of subjects and amount of information recorded, the efficiency of the frequency distribution as a method of data presentation also increases. A frequency polygon is a graphic representation of a frequency distribution. These are especially useful to facilitate comparisons of two or more data sets by constructing a number of frequency polygons on the same graph.

9-4. Three measures of central tendency that are encountered in the literature are the mean, median, and mode. The mean, or arithmetic average, is the most commonly used measure of central tendency. It forms the basis for a large proportion of statistical hypothesis tests. As a descriptive statistic, however, it is very sensitive to extreme values, or outliers. Consequently, if a distribution is asymmetrical, the mean is not the best measure of central tendency. The median, or centrally ranked value in the distribution, is not affected by extreme values, which makes it a better measure than the mean for describing asymmetrical distributions, though it is far less amenable to tests of statistical significance. The mode, or most common value encountered in a distribution, is rarely used as the sole descriptive measure and is even less amenable to statistical testing than the median.

With respect to measures of variability, one simple descriptive measure is the range. It is, however, neither stable nor a good description of the majority of the observations. Thus, the most frequently employed measures of variability are the variance and its square root, the standard deviation.

Chapter 10

10-1. The *P* value is a conditional probability statement representing the likelihood that the result observed in the data, or one more extreme, is due to chance, given that the null hypothesis is true. If the *P* value is low, conventionally less than 0.05, the null hypothesis of no association is rejected, chance is considered an unlikely explanation for the findings, and the results are termed statistically significant at that level. If the *P* value is greater than or equal to 0.05, the interpretation is that chance cannot be excluded as a likely explanation for the findings, the null hypothesis cannot be rejected, and the results are not statistically significant at the 0.05 level.

The confidence interval provides the range within which the true estimate of effect lies with a certain level of confidence. Thus, a 95-percent confidence interval around an observed relative risk estimate indicates that, with 95 percent confidence, the true relative risk will be no less than the lower bound and no greater than the upper bound.

10-2. There are two factors that affect the size of the *P* value: the magnitude of the difference between the study groups and the size of the sample. Consequently, even a small difference can be statistically significant if the sample size is sufficiently large, and conversely, a difference that may be of interest clinically may not achieve statistical significance if the sample size is small. The confidence interval is more informative than the *P* value, since it separates information about the magnitude of effect from that concerning the variability of the estimate. The width of the interval indicates the amount of variability inherent in the estimate of effect. The larger the sample size, the more stable the estimate, and the narrower the confidence interval. Moreover, the confidence interval indicates whether the findings are statistically significant at a given level. If, for example, the null value for a relative risk, 1.0, is included in the 95-percent confidence interval, the results are not statistically significant at the 0.05 level.

10-3. The power of a study is defined as the probability of detecting a difference between the study groups if one truly exists. This ability is dependent on two factors: the magnitude of the effect as well as the size of the study population. The issue of power needs to be considered both in the design of a study and in the interpretation of its findings. In designing any investigation, it is crucial to calculate the sample size necessary to ensure that the study has adequate power to detect the most likely magnitude of effect with the desired level of confidence. Moreover, in interpreting a finding that does not achieve statistical significance, it is necessary to consider whether the study had adequate ability to detect an effect of the observed magnitude. If not, the finding is not merely a null result, but a null result that is uninformative.

10-4. An overview is a statistical approach that combines all available data from a number of studies. As a result, it can provide the most precise estimate of effect from existing evidence. The main advantage of an overview is that it increases the statistical power to detect an effect, if one truly exists. This is especially useful in circumstances where individual randomized trials were of inadequate sample size to detect the small to moderate effects that are most likely to occur, so that the individual results did not achieve statistical significance. Overviews are of great practical utility in the planning of trials, by providing the best estimate of the magnitude of the treatment effect and, thus, of the sample size required to test the hypothesis definitively.

Chapter 11

11-1. Selection bias is a particular problem in case-control studies because both exposure and disease have occurred at the time individuals are chosen for study. In prospective cohort studies, this type of bias is virtually nonexistent because exposure is ascertained before the occurrence of disease. In retrospective cohort studies, however, the potential for selection bias is similar to that in case-control studies because both the exposure and disease have occurred at the start of the investigation.

Observation or information bias, which results from systematic differences in the way information on exposure or outcome is obtained from the different study groups, includes several specific types. Recall bias, which arises when individuals with a particular exposure or outcome remember and report their experiences differently from those who are not affected, is a particular problem in case-control studies and retrospective cohort studies. In contrast, loss of subjects to follow-up is the major source of bias in cohort studies. In addition, case-control studies can be affected by differential probing for exposure history on the basis of an observer's knowledge of a subject's disease status, while cohort studies may be affected by differential ascertainment of outcome due to awareness of exposure status.

11-2. Random misclassification, which increases the similarity between the exposed and nonexposed groups, will always tend to dilute the association between the exposure and disease, causing the relative risk estimate to move closer to 1.0, the null value. In contrast, nonrandom misclassification can bias the estimate of effect in the direction of being either more or less extreme than the true association, depending on the situation. Random misclassification should therefore always be considered in the interpretation of a null result.

11-3. The major approaches in the design of a study to eliminate the occurrence of bias include the selection of a study population on whom complete and accurate information is readily obtainable; the construction of objective, detailed data collection instruments that allow as little room for interpretation by the investigator as possible; the maintenance of blindness among study personnel with respect to the exposure and disease status of subjects; the implementation of rigorous, standardized protocols for data collection, whether this involves interviews, physical examinations, or abstraction of records; and the use of standard, uniform criteria for defining outcomes of interest.

Chapter 12

12-1. The use of matching in the design of a study does not in itself control confounding. To be correctly implemented, matching in the design must be accompanied by stratification in the analysis. Failure to do so may introduce bias in the estimate of the magnitude of the association between the exposure and disease, since matching on confounding factors may introduce a similarity in the exposure status of the groups that otherwise would not have occurred. If the results of analyses retaining the matched pairs and those ignoring the matching are similar, the matching can safely be disregarded.

12-2. While the same variable in a single study can be a confounder, an effect modifier, both, or neither, confounding and effect modification are actually very different conceptually. Confounding is a nuisance effect that is distorting the true relationship between the exposure and disease. The aim is therefore to control confounding and eliminate its effects. Effect modification provides information about how the association differs for varying levels of another factor. This information can provide insight into the interrelationships and mechanisms of these variables. Thus, the aim is to describe and report effect modification rather than to control it. Both confounding and effect modification are evaluated through the process of stratification. If the stratum-specific estimates differ, effect modification is present. If the crude estimate differs from the combination (through pooling or standardization) of the stratum-specific, unconfounded estimates, confounding was present.

12-3. The major advantage of multivariate analysis is that it allows for the efficient estimation of measures of association between exposure and disease while controlling simultaneously for a number of confounding factors, even in situations where stratification would fail because of insufficient numbers. The disadvantage is that this may occur at the expense of a familiarity with the data and a clear understanding and communication of the results. To overcome this, simple stratified analyses should always be examined prior to performing the multivariate analyses, and the results of both should be presented.

Chapter 13

13-1. For a disease to be suitable for screening, it must be serious, treatment given before symptoms develop must be more efficacious in terms of reducing morbidity or mortality than that given after the development of clinical manifestations of the disease, and the prevalence of preclinical disease must be high among the screened population.

13-2. Factors that can increase the positive predictive value of a screening test include screening a population at high risk of developing the disease and increasing the specificity of the screening test.

13-3. Two major types of bias that can occur in the evaluation of screening programs include lead-time bias and length bias. Lead time is the interval between diagnosis at screening and when the disease would have been detected due to the development of symptoms. If not taken into account, the survival of screen-detected cases will appear longer than that of symptom-diagnosed cases only because the diagnosis has been advanced. Length bias refers to overrepresentation among screen-detected cases of those with long preclinical phases of disease and thus a more favorable prognosis.

13-4. Evaluation of the effectiveness of a screening program involves questions of both feasibility and efficacy. Feasibility is evaluated by an examination of the screening process itself, including the acceptability of the test to the target screening population, the cost-effectiveness of the program, and the case yield. The appropriate measures to address these questions include the total cost of the program, the cost per case detected, the proportion of the target population screened, the rate of follow-up and treatment of those who test positive, and the predictive value of the screening test. While useful in assessing whether the screening program can realistically be carried out, these factors in no way address the crucial issue of whether the screening program results in lowered morbidity or mortality from the disease. The most clear-cut and objective outcome measure to evaluate the impact of the screening program on the disease is cause-specific mortality, taking into account factors such as the lead time introduced by the screening process itself.

INDEX

Index